Stem Cells in Endocrinology

CONTEMPORARY ENDOCRINOLOGY

P. Michael Conn, SERIES EDITOR

Stem Cells in Endocrinology, edited by LINDA B. LESTER, 2005
Office Andrology, edited by PHILLIP E. PATTON AND DAVID E. BATTAGLIA, 2005
Male Hypogonadism: Basic, Clinical, and Therapeutic Principles, edited by STEPHEN J. WINTERS, 2004
Androgens in Health and Disease, edited by CARRIE J. BAGATELL AND WILLIAM J. BREMNER, 2003
Endocrine Replacement Therapy in Clinical Practice, edited by A. WAYNE MEIKLE, 2003
Early Diagnosis of Endocrine Diseases, edited by ROBERT S. BAR, 2003
Type I Diabetes: Etiology and Treatment, edited by MARK A. SPERLING, 2003
Handbook of Diagnostic Endocrinology, edited by JANET E. HALL AND LYNNETTE K. NIEMAN, 2003
Pediatric Endocrinology: A Practical Clinical Guide, edited by SALLY RADOVICK AND MARGARET H. MACGILLIVRAY, 2003
Diseases of the Thyroid, 2nd ed., edited by LEWIS E. BRAVERMAN, 2003
Developmental Endocrinology: From Research to Clinical Practice, edited by ERICA A. EUGSTER AND ORA HIRSCH PESCOVITZ, 2002
Osteoporosis: Pathophysiology and Clinical Management, edited by ERIC S. ORWOLL AND MICHAEL BLIZIOTES, 2002
Challenging Cases in Endocrinology, edited by MARK E. MOLITCH, 2002
Selective Estrogen Receptor Modulators: Research and Clinical Applications, edited by ANDREA MANNI AND MICHAEL F. VERDERAME, 2002
Transgenics in Endocrinology, edited by MARTIN MATZUK, CHESTER W. BROWN, AND T. RAJENDRA KUMAR, 2001
Assisted Fertilization and Nuclear Transfer in Mammals, edited by DON P. WOLF AND MARY ZELINSKI-WOOTEN, 2001
Adrenal Disorders, edited by ANDREW N. MARGIORIS AND GEORGE P. CHROUSOS, 2001
Endocrine Oncology, edited by STEPHEN P. ETHIER, 2000
Endocrinology of the Lung: Development and Surfactant Synthesis, edited by CAROLE R. MENDELSON, 2000
Sports Endocrinology, edited by MICHELLE P. WARREN AND NAAMA W. CONSTANTINI, 2000
Gene Engineering in Endocrinology, edited by MARGARET A. SHUPNIK, 2000
Endocrinology of Aging, edited by JOHN E. MORLEY AND LUCRETIA VAN DEN BERG, 2000
Human Growth Hormone: Research and Clinical Practice, edited by ROY G. SMITH AND MICHAEL O. THORNER, 2000
Hormones and the Heart in Health and Disease, edited by LEONARD SHARE, 1999
Menopause: Endocrinology and Management, edited by DAVID B. SEIFER AND ELIZABETH A. KENNARD, 1999
The IGF System: Molecular Biology, Physiology, and Clinical Applications, edited by RON G. ROSENFELD AND CHARLES T. ROBERTS, JR., 1999
Neurosteroids: A New Regulatory Function in the Nervous System, edited by ETIENNE-EMILE BAULIEU, MICHAEL SCHUMACHER, AND PAUL ROBEL, 1999
Autoimmune Endocrinopathies, edited by ROBERT VOLPÉ, 1999
Hormone Resistance Syndromes, edited by J. LARRY JAMESON, 1999
Hormone Replacement Therapy, edited by A. WAYNE MEIKLE, 1999
Insulin Resistance: The Metabolic Syndrome X, edited by GERALD M. REAVEN AND AMI LAWS, 1999

STEM CELLS IN ENDOCRINOLOGY

Edited by

LINDA B. LESTER, MS, MD

Division of Endocrinology, Diabetes and Clinical Nutrition
Department of Medicine, Oregon Health and Sciences University
Portland, Oregon

HUMANA PRESS
TOTOWA, NEW JERSEY

999 Riverview Drive, Suite 208
Totowa, New Jersey 07512

humanapress.com

For additional copies, pricing for bulk purchases, and/or information about other Humana titles,contact Humana at the above address or at any of the following numbers: Tel: 973-256-1699;Fax: 973-256-8341; E-mail: humana@ humanapr.com.com or visit our website at humanapress.com

This publication is printed on acid-free paper. ∞
ANSI Z39.48-1984 (American National Standards Institute)
Permanence of Paper for Printed Library Materials.

Production Editor: Anne Peters
Cover Design: Patricia Cleary
Cover illustration from Fig. 5, Chapter 5, "Growth Conditions for Primate vs Murine Embryonic Stem Cells," by Gillian M. Beattie, Nathan Bucay, Rohan Humphrey, Ana D. Lopez, and Alberto Hayek

Printed in the United States of America. 10 9 8 7 6 5 4 3 2 1

e-ISBN:1-59259-900-1

Library of Congress Cataloging-in-Publication Data

Stem cells in endocrinology / edited by Linda B. Lester.
p. cm. -- (Contemporary endocrinology)
Includes bibliographical references and index.
ISBN 1-58829-407-2 (alk. paper)
1. Stem cells. 2. Endocrinology, Experimental. I. Lester, Linda B. II.
Series: Contemporary endocrinology (Totowa, N.J.)
QH588.S83S747 2005
616'.02774--dc22

2004017508

Dedication

The lights of stars that were extinguished ages ago still reach us.
So it is with great men who died centuries ago, but still reach us
with the radiations of their personalities.

— *Khalil Gibran*

The recent death of James R. Hansen, MD (August 24, 1951 to May 27, 2003) cut short a life dedicated to family, patients, and a cure for type 1 diabetes. After medical school at Oregon Health Sciences University, Jim completed a pediatric residency and pediatric endocrine fellowship at the University of Iowa. Upon returning to Portland, Oregon, Jim became medical director of the Emanuel Children's Diabetes and Endocrine Center. There he worked passionately to care for his patients with type 1 diabetes and continued to pursue novel diabetes therapies through ongoing clinical research. Jim was actively involved with the Juvenile Diabetes Research Foundation (JDRF) at both the local and international levels. He was very enthusiastic about the use of stem cells for endocrine therapies, particularly for treating patients with type 1 diabetes. Jim served as the committee chair for the JDRF's Human Stem Cell Research Committee up until a few weeks before his death.

This book is dedicated to Dr. James Hansen, in memory of his life, vision, and inspiration. He continues to shine for those of us he touched.

Preface

As the world population ages, health care costs are expected to escalate as a result of the increase in age-related, degenerative diseases. Regenerating the failing cells and organs associated with these diseases would preserve quality of life and help curtail the increase in health care costs. Medical scientists today are faced with the challenge of developing new and innovative regenerative therapies to meet this need. A major focus of this research is to identify sources of cells and tissues that can be used in regenerative therapies. Stem cells, by definition, can self-replicate and, under the right conditions, differentiate into mature cell phenotypes. Stem cells are a potential source of cells for regenerative medical therapies, and research on defined stem cell populations will facilitate the study of organ development ex vivo. Understanding stem cell growth and development will shed light on the biological process of tissue/organ development and likely lead to novel regenerative therapies.

Although all stem cells have a limited capacity for self-replication and differentiation, some stem cells are capable of differentiating into multiple cell types, a property known as plasticity. Embryonic stem (ES) cells are derived from the early blastocyst and contain stem cells capable of generating all adult tissues. This makes ES cells the most pluripotent, or plastic, of the available stem cells. Recently, ES cell lines were derived from animal and human blastocysts. These cell lines are capable of self-replication and can be expanded in culture to provide a renewable source of cells. Human ES cell lines are an invaluable research tool for the study of human development in vitro. In addition, human ES cells have the potential for direct use in therapies; thus, these cell lines represent a major advance in cell biology that will have a broad impact on subsequent medical research.

The study of stem cell biology is likely to have profound effects for the near future, affecting the current equilibrium in medical research. The evolution of science and medicine is punctuated by events that are clearly so significant that they alter the future course of scientific and medical discovery. The derivation of human ES cell lines, in my mind, is clearly such an event. Human ES cell lines, along with other stem cell lines, will have broad and long-lasting effects on developmental biology and translational research. However, the fundamental importance of ES cell lines does not necessarily imply that ES cells will become the cell source for regenerative medicine. The appropriate stem cells will need to be evaluated for each disease system that may benefit from regenerative therapy.

Many disease processes stand to benefit from regenerative medical therapies, including disorders of the central nervous system, cardiovascular, gastrointestinal, and hematologic systems. Currently, some of these disorders can be treated using whole organ transplantation. However, whole organ transplantation is limited to a small percent of patients because of the scarcity of organs for donation and the need for broad spectrum immunosuppressive therapies. As opposed to other systems, degenerative disorders of the endocrine system can currently be treated using exogenous hormonal therapies. These therapies, however, are frequently inadequate, resulting in significant morbidity and mortality to patients. The difficulty in treating endocrine disorders is developing a therapy that mimics the natural feedback mechanisms inherent to functional endocrine organs. Most current exogenous endocrine therapies fail to mimic the precise metabolic control of endogenous hormone release, resulting in under- or overtreatment and thereby leading to complications. This is clearly illustrated by the persistent complications of diabetes in patients on exogenous insulin therapy. Replacing endocrine organ function with functionally responsive cells will allow for the precise regulation of hormone release through natural feedback and should dramatically improve medical care. The recent success of islet transplantation indicates the potential for cell therapies to improve medical care for patients with diabetes. Again, the major drawback is the lack of tissue available for these procedures. The shortage of islets and other endocrine tissues could be overcome by developing alternative tissue sources such as the use of stem cells. Endocrine diseases, in particular diabetes, are therefore prime targets for stem cell therapeutics.

The objective of this text is to provide a primary source of information on basic stem cell biology and the application of stem cell research to endocrine diseases. As such, this book should be useful for both clinical endocrinologists and endocrine researchers alike. The information in this book is divided into two main sections: first, a basic stem cell biology section and second, translational stem cell research with endocrine applications. In the basic science section, each of the major sources of stem cells are discussed, including embryonic, cord blood, germ line, and adult stem cells tissues. Because it is not clear which stem cell types will eventually be used for endocrine therapies discussing all stem cells allows a side-by-side comparison of the different stem cell types and a full understanding of the pros and cons of each. The second section explores how stem cells may be employed to develop endocrine-related cells or tissues. This includes discussions on directed differentiation using transgenes and development of endocrine-specific phenotypes including β-cells, hepatocytes, bone, and sperm. Because many endocrine disorders are autoimmune mediated, we also include a discussion of stem cell therapy for the treatment of autoimmune disorders. In the future, stem cell therapies for thyroid and other endocrine disorders may be available, but these areas are not discussed given the limited amount of research currently available.

In closing, I would like to thank all the contributing authors for taking time from their research efforts to share their thoughts and ideas in this book. Their collective expertise provides an excellent starting point for the endocrine researcher, illuminating the complexity and potential of stem cell research in endocrinology. I also want to thank Drs. Laura Andrews and Brian Nauert for their thoughts, editorial comments, and efforts in my research lab while I was working on this project. Finally, I would like to thank Dr. Lynn Loriaux for his ongoing support of stem cell research at Oregon Health and Sciences University and my family, for enduring cold dinners and late nights with few complaints. I could not flourish without their support and encouragement. My accomplishments are clearly a reflection of all those around me.

Linda B. Lester, MS, MD

Contents

Contributors

GILLIAN M. BEATTIE, PhD • *Whittier Institute, University of California San Diego, La Jolla, CA*
ASA C. BLACK, JR., MD • *Division of Basic Medical Science, Department of Obstetrics and Gynecology, Mercer University School of Medicine, Macon, GA*
VICTORIA L. BROWNING, PhD • *Department of Surgery, University of Wisconsin, Madison, WI*
NATHAN BUCAY, PhD • *Whittier Institute, University of California San Diego, La Jolla, CA*
EWA CARRIER, MD • *Cancer Center, University of California San Diego, La Jolla, CA*
MICHAEL D. GRISWOLD, PhD, DVM • *School of Molecular Biosciences, Washington State University, Pullman, WA*
SANJEEV GUPTA, MD • *Marion Bessin Liver Research Center, Albert Einstein College of Medicine, Bronx, NY*
ALBERTO HAYEK, MD • *Whittier Institute, University of California San Diego, La Jolla, CA*
ROHAN HUMPHREY, PhD • *Whittier Institute, University of California San Diego, La Jolla, CA*
LINDA B. LESTER, MS, MD • *Division of Endocrinology, Diabetes and Clinical Nutrition, Department of Medicine, Oregon Health and Sciences University, Portland, OR*
ANA D. LOPEZ, PhD • *Whittier Institute, University of California San Diego, La Jolla, CA*
WILLIAM L. LOWE, JR., MD • *Feinberg School of Medicine, Northwestern University, Chicago, IL*
NADYA LUMELSKY, PhD • *Islet and Autoimmunity Branch, National Institute of Diabetes and Digestive and Kidney Diseases, National Institutes of Health, Bethesda, MD*
DEREK MCLEAN, PhD • *Department of Animal Sciences, Center for Reproductive Biology, Washington State University, Pullman, WA*
KATHY E. MITCHELL, PhD • *Department of Pharmacology and Toxicology, University of Kansas, Lawrence, KS*
MAKOTO C. NAGANO, PhD, DVM • *Department of Obstetrics and Gynecology, McGill University, Montreal, Quebec, Canada*

IREM NASIR, PhD • *Department of Anatomy, Downstate Medical Center, SUNY, Brooklyn, NY*

JON S. ODORICO, MD • *Department of Surgery, University of Wisconsin, Madison, WI*

K. Y. FRANCIS PAU, PhD • *Division of Reproductive Health, Oregon National Primate Research Center, Oregon Health & Sciences University, Beaverton, OR*

JODY SCHUMACHER, PhD • *Whittier Institute, University of California San Diego, La Jolla, CA*

GLADYS TEITELMAN, PhD • *Department of Anatomy, Downstate Medical Center, SUNY, Brooklyn, NY*

SHELLEY R. WINN, PhD • *Division of Plastic and Reconstructive Surgery, Department of Surgery, Oregon Health & Sciences University, Portland, OR*

DON P. WOLF, PhD • *Division of Reproductive Health, Oregon National Primate Research Center, Oregon Health and Sciences University, Beaverton, OR*

HENRY E. YOUNG, PhD • *Department of Pediatrics, Division of Basic Medical Science, Mercer University School of Medicine, Macon, GA*

I BASIC STEM CELL BIOLOGY

1 Embryonic Stem Cells

Derivation, Properties, and Therapeutic Implications

Victoria L. Browning and Jon S. Odorico

CONTENTS

1. INTRODUCTION

Stem cells, which have a great capacity for self-renewal and can differentiate into at least one committed cell type, exist in embryonic and adult organisms of many phyla. Although stem cells of various types from mice and other lower organisms have been studied for many years, it was not until the derivation of stem cell lines from human embryos in 1998 *(1,2)* that the idea of stem cell-based therapies became widespread for the treatment of a range of disorders from Alzheimer's disease to type I diabetes. Efforts to generate insulin-producing islet cells from murine and human embryonic stem (ES) cells followed the establishment of these ES cell lines. In this review we will discuss the derivation proce-

From: *Contemporary Endocrinology: Stem Cells in Endocrinology*
Edited by: L. B. Lester © Humana Press Inc., Totowa, NJ

dures and growth characteristics of ES cell lines from these two species and the status of research to promote their differentiation into cells of the endocrine pancreas lineage.

Recently, experiments in a number of laboratories have suggested that stem cell populations in adult somatic tissues may have a previously unimagined ability to become other cell types, making them a potential attractive source of material for in vitro growth or in vivo repair of a variety of damaged or diseased tissues. This chapter will also review recent reports of adult bone marrow–derived and pancreas-derived islet tissue. Despite the promise of both adult and embryonic stem cells, a great deal of work remains before an ideal cell therapy for treatment of human diabetes is devised.

2. DERIVATION OF EMBRYONIC STEM CELLS

Scientists have been studying mammalian pluripotent stem cells for more than a half century. Embryonal carcinoma (EC) cells, derived from teratocarcinomas, were the first pluripotent stem cells to be studied. Teratocarcinomas are gonadal tumors originating from germ cells that contain differentiated cell types from each of the three embryonic germ layers: endoderm, ectoderm, and mesoderm. Because teratocarcinomas also contain some undifferentiated, proliferating EC cells, tumors could be serially transplanted, although with considerable difficulty *(3)*, and EC cells were isolated from the propagated tumors and grown in vitro *(4)*. Because of their expandability in culture and capacity for differentiation into embryonic tissues, EC cells were used for many years as tools to study early embryonic development, despite the fact that many of the lines have abnormal karyotypes. It was shown subsequently that injection of whole preimplantation embryos into non-uterine sites of histocompatible animals also resulted in the formation of tumors *(5,6)*, suggesting the existence of a stem cell population residing within the early embryo that might be amenable to isolation.

Building on the work performed to generate EC cell lines, researchers described the first murine ES cells in 1981 *(7,8)*. These pluripotent cells, derived from the cells of the inner cell mass (ICM), have the ability to give rise to all cell lineages of the embryo and adult, but not to extraembryonic tissues such as the placenta. Only totipotent cells, such as a fertilized egg or an individual blastomere from a two-, four-, or eight-cell stage embryo can develop into both the embryo proper and all extra-embryonic tissues. ICM cells are not stem cells *per se*, because they are transitory and do not undergo proliferation and massive expansion in the embryo before they differentiate into the epiblast. ES cells can thus be considered to be ICM cells held in an uncommitted state by an ex vivo culture environment, poised to differentiate as they normally would during early embryogenesis.

These first-reported murine ES cell lines were shown to be karyotypically normal, had the capacity to grow in vitro in an undifferentiated state for relatively long periods, and were able to differentiate into a wide array of cell types both in vitro and in vivo. Later, it was shown that pluripotent ES cells cultured in vitro could contribute to all the tissues of the developing chimeric mouse, including the germline, when injected into a blastocyst that was then transferred to a pseudopregnant host female *(9,10)*. Shortly thereafter, homologous recombination was used to modify the genome of cultured ES cells *(11)*. This technique, in combination with blastocyst injection, allowed researchers to make animals carrying specifically designed genetic alterations. In conjunction with the advent of molecular biology, mouse ES cells revolutionized the study of mammalian development because of the combination of their pluripotential and the ease with which they could be genetically manipulated. ES cell lines were subsequently developed from nonhuman primates *(12–14)*, among other species *(16–19)*.

The derivation of ES cells is a relatively straightforward process *(20,21)*. Essentially, the ICM is removed from a blastocyst and grown in vitro under conditions designed to prevent differentiation. A percentage of the time, this will result in the production of a true pluripotent ES cell line. When considering the mouse as a model, it is widely known that the genetic background greatly influences the success of ES cell derivation. ES cell lines can be efficiently generated from animals with a high percentage of 129 DNA (including F1 hybrids). This is perhaps related to the fact that 129 animals are characterized by a high incidence of spontaneous testicular carcinomas *(22)*, but the precise reasons for these differences are not known. Although ES cell lines derived from animals of the 129 substrains are the most widely used (including R1, D3, and AB1), pluripotent cell lines capable of populating the germline have also been developed from other mouse strains, including C57BL/6 *(23,24)*, BALB/C *(24)*, and NODx129 F1 hybrids *(25)*; however, some strains appear to be refractory to ES cell line derivation.

Today, perhaps the most common protocol for the derivation of mouse ES cells is essentially a combination of the two original protocols published in 1981, including both in vivo delay and immunosurgery. Mice are set up in natural matings, and females are checked for vaginal plugs in the morning; this is considered 0.5 days postcoitum (dpc). At 2.5 dpc, females are ovariectomized and given an intramuscular injection of the synthetic progesterone Depo-Provera to prevent implantation of the blastocysts. This so-called in vivo delay has been demonstrated to increase the efficiency by which new pluripotent ES cell lines are derived *(26)*; whether this is through an increase in cell number, an arrest in development, or some other mechanism has not been determined. After 5–7 days, blastocysts are flushed from the uterus and plated, in the presence of leukemia inhibitory factor (LIF) (*see* Section 3) and fetal bovine serum (FBS), onto gelatinized plates containing mitotically inactivated mouse embryonic fibroblasts (MEFs), often referred to as feeder cells. ES cell lines have also been successfully derived without an in vivo delay period, by flushing the blastocysts from the uterus at 3.5 dpc and plating as described.

After plating intact blastocysts, a percentage of the embryos will hatch from the zona pellucida, attach to the feeder layer, and begin to grow. The cells of the ICM can be distinguished morphologically from other cell types that will grow from the blastocyst, including trophoblast cells and "epithelial-like" cells *(20)*. Within 4–5 days of initial culture, the ICM cells will form a small colony, similar in appearance to an ES cell colony; at this point, the colony is dislodged, disaggregated, and replated to another plate with fresh feeder cells. Cells that maintain an ES cell-like morphology are then characterized for cell-surface antigen expression, karyotype, and their ability to differentiate in vitro and in vivo, usually through examination of cell types present in tumors that form after ES cell injection into immunoincompetent mice. Typically, new mouse ES cell lines are tested for pluripotency in vivo by injecting them into blastocysts to generate chimeras and observing whether the injected cells have populated all cell lineages, including the germline. For obvious ethical reasons, parallel experiments with human ES cells are not carried out.

Both ICM-derived ES cell lines and trophoblast stem (TS) cells can be derived from blastocysts (reviewed in ref. *27)*. Despite the fact that the two cell types have different requirements for growth in culture, TS cells can often overgrow cultures of blastocysts that are intended for ES cell line derivation. Dissecting the ICM by immunosurgery or microdissection is a useful means for increasing the efficiency of ES cell line derivation. Immunosurgery was first described in the 1970s, when Solter and Knowles *(28)* published the technique for the efficient derivation of ICMs without trophoblastic cell contamination. In this protocol, blastocysts were incubated first with rabbit anti-mouse spleen serum and then with guinea pig serum as a source of complement. When the appropriate dilutions and lengths of incubation were used, trophoblastic cells were selectively killed, without harm to the cells of the ICM. This technique, using different initial antisera, was used to derive primate ES cell lines from rhesus monkeys *(12)* and humans *(1,15)*. Microdissection, an alternate technique to isolate ICMs, was described by Brook and Gardner *(26)* and entails tearing open the blastocyst and pinning down the trophectoderm. With the cells of the ICM exposed, the primitive endoderm, which surrounds the epiblast (pluripotent cells that will grow into the fetus), can be removed, after which the epiblast is removed from the trophectoderm, dissociated, and plated. Both immunosurgery and microdissection are routinely used to minimize contamination of new ES cell cultures with other cell types.

3. GENERAL GROWTH CHARACTERISTICS OF ES CELLS

Mouse ES cells are typically grown on gelatin-coated plates in media containing FBS on a feeder layer of MEFs. The quality of the FBS is of great importance, and serum should be tested for its ability to promote ES cell growth in an undifferentiated state *(20)*. The requirement for the feeder layer can be eliminated if exogenous LIF is added to the culture media. In maintaining cells in an undifferentiated state, LIF is thought to act through a LIF receptor/gp130 receptor complex that regulates the activity of two parallel signaling pathways: the JAK/STAT and Shp2/Ras-dependent ERK pathway *(29,30)*. The relative balance of activity of these two pathways may prompt the decision for either self-renewal or differentiation. Recently, it has been shown that murine ES cells can be grown in an undifferentiated state in serum-free, feeder-free conditions provided that LIF and bone morphogenetic protein 4 (BMP4) are added exogenously *(31)*. BMP4 appears to induce expression of the Id genes through the Smad pathway, and the LIF/STAT and BMP/Smad pathways act in combination to maintain self-renewal and undifferentiated growth *(31)*.

Most mouse ES cell lines are quite robust and easy to culture, though they do require media replenishment on a daily basis. Cells have a doubling time of roughly 12–16 hours, are maintained at relatively high density, and are passaged every 2–3 days using trypsin to disrupt colonies to a single cell suspension that can be replated or frozen in media containing serum and DMSO. The cells are amenable to electroporation, and colonies representing stably transfected lines are simple to isolate and expand. There exist a great variety of constructs and techniques designed for alteration of mouse genomic DNA (*see* ref. *32,* for example), and the procedures are well within the grasp of nearly all modern laboratories.

The conditions for growing human ES cells vary somewhat in comparison with mouse ES cells. In the original derivation protocols, human ICMs were isolated by immunosurgery and plated onto MEF feeder layers with *(1)* or without *(15)* addition of human basic fibroblast growth factor (bFGF). Although it is clear that the MEF layer provides some critical factors required to maintain the cells in an undifferentiated state, it has been demonstrated that for human ES cells, LIF is not the factor *(1,15)*. To eliminate any potential contamination with murine retroviruses, some groups have switched to human fibroblasts as feeder layers *(33–35)*. Feeder-free growth of human ES cells has been developed by using tissue culture plates coated with Matrigel (a commercially available extracellular matrix, essentially a mixture of laminin, collagen IV, and heparin sulfate proteoglycan) and feeding cells with MEF-conditioned media containing human bFGF *(36)*. Human ES cells can be grown either with FBS, serum replacement (a synthetic, commercially available product), or a combination of the two. In general, human ES cells do not thrive when made into a single cell suspension, though clonal lines have been derived *(37)* and electroporation protocols have been devised *(38)*. Human ES cells have a doubling time of roughly 35–40 hours *(36,37)* and are passaged approximately once per week using collagenase to dislodge and disrupt colonies.

Regardless of the species, undifferentiated ES cells express several cell surface markers; these include stage-specific embryonic antigens, SSEA-1 in mouse and SSEA-3 and SSEA-4 in human, and well as tumor-recognition antigens TRA-1-60 and TRA-1-81 in human. In the uncommitted state both mouse and human ES cells express alkaline phosphatase, the POU-domain transcription factor Oct-4, and telomerase. When removed from the specific culture conditions required to maintain an undifferentiated state, ES cell lines from both species can spontaneously differentiate in vitro to form a wide variety of cell types derived from each of the three germ layers. Often, differentiation is achieved by growing cells in suspension in the absence of a feeder layer, LIF, bFGF, and conditioned media, which allows them to form multilayered structures known as embryoid bodies (EBs) because of their resemblance to preimplantation embryos. After some time in this state, the EBs can be allowed to adhere and to continue their growth and differentiation. Even without the addition of any exogenous growth factors, ES cells allowed to differentiate will spontaneously form neurons, cardiomyocytes, epithelial cells, pancreatic precursors, and many other cell types (*39–47; see* ref. *48* for a recent review). Although EB formation is not required, differentiation of some cell types may be enhanced and others reduced through this process.

4. DIFFERENTIATION OF ES CELLS INTO PANCREATIC LINEAGES

Isolated islet and whole-organ pancreas transplants are accepted therapies for some patients with type I diabetes. Fewer than 100 islet cell transplants and approximately 1400 pancreas transplants are performed annually in the United States, and cadaver donor shortages severely limit more widespread application. The generation of glucose-responsive, insulin-secreting β cells from a renewable human source would thus be an ideal alternative to organs procured through donation. Unfortunately, current technology does not allow precise directed differentiation of ES cells, whether from mouse or human, into islet lineages. Several approaches have been taken toward the generation of cells of pancreatic lineage from mouse and human ES cells.

Work in our own lab *(39)* and others *(49)* has shown that, under nonselective conditions, ES cells are capable of differentiation into pancreatic endocrine cell lineages. Using murine ES cells, we followed a two-step nonselective culture protocol including EB formation for 5–7 days followed by plating and further differentiation in the presence of FBS. In these differentiated cultures, foci of pancreatic lineage cells emerge, including cells that stain positively for PDX1 (pancreatic duodenal homeobox 1, a homeodomain protein absolutely required for pancreas development in both humans and mice *[50–52]*), peptide YY (a marker of early endocrine cells), and endocrine hormones including insulin, glucagon, and somatostatin *(39)*. Although lineage tracing has yet to be performed on cells grown under these experimental conditions, it appears that the culture system recreates the classical developmental stages of islet cytodifferentiation, because the timing of appearance of specific cell types is compatible with the derivation of islet cell types from pancreatic progenitor cells. For example, hormone-positive cells emerge from within PDX1-positive foci. In addition, the primary to secondary transition pattern seen in pancreas development in vivo appears to be recapitulated in these cultures, because there is an abrupt transition from cells that stain for both insulin and glucagon in early stage cultures to single hormone-positive cells found in later cultures. Ultimately, cells that are reminiscent of true β cells emerge in the cultures *(39)*.

Under the same nonselective culture conditions used for mouse ES cells, we have obtained similar results with human ES cells. Given the longer doubling time of human ES cells, we empirically increased the lengths of both the EB formation step and the subsequent differentiation after plating EBs. As in the mouse cultures, discrete foci of PDX1-positive cells are observed, followed by the emergence of hormone-positive cells (unpublished data). The nonselective culture conditions allow, but importantly, do not appear to promote, directed differentiation toward a pancreas fate. The frequency with which pancreatic-lineage cells are generated under these conditions is less than 0.1%; however, modification of culture conditions using a growth factor addition scheme based on developmental mechanisms is likely to promote pancreatic fate determination from ES cell-derived endoderm, ultimately producing the desired pancreatic cell types including islet endocrine cells. Such a strategy has been effective in producing enriched populations of motor neurons *(53)*, cardiomyocytes *(54)*, and hematopoietic lineages *(55)*.

5. RECAPITULATING DEVELOPMENTAL MECHANISMS TO DIRECT DIFFERENTIATION TO PANCREATIC LINEAGES

A thorough understanding of the mechanisms involved in pancreas and islet differentiation from endoderm is critical in developing tools required for effective differentiation of stem cells to these fates in vitro. Classical developmental biology studies, such as explant coculture studies in mice and chickens, have begun to define the initiating events that pattern foregut endoderm to a pancreatic fate. The downregulation of *hedgehog (hh)* expression in this region of gut epithelium appears to be important *(56,57)*, and notochord-derived factors such as FGF2 and activin β have been implicated in the initial repression of *hh* expression in the presumptive dorsal pancreatic endoderm *(58)*. Coculture of dissected dorsal aortae with prepancreatic epithelium promotes pancreatic fate suggesting a role for vascular epithelium and vascular epithelial growth factor in addition to the permissive signals of the notochord *(59)*. Whereas vascular epithelium and notochord are able to promote pancreatic differentiation in foregut endoderm destined to become pancreas, lateral plate mesoderm can provide instructive signals directing non-pancreatic endoderm to initiate pancreatic differentiation including *pdx*1 gene expression *(60)*. In addition, factors such as BMP4, BMP7, and activin A are capable of inducing *pdx*1 gene expression in anterior chick endoderm when combined with appropriate mesoderm, suggesting that these factors may be mediating the inductive signals of the lateral plate mesoderm.

After pancreas specification has been initiated in the previously uncommitted endoderm, other factors, such as FGFs, which are known to regulate branching morphogenesis of many endodermally derived organs, are involved in growth of the pancreatic epithelium. FGF10, normally present in the pancreatic mesenchyme, is required for normal pancreatic development *(61)* and may mediate inductive mesenchymal-to-epithelial interactions. In one report, ectopic FGF10 expression in the foregut epithelium increased proliferation of a pool of undifferentiated pancreatic stem cells and resulted in a hyperplastic pancreas *(62)*. Together, these studies provide important insights into the early patterning events of the embryonic endoderm and begin to define the molecular control of epithelial-mesenchymal interactions occurring in pancreatic development.

6. NESTIN AS A MARKER OF ISLET PROGENITOR CELLS?

Identification of a pancreas progenitor cell would be an important step in our ability to isolate large numbers of cells that could be readily differentiated into islets or β cells. Based on expression of many neuronal cell markers, a neuroectodermal origin of pancreatic endocrine cells has been hypothesized for many years. It was suggested that the intermediate filament protein nestin, which is expressed in neuronal precursors, might be a marker of islet progenitor cells *(63)*. This speculation was enforced when it was shown that a subset of nestin-positive adult rat pancreatic cells that do not express any of the four islet hormones, could be expanded in vitro and appeared to have the capacity to differentiate into cells expressing PDX1, insulin, and glucagon *(64)*. Several groups have used protocols designed to enrich for neural precursors, characterized by the expression of nestin, in attempts to coax ES cells to adopt a pancreatic islet fate. Lumelsky and coworkers *(65)* generated a population of nestin-expressing cells from mouse ES cells through growth of EBs in serum-free media containing insulin, transferrin, selenium, fibronectin. The cells were then grown in N2 serum-free medium with the addition of bFGF and B27 to expand the pancreatic progenitor cells, and the final step was induction of differentiation through removal of bFGF and addition of nicotinamide. Cells obtained at the end of this multistep differentiation protocol stained positively for several islet marker proteins, including insulin, but were not functional in vitro or in vivo at the levels expected of normal isolated islets.

Using the same protocol, another group *(66)* subsequently demonstrated that although a number of nestin-positive ES cells did form clusters that stained positively for insulin, these clusters neither accumulated insulin transcript nor showed staining with an antibody specific for C-peptide, a protein that results from the cleavage of proinsulin to insulin. In addition, many of the insulin-positive cells were positive in the TUNEL assay, suggesting that they were undergoing apoptosis. Finally, it was demonstrated that cells were capable of taking up exogenous insulin from the medium, perhaps explaining their staining patterns and their failure to reverse hyperglycemia in streptozotocin-induced diabetic animals.

Other investigators have used a similar differentiation protocol involving insulin, transferrin, selenium, fibronectin serum-free media and bFGF, B27, and nicotinamide *(67,68)*. Hori et al. *(67)* used similar conditions for the initial stages of differentiation, but in the last stage replaced B27 with a PI3 kinase inhibitor (LY294002) to reduce the growth of neuronal cells and promote terminal differentiation to insulin-positive cells. The results of these growth conditions were so-called insulin-producing cell clusters, which appear to express insulin, C-peptide, PDX1, GLUT2, and glucokinase and exhibit better insulin release than cells derived through the B27-supplemented protocol. Insulin-producing cell clusters were grafted into the kidney capsules of streptozotocin-induced diabetic NOD *scid* mice, but these animals did not display markedly improved glycemic control. Histological analysis of engrafted insulin-producing cell clusters revealed many pyknotic nuclei, indicative of ongoing apoptosis. This and another study *(68)* suggest that a culture protocol that promotes enrichment of nestin-positive precursors does not result in the production of robust glucose-responsive insulin-secreting cells.

Aside from the question of whether ES cell-derived nestin-positive cells can differentiate into insulin-secreting cells, there has been a great deal of debate as to whether nestin is a marker of islet endocrine progenitors in vivo. Lineage tracing experiments have recently readdressed this question *(69–72)*. In these lineage tracing studies, three independent groups used the *cre*-loxP system to genetically mark cells that activated the nestin promoter *(69–72)*. Although the results varied somewhat among the three studies, none of the investigators found any evidence that nestin-positive cells contribute to the endocrine pancreas, and instead found that these cells can contribute to mesenchymal and epithelial cells of the exocrine lineage, as well as acinar and ductal tissue. Humphrey et al. *(70)* constructed a vector containing nestin regulatory elements driving the neomycin-resistance gene, transduced primary human fetal pancreas tissue, and selected a nestin-positive cell population. They found that nestin was not a specific marker of β cell precursors based on their observation that nestin colocalized with PECAM, α smooth muscle actin, and vimentin but was not present in insulin-positive cells or ductal epithelium positive for pan cytokeratin. They also found that growth factors known to aid maturation of fetal pancreatic tissue, such as Exendin 4, nicotinamide, and hepatocyte growth factor did not induce expression of pancreatic lineage markers in the isolated nestin-positive population. Selected nestin-positive cells transplanted into immunoincompetent mice failed to develop into β cells, as judged by lack of synthesis and release of human C-peptide after stimulation with glucose. These and other studies *(73)*, which are consistent with previous immunohistochemical data *(74)*, suggest that nestin is not a marker of islet progenitors (*see also* ref. *75* and references therein).

7. TRANSDIFFERENTIATION OF ADULT STEM CELLS

Several adult tissues, including blood, epidermis, liver, enterocytes, and spermatogonia, are replenished throughout life by tissue-specific stem cells. Unlike pluripotent stem cells derived from germ cells or the ICM, these somatic stem cells present within organs have not been shown to be capable of differentiating into germ cells. However, somatic stem cells may be multipotent, wherein their progeny can differentiate into multiple discrete cell types, as in the case of hematopoietic stem cells, or unipotent, such as spermatogonia, whose progeny can develop only into the sperm-producing lineage (spermatocytes, spermatids, and spermatozoa). It has been appreciated for many years that the long-lived developmental potential of these somatic stem cells in vivo is critical to organ function. Recently, the question of whether these somatic stem cells may have the capacity for transdifferentiating into cell types specific to other organs, a concept that is counter to the basic tenets of biology, has been discussed.

Indeed, some studies suggest that there may be a greater degree of plasticity, perhaps even pluripotency, associated with adult stem cells than was previously believed. A great deal of excitement ensued when, in 1998, Ferrari et al. *(76)* showed the incorporation of transplanted bone marrow cells into injured skeletal muscle. Subsequently, numerous publications (reviewed in refs. *77–79*) have described various transdifferentiation events, in which adult stem cells from one organ give rise to cell types characteristic of a different organ. These include: bone marrow cells apparently changing their fate into skeletal muscle, cardiac myocytes, endothelial cells, neurons, hepatocytes, and pancreas; and neuronal cells transdifferentiating into blood and skeletal muscle. The fervor accompanying these reports was understandable, particularly with regard to their potential therapeutic value. In particular, adult bone marrow-derived cells have many attractive features as a source of functional, transplantable cellular material. First, they are relatively easy to isolate, and their putative ability to differentiate into cells from a multitude of lineages suggests their use in treating a variety of diseases. Second, ethical questions surrounding the use of human embryonic stem cells are essentially absent from the discussion of adult stem cells. Third, because they can be isolated from the prospective patient, they would be genetically matched, thus eliminating the need for immunosuppressive therapies.

There is, however, a great deal of controversy surrounding the reports of transdifferentiation, and questions remain as to whether adult bone marrow-derived cells will fulfill their promise, and for which cell lineages or diseases they will ultimately be useful. In several cases, efforts to reproduce published results failed *(80–82)* though often these efforts were not exact replications of the original experiments. Minor experimental details notwithstanding, it now appears that many reports of adult stem cell plasticity were likely demonstrations of cell fusion *(83–85)*, which had not been ruled out as a mechanism in any of the early transdifferentiation papers. That differentiated cells are capable of fusion with cells from bone marrow is still an interesting phenomenon, especially in cases in which both nuclei remain intact and at least partly functional (for example, *see* ref. *86*). However, the description of these cells as pluripotent adult stem cells now seems inappropriate.

With specific regard to pancreatic lineages there has been a report of transdifferentiation in the absence of cell fusion by Ianus and colleagues *(87)* who studied in vivo differentiation of adult bone marrow-derived cells into pancreatic endocrine cells. Bone marrow was isolated from male mice carrying insulin-*cre* and a stop codon-floxed EGFP, and then transplanted into unmarked irradiated female mice. The recipients were shown to have EGFP-marked islets, demonstrating that transplanted bone marrow had differentiated into cells that populated the islets; these green-fluorescing cells also displayed other markers of endocrine pancreas, including expression of PDX1 and insulin secretion in response to glucose. To test the frequency with which donor cells fused with host cells in vivo, a second set of experiments was performed in which marrow from male insulin-*cre* mice was transplanted into female mice harboring a stop codon-floxed EGFP. In the analysis, islet cells carrying a Y chromosome were identified, but none of these cells expressed EGFP, demonstrating that fusion had not occurred; in a separate experiment it was shown that fusion of *cre* and stop floxed-EGFP cells in vitro did result in EGFP expression after removal of the floxed stop codon. These results suggest that a population of cells within the bone marrow has the capacity to transdifferentiate into cells that can populate, and perhaps function within, the endocrine pancreas. The extent to which injury plays a role in this phenomenon has yet to be addressed.

Many of the transdifferentiation experiments have been criticized because heterogeneous populations of cells, not single cells or clonal cells, were used for transplantation, making it impossible to determine conclusively that the observed engrafted cell was the progeny of a unique transdifferentiated adult stem cell, and not a previously differentiated cell that existed within the original population. Several protocols included an in vitro culture step, which could potentially result in genetic or epigenetic changes that might promote otherwise rare or "unnatural" differentiation events. One study using streptozotocin-induced pancreas damage demonstrated that pancreatic cell proliferation was induced after bone marrow transplantation *(88)*. These results raise the question of whether the described instances of transdifferentiation may be extremely rare events that are experimental artifacts promoted by induction of tissue injury.

Although these are valid concerns in terms of addressing the question of transdifferentiation and adult stem cell plasticity, they may not be specifically relevant to the discussion of using adult stem cells in the development of transplantable cell populations. Indeed, Verfaillie and colleagues described the isolation of multipotent adult progenitor cells (MAPCs) through ex vivo culture of adult bone marrow *(89,90)*. These rare cells have a life-span in culture upwards of 100 doublings, and can thus be expanded many-fold in vitro. MAPCs express telomerase, retain a wild-type karyotype through many passages, and when derived from mice, require exogenous LIF to retain their undifferentiated proliferative capacity, reminiscent of mouse ES cells. MAPCs have been shown to have the capacity to differentiate into endodermal, ectodermal, and mesodermal/endothelial cell types both in vitro and in vivo *(89)*. An experiment in which the early culture was retrovirally infected suggests that a single isolated cell gave rise to the MAPC cell line. These cells could potentially be isolated from the bone marrow of the patient that requires treatment, thus providing a source of isogenic material for transplantation that would not be immunologically rejected. Although these cells may be pluripotent, islet lineage differentiation from MAPCs has not been demonstrated.

8. PANCREAS-DERIVED STEM CELLS

The prospect of treating human diseases with stem cell-based therapies has stimulated intensive study of organ-specific stem cells. For some tissues, such as intestine and skin, robust stem cells have been known to exist for many years, and clearly contribute to normal cellular turnover and tissue regeneration, as well as repair in pathologic states. Because β-cell mass continues to increase after birth

(91), and the adult pancreas has regenerative capacity after partial pancreatectomy *(92)* and inflammation *(93)* at least in rodents, there has long been speculation as to the existence of a progenitor cell within the pancreas (recently reviewed in refs. *75* and *94*). In concert with these in vivo findings, several groups have demonstrated that culture of pancreatic ductal tissue can result in growth of islet-like tissues from both mice *(95)* and humans *(96,97)*. In each case, an expansion of β cell-like tissue was observed, as demonstrated by expression of *pdx1* and insulin, as well as insulin secretion in response to glucose. Ramiya and colleagues showed that their in vitro generated islets could reverse insulin-dependent diabetes in an NOD mouse model *(95)*. Most evidence suggests ductal or acinar tissue as the source of putative islet stem cells; unfortunately, however, the characterization and isolation of an islet stem cell has been hindered by the absence of specific cell surface markers. Thus none of these studies were able to identify a stem cell population that is responsible for the regenerative growth of islet tissues.

Much of the impetus to isolate a pancreatic islet stem cell is for the development of a therapy for patients with type I diabetes, whose insulin-secreting β cells are destroyed by a poorly understood autoimmune response. Today, some of these patients are eligible for whole organ or islet cell transplantation, but the number of cadaver organs available is limiting. If islet stem cells could be isolated from cadaver organs that were capable of unrestricted growth and differentiation in vitro, it would facilitate the treatment of many more patients than is currently possible. One might envision a scenario in which a bank of pancreatic islet stem cells derived from nondiabetic cadaver donors was created, each line with a different histocompatibility. Similar to the current situation with human ES cell lines, there are ethical and scientific considerations for the development of such a group of cell lines; however, the isolation of an endocrine pancreatic stem cell would be a major advance toward a viable treatment for insulin-dependent diabetes. If pancreatic islet stem cells could be easily isolated from parts of the pancreas that are not destroyed in type I diabetes, such as ductal tissue, it might be possible to isolate autologous cells from the prospective patient. In the case of autoimmune diabetes, however, patients generally retain the destructive autoimmunity and would likely destroy any histocompatible transplant without immunosuppression or immune modulation.

9. POTENTIAL PITFALLS OF STEM CELL-BASED THERAPIES FOR DIABETES IN HUMANS

Both embryonic and adult stem cells represent an underdeveloped resource for the treatment and potential cure for a host of diseases, including type I diabetes. As efforts are made to develop transplantable tissue from each stem cell source, it is important to keep in mind potential pitfalls. Somatic stem cells, either from the bone marrow or ductal elements of the pancreas itself, could be obtained from a cadaver donor, related or unrelated live donor, or directly from the patient. In this final case, the need for immunosuppressive therapy to prevent graft rejection would be eliminated; however, autoimmune destruction of newly generated isogenic islet tissue would likely occur in the type I diabetic. Currently, the ability to expand ex vivo an islet progenitor cell population from ductal or discarded pancreatic tissue is quite limited, and a significant amount of scale-up would be required to make this a feasible therapeutic option. As with pancreas-derived stem cells, stem cells from bone marrow could be isolated from a number of different donors. These cells exhibit capacity for prolonged self-renewal in vitro, making them an attractive option. However, there are no data on the ex vivo differentiation of these cells to pancreas progenitors, and differentiation of these cells into islet-like cell types in vivo is a rare occurrence and may be dependent on acute injury. Much work must be carried out to develop protocols that allow the directed in vitro differentiation of bone marrow-derived stem cells or MAPCs to pancreatic islet lineages.

Embryonic stem cells have been shown to differentiate into various cell types, both in vitro and in vivo, including pancreatic islet lineages *(39,49,98)*. However, functional islet tissue has not been derived from human ES cells to date, and whether ES cell-derived islet tissue will exhibit mature glucose-stimulated insulin secretion or immature function akin to fetal islets remains to be determined. Because theoretically there is no limit to the number of undifferentiated ES cells that can be grown in vitro, the amount of tissue for therapy generated from these cells is also potentially unlimited.

Recently, derivation of a human ES cell line derived from a blastocyst cloned using somatic cell nuclear transfer was reported *(99)*, suggesting that it might some day be possible to grow tissues from isogenic cell lines from all prospective patients, though currently the extremely low efficiency of this process is prohibitive. Another option to prevent rejection without immunosuppressive therapy is to genetically engineer ES cells to be less immunogenic by adding immunomodulatory genes, removing costimulatory molecules, or removing or altering non-self major histocompatibility complex proteins.

Protocols designed to prompt ES cells to differentiate into specific cell types en masse are required before these cells can be used in therapeutic settings. The tumorigenicity of ES cells is a potential caveat, even in situations where the vast majority of cultured cells undergo differentiation to the correct cell fate. While still in culture, genetic selection can be applied to ES cells both to increase the numbers of lineage-specific cell types *(98,100–102)* and to eliminate residual undifferentiated cells prior to transplantation *(102)*.

10. SUMMARY

Although much potential has been ascribed to bone marrow-, pancreas-, and embryo-derived stem cells, there are still significant challenges ahead before a stem cell-based therapy for type I diabetes will be able to enter clinical trials. A more thorough understanding of the nature of pancreatic precursor cells and islet progenitor cells is necessary to identify conditions that will allow their large-scale purification from stem cell sources. Still, the plasticity and inherent developmental potential of these cell populations promises many advances in regenerative medicine that the scientific community has only begun to realize.

ACKNOWLEDGMENTS

The authors would like to thank Drs. Brenda Kahan and David Aceti for a critical reading of the manuscript. Work in the Odorico lab is funded by the Juvenile Diabetes Research Foundation, the National Institutes of Health—NIDDK, the Roche Organ Transplant Research Foundation, and Geron, Inc.

REFERENCES

1. Thomson JA, Itskovitz-Eldor J, Shapiro SS, et al. Embryonic stem cell lines derived from human blastocysts. Science 1998;282:1145–1147.
2. Shamblott MJ, Axelman J, Wang S, et al. Derivation of pluripotent stem cells from cultured human primordial germ cells. Proc Natl Acad Sci USA 1998;95:13726–13731.
3. Stevens LC. Studies on transplantable testicular teratomas of strain 129 mice. J Natl Cancer Inst 1958;20:1257–1275.
4. Kahan BW, Ephrussi B. Developmental potentialities of clonal in vitro cultures of mouse testicular teratoma. J Natl Cancer Inst 1970;44:1015–1036.
5. Stevens LC. The development of transplantable teratocarcinomas from intratesticular grafts of pre- and postimplantation mouse embryos Dev Biol 1970;21:364–382.
6. Solter D, Dominis M, Damjanov I. Embryo-derived teratocarcinoma. II. Teratocarcinogenesis depends on the type of embryonic graft. Int J Cancer 1980;25:341–343.
7. Martin GR. Isolation of a pluripotent cell line from early mouse embryos cultured in medium conditioned by teratocarcinoma stem cells. Proc Natl Acad Sci USA 1981;78:7634–7638.
8. Evans MJ, Kaufman MH. Establishment in culture of pluripotential cells from mouse embryos. Nature 1981;292:154–156.
9. Bradley A, Evans M, Kaufman MH, Robertson E. Formation of germ-line chimaeras from embryo-derived teratocarcinoma cell lines. Nature 1984;309:255–256.
10. Nagy A, Rossant J, Nagy R, Abramow-Newerly W, Roder JC. Derivation of completely cell culture-derived mice from early-passage embryonic stem cells. Proc Natl Acad Sci USA 1993;90:8424–8428.
11. Thomas KR, Capecchi MR. Site-directed mutagenesis by gene targeting in mouse embryo-derived stem cells. Cell 1987;51:503–512.
12. Thomson JA, Kalishman J, Golos TG, et al. Isolation of a primate embryonic stem cell line. Proc Natl Acad Sci USA 1995;92:7844–7848.

13. Thomson JA, Kalishman J, Golos TG, Durning M, Harris CP, Hearn JP. Pluripotent cell lines derived from common marmoset (Callithrix jacchus) blastocysts. Biol Reprod 1996;55:254–259.
14. Suemori H, Tada T, Torii R, et al. Establishment of embryonic stem cell lines from cynomolgus monkey blastocysts produced by IVF or ICSI. Dev Dyn 2001;222:273–279.
15. Reubinoff BE, Pera MF, Fong CY, Trounson A, Bongso A. Embryonic stem cell lines from human blastocysts: somatic differentiation in vitro. Nat Biotechnol 2000;18:399–404.
16. Pain B, Clark ME, Shen M, et al. Long-term in vitro culture and characterisation of avian embryonic stem cells with multiple morphogenetic potentialities. Development 1996; 122:2339–2348.
17. Doetschman T, Williams P, Maeda N. Establishment of hamster blastocyst-derived embryonic stem (ES) cells. Dev Biol 1988;127:224–227.
18. Schoonjans L, Albright GM, Li JL, Collen D, Moreadith RW. Pluripotential rabbit embryonic stem (ES) cells are capable of forming overt coat color chimeras following injection into blastocysts. Mol Reprod Dev 1996;45:439–443.
19. Vassilieva S, Guan K, Pich U, Wobus AM. Establishment of SSEA-1- and Oct-4-expressing rat embryonic stem-like cell lines and effects of cytokines of the IL-6 family on clonal growth. Exp Cell Res 2000;258:361–373.
20. Nagy A, Gertsenstein M, Vintersten K, Behringer R. Manipulating the Mouse Embryo: A Laboratory Manual, 3rd ed. Cold Spring Harbor Laboratory Press, Cold Spring Harbor, NY, 2002.
21. Robertson EJ. Teratocarcinomas and embryonic stem cells: a practical approach. IRL Press, Oxford, 1987.
22. Stevens LC. A new inbred subline of mice (129-terSv) with a high incidence of spontaneous congenital testicular teratomas. J Natl Cancer Inst 1973;50:235–242.
23. Ledermann B, Burki K. Establishment of a germ-line competent C57BL/6 embryonic stem cell line. Exp Cell Res 1991;197:254–258.
24. Kawase E, Suemori H, Takahashi N, Okazaki K, Hashimoto K, Nakatsuji N. Strain difference in establishment of mouse embryonic stem (ES) cell lines. Int J Dev Biol 1994;38:385–390.
25. Brook FA, Evans EP, Lord CJ, et al. The derivation of highly germline-competent embryonic stem cells containing NOD-derived genome. Diabetes 2003;52:205–208.
26. Brook FA, Gardner RL. The origin and efficient derivation of embryonic stem cells in the mouse. Proc Natl Acad Sci USA 1997;94:5709–5712.
27. Rossant J. Stem cells from the mammalian blastocyst. Stem Cells 2001;19:477–482.
28. Solter D, Knowles BB. Immunosurgery of mouse blastocyst. Proc Natl Acad Sci USA 1975;72:5099–5102.
29. Niwa H, Burdon T, Chambers I, Smith A. Self-renewal of pluripotent embryonic stem cells is mediated via activation of STAT3. Genes Dev 1998;12:2048–2060.
30. Burdon T, Stracey C, Chambers I, Nichols J, Smith A. Suppression of SHP-2 and ERK signalling promotes self-renewal of mouse embryonic stem cells. Dev Biol 1999;210:30–43.
31. Ying QL, Nichols J, Chambers I, Smith A. BMP induction of Id proteins suppresses differentiation and sustains embryonic stem cell self-renewal in collaboration with STAT3. Cell 2003;115:281–292.
32. Joyner AL. Gene Targeting, 2nd ed. Oxford University Press, New York, 2000.
33. Amit M, Margulets V, Segev H, et al. Human feeder layers for human embryonic stem cells. Biol Reprod 2003;68:2150–2156.
34. Richards M, Tan S, Fong CY, Biswas A, Chan WK, Bongso A. Comparative evaluation of various human feeders for prolonged undifferentiated growth of human embryonic stem cells. Stem Cells 2003;21:546–556.

35. Richards M, Fong CY, Chan WK, Wong PC, Bongso A. Human feeders support prolonged undifferentiated growth of human inner cell masses and embryonic stem cells. Nat Biotechnol 2002;20:933–936.
36. Xu C, Inokuma MS, Denham J, et al. Feeder-free growth of undifferentiated human embryonic stem cells. Nat Biotechnol 2001;19:971–974.
37. Amit M, Carpenter MK, Inokuma MS, et al. Clonally derived human embryonic stem cell lines maintain pluripotency and proliferative potential for prolonged periods of culture. Dev Biol 2000;227:271–278.
38. Zwaka TP, Thomson JA. Homologous recombination in human embryonic stem cells. Nat Biotechnol 2003;21:319–321.
39. Kahan BW, Jacobson LM, Hullett DA, Oberley TD, Odorico JS. Pancreatic precursors and differentiated islet cell types from murine embryonic stem cells: an in vitro model to study islet differentiation. Diabetes 2003;52:2016–2024.
40. Doetschman TC, Eistetter H, Katz M, Schmidt W, Kemler R. The in vitro development of blastocyst-derived embryonic stem cell lines: formation of visceral yolk sac, blood islands and myocardium. J Embryol Exp Morphol 1985;87:27–45.
41. Keller GM. In vitro differentiation of embryonic stem cells. Curr Opin Cell Biol 1995;7:862–869.
42. Baker RK, Lyons GE. Embryonic stem cells and in vitro muscle development. Curr Top Dev Biol 1996;33:263–279.
43. Bain G, Kitchens D, Yao M, Huettner JE, Gottlieb DI. Embryonic stem cells express neuronal properties in vitro. Dev Biol 1995;168:342–357.
44. Risau W, Sariola H, Zerwes HG, et al. Vasculogenesis and angiogenesis in embryonic-stem-cell-derived embryoid bodies. Development 1998;102:471–478.
45. Maltsev VA, Wobus AM, Rohwedel J, Bader M, Hescheler J. Cardiomyocytes differentiated in vitro from embryonic stem cells developmentally express cardiac-specific genes and ionic currents. Circ Res 1994;75:233–244.
46. Rohwedel J, Maltsev V, Bober E, Arnold HH, Hescheler J, Wobus AM. Muscle cell differentiation of embryonic stem cells reflects myogenesis in vivo: developmentally regulated expression of myogenic determination genes and functional expression of ionic currents. Dev Biol 1994;164:87–101.
47. Yamane T, Hayashi S, Mizoguchi M, Yamazaki H, Kunisada. Derivation of melanocytes from embryonic stem cells in culture. Dev Dyn 1999;216:450–458.
48. Czyz J, Wiese C, Rolletschek A, Blyszczuk P, Cross M, Wobus AM. Potential of embryonic and adult stem cells in vitro. Biol Chem 2003;384:1391–1409.
49. Assady S, Maor G, Amit M, Itskovitz-Eldor J, Skorecki KL, Tzukerman M. Insulin production by human embryonic stem cells. Diabetes 2001;50:1691–1697.
50. Offield MF, Jetton TL, Labosky PA, et al. PDX-1 is required for pancreatic outgrowth and differentiation of the rostral duodenum. Development 1996;122:983–995.
51. Jonsson J, Carlsson L, Edlund T, Edlund H. Insulin-promoter-factor 1 is required for pancreas development in mice. Nature 1994;371:606–609.
52. Stoffers DA, Zinkin NT, Stanojevic V, Clarke WL, Habener JF. Pancreatic agenesis attributable to a single nucleotide deletion in the human IPF1 gene coding sequence. Nat Genet 1997;15:106–110.
53. Wichterle H, Lieberam I, Porter JA, Jessell TM. Directed differentiation of embryonic stem cells into motor neurons. Cell 2002;110:385–397.
54. Wobus AM, Kaomei G, Shan J, et al. Retinoic acid accelerates embryonic stem cell-derived cardiac differentiation and enhances development of ventricular cardiomyocytes. J Mol Cell Cardiol 1997;29:1525–1539.

55. Kaufman DS, Hanson ET, Lewis RL, Auerbach R, Thomson JA. Hematopoietic colony-forming cells derived from human embryonic stem cells. Proc Natl Acad Sci USA 2001;98:10716–10721.
56. Hebrok M. Hedgehog signaling in pancreas development. Mech Dev 2003;120:45–57
57. Hebrok M, Kim SK, St Jacques B, McMahon AP, Melton DA. Regulation of pancreas development by hedgehog signaling. Development 2000;127:4905–4913.
58. Hebrok M, Kim SK, Melton DA. Notochord repression of endodermal Sonic hedgehog permits pancreas development. Genes Dev 1998;12:1705–1713.
59. Lammert E, Cleaver O, Melton D. Induction of pancreatic differentiation by signals from blood vessels. Science 2001;294:564–567.
60. Kumar M, Jordan N, Melton D, Grapin-Botton A Signals from lateral plate mesoderm instruct endoderm toward a pancreatic fate. Dev Biol 2003;259:109–122.
61. Bhushan A, Itoh N, Kato S, et al. Fgf10 is essential for maintaining the proliferative capacity of epithelial progenitor cells during early pancreatic organogenesis. Development 2001;128: 5109–5117.
62. Norgaard GA, Jensen JN, Jensen J. FGF10 signaling maintains the pancreatic progenitor cell state revealing a novel role of Notch in organ development. Dev Biol 2003;264:323–338.
63. Hunziker E, Stein M. Nestin-expressing cells in the pancreatic islets of Langerhans. Biochem Biophys Res Commun 2000;271:116–119.
64. Zulewski H, Abraham EJ, Gerlach MJ, et al. Multipotential nestin-positive stem cells isolated from adult pancreatic islets differentiate ex vivo into pancreatic endocrine, exocrine, and hepatic phenotypes. Diabetes 2001;50:521–533.
65. Lumelsky N, Blondel O, Laeng P, Velasco I, Ravin R, McKay R. Differentiation of embryonic stem cells to insulin-secreting structures similar to pancreatic islets. Science 2001;292:1389–1394.
66. Rajagopal J, Anderson WJ, Kume S, Martinez OI, Melton DA. Insulin staining of ES cell progeny from insulin uptake. Science 2003;299:363.
67. Hori Y, Rulifson IC, Tsai BC, Heit JJ, Cahoy JD, Kim SK. Growth inhibitors promote differentiation of insulin-producing tissue from embryonic stem cells. Proc Natl Acad Sci USA 2002;99:16105–16110.
68. Blyszczuk P, Czyz J, Kania G, et al. Expression of Pax4 in embryonic stem cells promotes differentiation of nestin-positive progenitor and insulin-producing cells. Proc Natl Acad Sci USA 2003;100:998–1003.
69. Treutelaar MK, Skidmore JM, Dias-Leme CL, et al. Nestin-lineage cells contribute to the microvasculature but not endocrine cells of the islet. Diabetes 2003;52:2503–2512.
70. Humphrey RK, Bucay N, Beattie GM, Lopez A, Messam CA, Cirulli V, Hayek A. Characterization and isolation of promoter-defined nestin-positive cells from the human fetal pancreas. Diabetes 2003;52:2519–2525.
71. Delacour A, Nepote V, Trumpp A, Herrera PL. Nestin expression in pancreatic exocrine cell lineages. Mech Dev 2004;121:3–14.
72. Esni F, Stoffers DA, Takeuchi T, Leach SD. Origin of exocrine pancreatic cells from nestin-positive precursors in developing mouse pancreas. Mech Dev 2004;121:15–25.
73. Street CN, Lakey JR, Seeberger K, et al. Heterogenous expression of nestin in human pancreatic tissue precludes its use as an islet precursor marker. J Endocrinol 2004;180:213–225.
74. Edlund H. Pancreatic organogenesis—developmental mechanisms and implications for therapy. Nat Rev Genet 2002;3:524–532.
75. Zhang YQ, Sarvetnick N. Development of cell markers for the identification and expansion of islet progenitor cells. Diabetes Metab Res Rev 2003;19:363–374.

76. Ferrari G, Cusella-De Angelis G, Coletta M, et al. Muscle regeneration by bone marrow-derived myogenic progenitors. Science 1998;279:1528–1530.
77. Goodell MA. Stem-cell "plasticity:" befuddled by the muddle. Curr Opin Hematol 2003;10:208–213.
78. Raff M. Adult stem cell plasticity: fact or artifact? Annu Rev Cell Dev Biol 2003;19:1–22
79. Joshi CV, Enver T. Plasticity revisited. Curr Opin Cell Biol 2002;14:749–755.
80. Castro RF, Jackson KA, Goodell MA, Robertson CS, Liu H, Shine HD. Failure of bone marrow cells to transdifferentiate into neural cells in vivo. Science 2002;297:1299.
81. Wagers AJ, Sherwood RI, Christensen JL, Weissman IL. Little evidence for developmental plasticity of adult hematopoietic stem cells. Science 2002;297:2256–2259.
82. Choi JB, Uchino H, Azuma K, et al. Little evidence of transdifferentiation of bone marrow-derived cells into pancreatic beta cells. Diabetologia 2003;46:1366–1374.
83. Ying QL, Nichols J, Evans EP, Smith AG. Changing potency by spontaneous fusion. Nature 2002;416:545–548.
84. Terada N, Hamazaki T, Oka M, et al. Bone marrow cells adopt the phenotype of other cells by spontaneous cell fusion. Nature 2002;416:542–545.
85. Wang X, Willenbring H, Akkari Y, et al. Cell fusion is the principal source of bone-marrow-derived hepatocytes. Nature 2003;422:897–901.
86. Weimann JM, Johansson CB, Trejo A, Blau HM. Stable reprogrammed heterokaryons form spontaneously in Purkinje neurons after bone marrow transplant. Nat Cell Biol 2003;5:959–966.
87. Ianus A, Holz GG, Theise ND, Hussain MA. In vivo derivation of glucose-competent pancreatic endocrine cells from bone marrow without evidence of cell fusion. J Clin Invest 2003;111:843–850.
88. Hess D, Li L, Martin M, et al. Bone marrow-derived stem cells initiate pancreatic regeneration. Nat Biotechnol 2003;21:763–770.
89. Jiang Y, Jahagirdar BN, Reinhardt RL, et al. Pluripotency of mesenchymal stem cells derived from adult marrow. Nature 2002;418:41–49.
90. Reyes M, Lund T, Lenvik T, Aguiar D, Koodie L, Verfaillie CM. Purification and ex vivo expansion of postnatal human marrow mesodermal progenitor cells. Blood 2001;98:2615–2625.
91. Montanya E, Nacher V, Biarnes M, Soler J. Linear correlation between beta-cell mass and body weight throughout the lifespan in Lewis rats: role of beta-cell hyperplasia and hypertrophy. Diabetes 2000;49:1341–1346.
92. Bonner-Weir S, Baxter LA, Schuppin GT, Smith FE. A second pathway for regeneration of adult exocrine and endocrine pancreas. A possible recapitulation of embryonic development. Diabetes 1993;42:1715–1720.
93. Rosenberg L, Vinik AI. In vitro stimulation of hamster pancreatic duct growth by an extract derived from the "wrapped" pancreas. Pancreas 1993;8:255–260.
94. Bonner-Weir S, Sharma A. Pancreatic stem cells. J Pathol 2002;197:519–526.
95. Ramiya VK, Maraist M, Arfors KE, Schatz DA, Peck AB, Cornelius JG. Reversal of insulin-dependent diabetes using islets generated in vitro from pancreatic stem cells. Nat Med 2000;6:278–282.
96. Bonner-Weir S, Taneja M, Weir GC, et al. In vitro cultivation of human islets from expanded ductal tissue. Proc Natl Acad Sci U S A 2000;97:7999–8004.
97. Gao R, Ustinov J, Pulkkinen MA, Lundin K, Korsgren O, Otonkoski T Characterization of endocrine progenitor cells and critical factors for their differentiation in human adult pancreatic cell culture. Diabetes 2003;52:2007–2015.

98. Soria B, Roche E, Berna G, Leon-Quinto T, Reig JA, Martin F. Insulin-secreting cells derived from embryonic stem cells normalize glycemia in streptozotocin-induced diabetic mice. Diabetes 2000;49:157–162.
99. Hwang WS, Ryu YJ, Park JH, et al. Evidence of a pluripotent human embryonic stem cell line derived from a cloned blastocyst. Science 2004;303:1669–1674.
100. Klug MG, Soonpaa MH, Koh GY, Field LJ. Genetically selected cardiomyocytes from differentiating embryonic stem cells form stable intracardiac grafts. J Clin Invest 1996;98:216–224.
101. Li M, Pevny L, Lovell-Badge R, Smith A. Generation of purified neural precursors from embryonic stem cells by lineage selection. Curr Biol 1998;8:971–974.
102. Billon N, Jolicoeur C, Ying QL, Smith A, Raff M. Normal timing of oligodendrocyte development from genetically engineered, lineage-selectable mouse ES cells. J Cell Sci 2002;115:3657–3665.

2 Germ Line Stem Cells

Makoto C. Nagano

CONTENTS

1. INTRODUCTION

Stem cells are a unique cell population in both biological and clinical contexts. Stem cells are defined by their function to reproduce themselves (self-renewal) and concurrently generate daughter cells that are committed to differentiation *(1)*. The differentiation of stem cells leads to the production of all cell types in a given cell lineage. Furthermore, stem cells conduct this dual function for a lifetime, thereby continuously providing specialized cells that perform normal functions of self-renewing tissues/organs (e.g., bone marrow, intestinal epithelium; *see* ref. *2*). Clinically, these characteristics of stem cells allow them to be a potentially powerful resource for various applications, such as regenerative medicine and gene therapy *(3)*. Our ability to understand stem cell biology is therefore crucial for such practical applications.

In general, stem cells can be categorized into three types. One type is a stem cell population of embryonic origin, and the other two are postnatal stem cells in

From: *Contemporary Endocrinology: Stem Cells in Endocrinology*
Edited by: L. B. Lester © Humana Press Inc., Totowa, NJ

somatic and germ cell lineages. Each of these three stem cell types has a unique property. Whereas somatic stem cells (e.g., hematopoietic stem cells) are indispensable for the survival of an individual, germ line stem cells are essential for the survival of a species. Thus germ line stem cells are the foundation for the manifestation of evolutionary processes, whereas somatic stem cells function as receptors of the selection pressure exerted by their environment. Stem cells derived from embryos have the broadest differentiation potential among the three and can produce all cell types in the body, including somatic and germ cell lineages. On the other hand, postnatal stem cells are essentially tissue-specific and produce only cells of the corresponding cell lineage *(4)*.

Among these three types of stem cells, somatic and embryonic stem cells have been more intensively investigated than germ line stem cells. However, because all embryonic and somatic cells originate from gametes, studies of germ line stem cells may facilitate understanding the biology of other two stem cell types. Alternatively, because the development of germ cells is initiated in embryos separately from that of somatic cells (*see* the following section), germ line stem cells might possess unique properties that distinguish them from other types of stem cells.

In this chapter, the current state of germ line stem cell research and knowledge accumulated during the past decade almost exclusively using a mouse model is discussed. Although some clinical perspectives are discussed in the last section of this chapter, readers are advised to refer elsewhere (Chapter 11 and ref. *5*) for more detailed discussions on applications of germ line stem cells. After brief descriptions on fetal germ cells, the main focus of this chapter will be stem cells of the postnatal male germ line, because using the strictest definition of stem cells, no stem cells exist in the fetal and female germ lines in mammals. In addition, the discussion in this chapter will focus on studies in which stem cells were analyzed by functional assays, even though extensive morphologic studies have historically provided important knowledge on germ line stem cells *(6)*. This is because stem cells are defined essentially by their functions and not by their morphology.

2. DEVELOPMENT OF GERM CELLS AND THEIR RELATIONS TO EMBRYONIC STEM CELLS

During embryonic development, germ cells first emerge at a specific location segregated from somatic cell development in both vertebrates and invertebrates *(7–9)*. This physical segregation of germ cells has been hypothesized to allow germ line specification to occur with a minimal influence from somatic cell development *(8)*. In mammals, germ cell development has been best studied in mice. Mouse germ cells are first recognized at the base of allantois in the extraembryonic mesoderm at approximately 7 days postcoitum (dpc) as a cluster of approximately 50 cells that exhibit the alkaline phosphatase activity *(7–9)*. These fetal germ cells are called primordial germ cells (PGCs). PGCs are then transferred from the extraembryonic tissue to the embryo *per se* at approximately 8.5 dpc and migrate through the hindgut while rapidly proliferating. These cells further migrate through the dorsal mesentery into the genital ridges (fetal gonads) at approximately 10.5 dpc. PGCs continue to proliferate in the genital ridge until approximately 12.5 dpc when the sex differentiation becomes morphologically evident. On 13.5 dpc, approximately 25,000 PGCs can be found in the genital ridge *(10)*; thus, PGCs increase 500-fold in number from the time of their emergence. At the initiation of sex differentiation, female and male germ cells take different developmental pathways (Fig. 1). In females, PGCs enter meiosis and then become arrested at meiotic prophase. In males, PGCs encapsulated in the testicular cords (fetal seminiferous tubules) become mitotically arrested. The arrested stage continues until birth in both sexes. After birth, female germ cells are periodically recruited for meiotic maturation, whereas male germ cells initiate mitosis. In the male, these diploid postnatal germ cells are called *spermatogonia*. Spermatogonia undergo mitosis and sequentially differentiate before committing to meiosis *(11)*. In mice, first meiotic male germ cells (spermatocytes) appear around 10 days of age and first spermatozoa, approximately 35 days of age *(12,13)*. The male gametogenesis (spermatogenesis) continues throughout life.

The mechanism of germ cell specification, migration, proliferation/survival, and sex-dependent differentiation during embryonic development remains elusive and is beyond the scope of this chapter (*see* refs. *8,9,14–17* for detail). However, the process of germ cell development depicts a unique characteristic of germ line stem cells. Because all female germ cells enter meiosis on sex differentiation, they lose self-renewal potential before birth, resulting in the loss of stem cells in the postnatal female germ line. In contrast, a population of self-renewing cells (stem cells) remains in the male germ line throughout life. This is the foundation of continuous spermatogenesis and the regeneration of spermatogenesis following testicular insults, including sterilizing cancer therapy *(5,18)*. Consequently, the number of gametes during the reproductively active periods in males far exceeds that in females. Such a sex-dependent difference in the existence of stem cells cannot be seen in other types of stem cells.

PGCs are a transient cell type and are not true stem cells under a strict stem cell definition. These cells are rather "precursors" of germ line stem cells, because the cells that have characteristics identical to PGCs do not exist in normal postnatal mammals, reflecting the lack of extended self-renewal activity of PGCs. If fact, many embryonic cells are precursors. For example, although the cells in the inner cell mass of blastocysts are the origin of embryonic stem cells

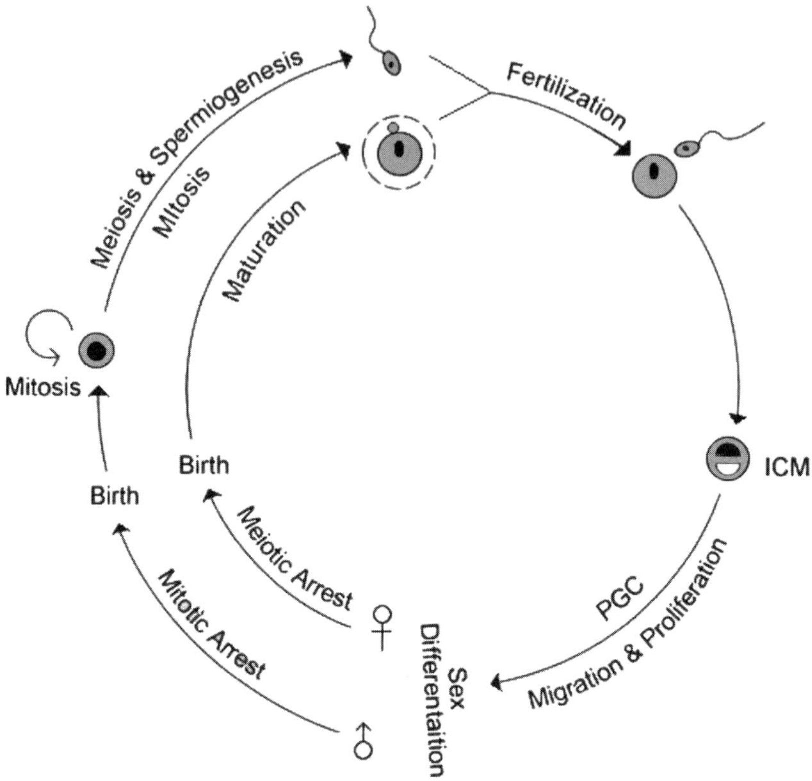

Fig. 1. The life cycle of germ cells. Fertilization of an egg by a sperm triggers the embryonic development. The cells in the ICM (shown as a dark part) of the blastocyst are the origin of all cell types in the body as well as ES cells. PGCs are first found in the extraembryonic mesoderm and translocate into the embryo *per se*. Then, they migrate toward the embryonic gonads while actively proliferating. These proliferating PGCs are capable of transforming to totipotent EG cells. After the migration into the gonads, male germ cells enter mitotic arrest, whereas all female germ cells enter meiosis, followed by the arrest at the meiotic prophase. After birth, male germ cells reinitiate mitosis and undergo meiosis and spermiogenesis, which is a complex morphologic transformation of haploid spermatids to sperm. Mitosis, meiosis, and spermiogenesis continue throughout life in the male germ line (spermatogenesis). It is important to note that a population of stem cells exists in the male germ line, whereas it is absent in the female germ line. (Modified from ref. *95* with permission.)

(ES cells; Chapter 1), they do not self-renew but rather disappear during normal embryonic development.

Although PGCs are a transient cell population, these cells have significant potential to be a source of stem cells, not only for male germ line stem cells but also for pluripotent embryonal carcinoma (EC) cells and totipotent embryonic germ (EG) cells (*see* Chapter 1). From the 1950s to the 1970s (reviewed in ref. *19*), Leroy Stevens at the Jackson Laboratory intensively studied teratomas/teratocarcinomas (hereafter, only the term "teratocarcinomas" will be used for simplicity). Using mice, he showed that the implantation of blastocysts or of the genital ridge (10.5–12.5 dpc) into adult testes resulted in the formation of teratocarcinomas, in which a wide range of differentiated tissues can be observed (*see* Chapter 1). He identified PGCs as the origin of teratocarcinomas that arise after implanting genital ridges into adult testes *(20)*. Teratocarcinomas were found to contain the stem cells that were later isolated and called EC cells (*see* Chapter 1). The self-renewal potential and pluripotency (potential to differentiate into multiple, *but not all*, cell types) of EC cells was proven by Barry Pierce, thus confirming the stem cell properties of these cells *(21)*. Ralph Brinster later demonstrated by injecting EC cells into blastocysts that these tumor stem cells could be integrated into the normal developmental process to produce chimeric mice without causing tumorigenesis *(22)*, although EC cells do not enter the germ line. Therefore, PGCs are the source of pluripotent EC cells that can contribute to the generation of chimeric mice.

In 1992, Matsui et al. *(23)* and Resnick et al. *(24)* reported that mouse PGCs transformed to cells that morphologically resembled ES cells when cultured in vitro with a cocktail of growth factors. These cells, called EG cells, were derived by culturing proliferating PGCs (8.5–12.5 dpc) with leukemia inhibitory factor (LIF), Steel factor (also called c-Kit ligand), and basic fibroblast growth factor (bFGF). Using similar culture techniques, EG cells have also been obtained from pigs and humans *(25,26)*. The studies using mice have shown that EG and ES cells are similar not only in their morphology, but also in their function. As with ES cells, EG cells can be maintained in undifferentiated states indefinitely in vitro and will generate teratocarcinomas in vivo *(23)*. When injected into blastocysts, both ES and EG cells are integrated into the normal developmental process of host mice and contribute to both somatic and germ cell lineages *(27)*. Therefore, ES and EG cells are both totipotent (differentiate into *all* cell types), although they are apparently not identical *(28)*. Another characteristic shared by both of these tumor stem cells is that they are derived from transient cell types that express Oct-3/4 transcription factor: ES cells from the inner cell mass/epiblast and EG cells from PGCs *(8,9,29,30)* (*see* Chapter 1).

Although mouse PGCs have the potential to transform into totipotent stem cells, ironically these cells have never been successfully used for cloning by nuclear transplantation *(31,32)*. Mice can be successfully cloned using the nuclei of many somatic cell types *(33)*. However, no reports have shown live birth of offspring cloned from PGC nuclei *(31,32)*. Yamazaki et al. have shown that embryos cloned using nuclei of 10.5-dpc PGCs can develop normally until midgestation but die shortly thereafter *(32)*. Furthermore, embryos cloned from later-stage PGCs never develop normally *(32)*. These results might indicate that the genomes of germ cells may be programmed in a specific manner. For example, it is well known that the patterns of DNA methylation and imprinting in the germ line are distinct from those of somatic cell lineages *(34,35)*. Therefore, it is possible that genomic modifications specific to the germ line render the reprogramming of the germ cell genome difficult in cloning by nuclear transplantation.

3. SPERMATOGONIAL TRANSPLANTATION—FUNCTIONAL ASSAY TO DETECT STEM CELL ACTIVITY

Postnatal male germ line stem cells, also called spermatogonial stem cells (SSCs), are a small fraction of spermatogonia *(6,18)*. SSCs and spermatogonia reside at the periphery of the seminiferous tubules on the basement membrane surrounded by Sertoli cells, which are somatic regulatory and supportive cells for spermatogenesis (Fig. 2).

Because stem cells are defined by their dual functions, studies of stem cells require a functional assay to detect stem cell *activity* (long-term self-renewal and differentiation). The unequivocal detection system for stem cells is a transplantation assay, in which the presence of stem cells is retrospectively confirmed by their ability to replenish a complete cell lineage in a damaged tissue. For example, the presence of hematopoietic stem cells (HSCs) in the bone marrow can be inferred when transplantation of marrow cells into lethally irradiated recipients results in a complete regeneration and long-term maintenance of hematopoiesis of donor origin *(1)*. Likewise, SSCs can be detected by a transplantation assay (spermatogonial transplantation). In fact, HSCs and SSCs are the only stem cell populations for which a transplantation assay has been established. The detection of other stem cells relies on more equivocal assay systems, such as an in vitro differentiation assay for neural stem cells *(36)*.

The spermatogonial transplantation assay was developed in 1994 using the mouse as a model species (Fig. 3; refs. *37,38*). In this assay system, a single cell suspension is first prepared from the testes of donor mice *(39,40)*. These cells are injected into the lumen of recipient mouse seminiferous tubules using a microinjection needle. The recipient mice are pretreated with an alkylating reagent, busulfan, to ablate endogenous spermatogenesis, thereby providing access and space for donor stem cells to colonize on the basement membrane and to develop spermatogenesis *(39–41)*. On transplantation, SSCs migrate from the tubular lumen to the basement membrane, settle in the microenvironment surrounded by recipient Sertoli cells, and regenerate spermatogenesis. The donor origin of regenerated spermatogenesis is readily confirmed by using transgenic mice as donors and wild-type mice as recipients. In an experiment shown in Fig. 3, donors were ROSA26 transgenic mice that ubiquitously express β-galactosi-

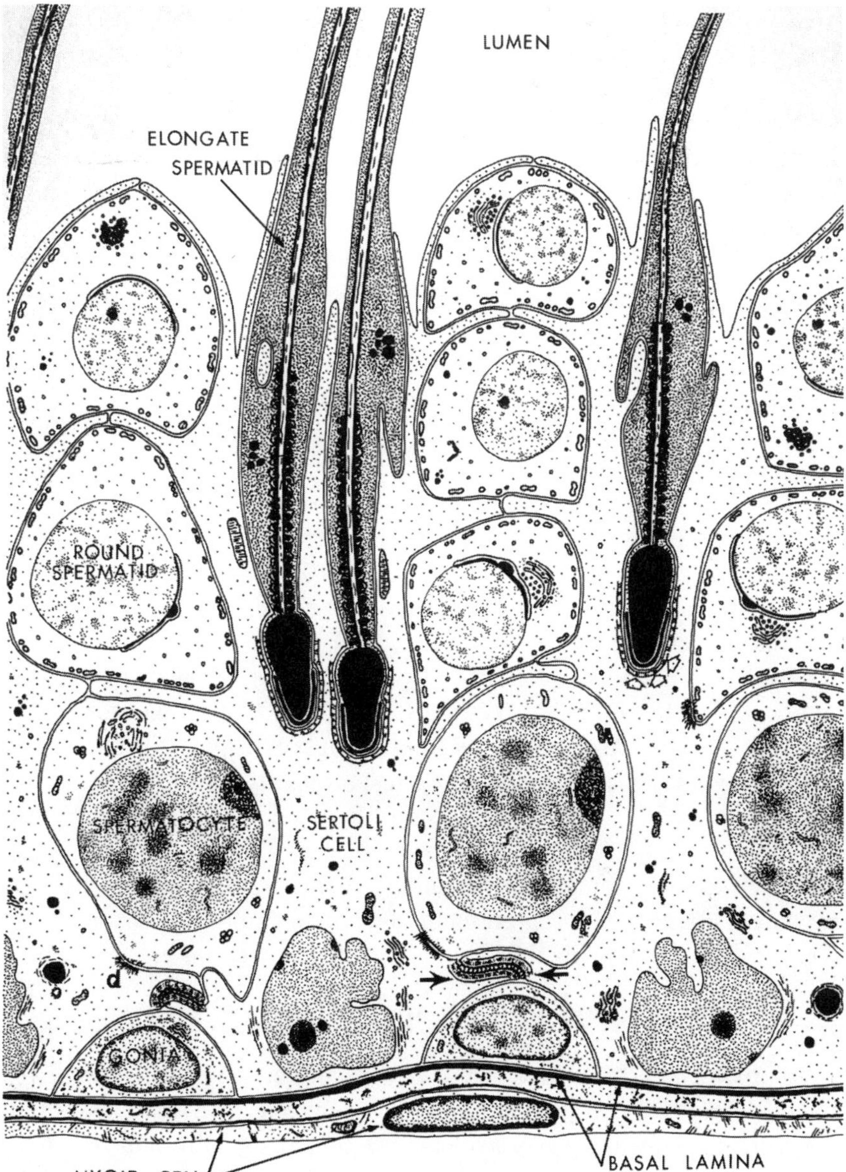

Fig. 2. A schematic representation of seminiferous epithelium. Diploid spermatogonia reside on the basement membrane at the periphery of seminiferous tubules, surrounded by Sertoli and peritubular myoid cells. Meiotic and haploid germ cells are located in the adlumenal compartment and migrate toward the lumen during their development. The final product of spermatogenesis, spermatozoa, is released into the lumen. Spermatogonial stem cells are a small fraction of spermatogonia. (From ref. *11* with permission.)

dase, and recipients were immunocompatible wild-type mice pretreated with busulfan. Thus donor-derived spermatogenesis can be detected as a blue segment (colony) in seminiferous tubules by staining recipient testes with X-gal. After transplantation, recipient mice can regain fertility and produce offspring carrying the donor genotype (*see* Fig. 3). Because such a complete recovery and long-term maintenance of spermatogenesis can be achieved only by stem cell activity, spermatogonial transplantation is the unequivocal assay for SSCs.

Spermatogonial transplantation has provided a unique opportunity to study the role of hormones in spermatogenesis. Although testosterone is essential to spermatogenesis, the target of its action (germ cells or somatic cells) was elusive for decades. This question was addressed using transplantation of testis cells obtained from the *tfm* (i.e., testicular feminization) mutant mice, which lacked functional testosterone receptors *(42)*. Transplantation of these cells into the testes of immunocompatible wild-type mice resulted in the complete regeneration of spermatogenesis in recipient testes. The result thus demonstrated that SSCs exist in the *tfm* mice and that the testosterone receptor is not required in germ cells but is essential in their environment *(42)*. Similarly, a transplantation study has demonstrated that the estrogen receptor α is not required in germ cells for complete spermatogenesis *(43)*.

Spermatogonial transplantation is not only a qualitative but also a quantitative assay for SSCs. Recent transplantation studies have shown that each colony of donor-derived spermatogonia arises from a single SSC *(44,45)*. Therefore, the number of colonies observed in recipient testes directly correlates with the number of functional SSCs that have successfully colonized the recipient environment and regenerated spermatogenesis.

Although spermatogonial transplantation is a time-consuming assay that detects SSCs only retrospectively, it is currently the only definitive assay for SSCs, and studies of SSCs have heavily relied on the development of this assay system.

4. THE FREQUENCY OF SSCs

A common characteristic observed in virtually all stem cell systems is that stem cells are a rare cell population in a cell lineage. For example, definitive HSCs represent only 0.007% of nucleated bone marrow cells in mice *(1)*. Using spermatogonial transplantation as a SSC bioassay, a recent study has demonstrated that adult mouse SSCs represent 0.01% of total testis cells (approximately 3000 SSCs/testis, ref. *46*). Thus 1 in 10,000 cells in an adult testis is a stem cell, a similar frequency to that observed with mouse HSCs in the bone marrow.

However, the number of SSCs appears to vary during postnatal development and between species. It has been shown that the total number of functional SSCs in a testis (those capable of regenerating spermatogenesis in recipient testes after

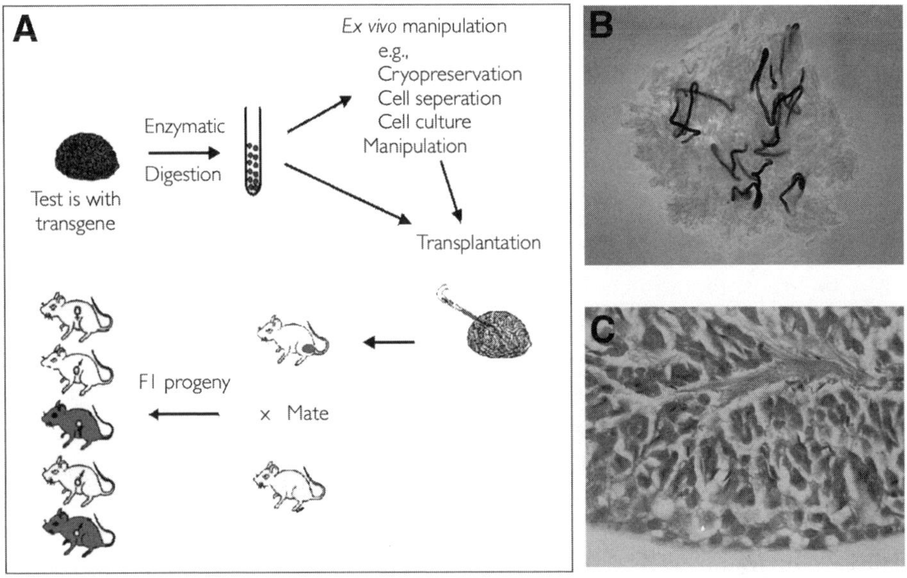

Fig. 3. **(A)** A flow chart of the spermatogonial transplantation procedure. Donor testes are enzymatically digested to a single cell suspension. These cells can be used for ex vivo manipulations, such as cryopreservation, cell selection, cell culture, and genetic modification. Donor cells are introduced into the lumen of seminiferous tubules. Spermatogonial stem cells included in the donor cell preparation colonize recipient testes and develop donor-derived spermatogenesis. Recipient males can become fertile and produce offspring carrying the donor genotype. Because such a complete and long-term regeneration of spermatogenesis cannot be accomplished without stem cells, spermatogonial transplantation is the unequivocal assay to detect stem cell activity. **(B)** When donor cells are derived from the testes of transgenic mice that express a marker gene (*lacZ* in this example) in germ cells, donor-derived spermatogenesis can be readily observed as blue-stained segments in seminiferous tubules (colonies; dark segments in this panel). The formation of morphologically distinct colonies allows quantitative analyses of stem cells by counting the number of colonies. **(C)** At 2 months posttransplantation, complete spermatogenesis is established in a colony. (From ref. *96* with permission.)

transplantation) increases up to 40-fold from the day of birth to adulthood in mice *(47)*. In the rat, the total number of functional SSCs also dramatically increases (70-fold) during postnatal development *(41,48)*. However, compared with mouse SSCs, rat SSCs are 2- to 10-fold higher in their concentration (frequency) and 30- to 120-fold higher in their total number per testis, depending on the stage of postnatal development *(41,47,48)*. Thus the frequency and the number of SSCs appear to differ greatly with age and between species.

5. KINETICS AND REGULATION OF SSC PROLIFERATION

Although proliferation kinetics of SSCs in the steady state (i.e., in intact testes) are unknown, some data are available on the SSC proliferation kinetics under experimental conditions in vivo and in vitro.

5.1 In Vivo Studies

SSC proliferation activity after transplantation has recently been characterized. On transplantation, adult mouse SSCs migrate to the basement membrane and settle in the recipient seminiferous epithelium in the first week *(46)*. During this period, the proliferation of SSCs is undetectable. From 1 to 4 weeks posttransplantation, SSCs rapidly proliferate (approximately eightfold), but thereafter, their proliferation activity significantly diminishes *(46,49)*. SSCs divide slowly from 1 month to more than 1 year after transplantation, and their population doubling time has been estimated to be approximately 80 days during this period *(49)*. Although SSCs slowly divide after 1 month posttransplantation, colonies of donor-derived spermatogonia continue to expand in a linear fashion. Interestingly, during this linear growth period, the concentration of SSCs in a colony appears to stay constant at approximately 8 SSCs per 2 mm of colony *(46,49)*. This consistent stem cell concentration during the colony growth phase suggests that the proliferation of SSCs is tightly regulated in coordination with the progress of spermatogenic regeneration and the number of differentiating germ cells produced by SSCs.

It is well known that spermatogenesis takes place in a species-specific cycle duration *(11)*. For example, one cycle of spermatogenesis takes 35 days in the mouse and 52 days in the rat. Such a species-specific cycle of spermatogenesis could be related to regulation of balance between the activity of SSCs and the progress of spermatogenesis described previously. A long-standing question was whether the spermatogenic cycle length is determined by germ cells, supporting Sertoli cells, or by both. This question was addressed by using xenogeneic spermatogonial transplantation, in which SSCs derived from transgenic rats were transplanted into the testes of immunodeficient mice *(50)*. The results showed that regenerated rat spermatogenesis exhibited spermatogenic cycle length characteristics of the rat (52 days), even though rat SSCs and spermatogenesis were supported by mouse Sertoli cells. Therefore, it was concluded that the cycle length of spermatogenesis is predominantly regulated by germ cells, rather than by Sertoli cells *(50)*. Because the progress of spermatogenesis apparently depends on the activity of SSCs to self-renew and supply differentiating germ cells *(46,49)*, the difference in the spermatogenic cycle length observed in various species might correlate with a species-specific SSC activity.

The proliferation of SSCs must also be regulated in concert with their differentiation and death *(6)*. For example, if one cell division of a SSC results in the production of one daughter stem cell and one differentiating spermatogonium (50% probability each for self-renewal and differentiation), the size of SSC population should be maintained at constant. If the probability is distorted to 100% self-renewal or 100% differentiation, it should result in the expansion of SSCs and the loss of differentiating cells or vice versa. Likewise, the death of daughter cells should result in a decrease in stem and/or differentiating cells. The pattern and mechanism of such stem cell regulation are unknown for SSCs *(6)*. However, observations of spermatogenesis in mutant mice suggest that the differentiation of spermatogonia/SSCs is less stable than their proliferation.

Mutant mice that lack functional Steel factor are devoid of spermatogenesis and infertile because Sertoli cells cannot support spermatogenesis. However, SSCs are retained in their testes and are capable of regenerating complete spermatogenesis when transplanted into the testes of wild-type mice *(51)*. A detailed study of spermatogenesis in Steel factor mutant mice has demonstrated that the loss of spermatogenesis results from defective differentiation of spermatogonia *(52)*. Provided with no functional Steel factor, SSCs can still proliferate and produce daughter spermatogonia, but these spermatogonia cannot proceed through further differentiation events and die by apoptosis. Similarly, adult *jsd* (juvenile spermatogonial deficiency) mice lack spermatogenesis and are infertile because of the intrinsic inability of spermatogonia produced by SSCs to complete differentiation, which results in spermatogonial death *(52,53)*. In another mutant mouse strain that overexpresses glial cell line-derived neurotrophic factor (GDNF), primitive spermatogonia accumulate in the seminiferous tubules, probably because of the blockade in spermatogonial differentiation while spermatogonial proliferation continues *(54)*. A similar pattern of spermatogonial accumulation caused by the differentiation blockade has also been observed in mutant mice that misexpress the anti-apoptotic *bcl-2* gene in germ cells *(55)*.

In contrast, despite the production of numerous mutant strains of infertile mice to date *(56)*, specific defects in the proliferation of spermatogonia or SSCs have not clearly been demonstrated. These studies thus suggest that the proliferation of spermatogonia and possibly SSCs is a rather autonomous function of these cells; whereas their differentiation is the vulnerable and potentially manipulative process during early spermatogenesis.

5.2 In Vitro Studies

Proliferation characteristics of SSCs have also been studied in vitro using retroviral vectors. These viral vectors can deliver and integrate a target gene into the genome of host cells. Because stem cells are retrospectively detected by their function, retroviruses are particularly powerful vectors to place a marker in stem cells before they exhibit their regeneration activity. In addition, retroviruses require host cell division for a successful gene delivery; thus, stem cell proliferation can be detected using these vectors. To evaluate the activity of SSC proliferation in vitro, a marker gene (*lacZ*) was delivered into SSCs using retroviral vectors in culture, followed by transplantation of cultured cells *(57)*. After 7 days of culture, the marker gene was found in 0.3% of total stem cells cultured. Therefore, at least 1 of 300 SSCs entered self-renewal during 1 week of culture. It has also be shown that the self-renewal activity of prepubertal SSCs derived from 1-week-old mice is approximately 10-fold higher than that of adult SSCs *(58)*, corresponding well with the behavior of prepubertal SSCs observed in vivo. Although adult SSCs are believed to be mostly quiescent, prepubertal spermatogonia and SSCs proliferate more actively during the first postnatal week in mice *(6)*.

Although the studies using retroviruses demonstrated that SSCs could divide in vitro, it has also been shown that the total number of mouse SSCs continuously decreases during 1 week of culture *(59)*. About half of SSCs placed in culture are lost within the first 2 days and only 12% of SSCs remain for 1 week. However, this continuous decrease in SSC numbers should not be a simple loss of SSCs during culture because SSCs undergo self-renewal in vitro. Because the number of SSCs detected by spermatogonial transplantation reflects a cumulative result of stem cell division, differentiation, and death, the observed decrease in the number of SSCs should imply that the differentiation or the death of SSCs exceeded their self-renewal under the culture conditions employed.

Using the same culture system, effects of soluble factors on the in vitro SSC maintenance have been examined *(59)*. Activin A is a member of transforming growth factor-β (TGF-β) family and has been shown to stimulate the proliferation of spermatogonia in vitro *(60)*. However, transplantation experiments using testis cells cultured with activin A have demonstrated a marked decrease in SSC numbers to 30% of those in control culture with no factors. The results thus suggest that activin A may act on differentiating spermatogonia, rather than SSCs *(59)*. Because spermatogenesis is a one-way differentiation cascade from stem cells to spermatozoa (Fig. 4), it may be reasonable to speculate that the proliferation of advanced spermatogonia stimulated by activin A might induce the recruitment of SSCs into differentiation at a rate that exceeds the self-renewal of SSCs to support expanding nonstem spermatogonia, thereby diminishing stem cell population in vitro.

In contrast to the effect of activin A, GDNF, which is another member of the TGF-β family, stimulates the maintenance of SSCs in vitro *(59)*. It has been shown that GDNF blocks the differentiation of spermatogonia in transgenic mice that constitutively express the factor, and undifferentiated spermatogonia accu-

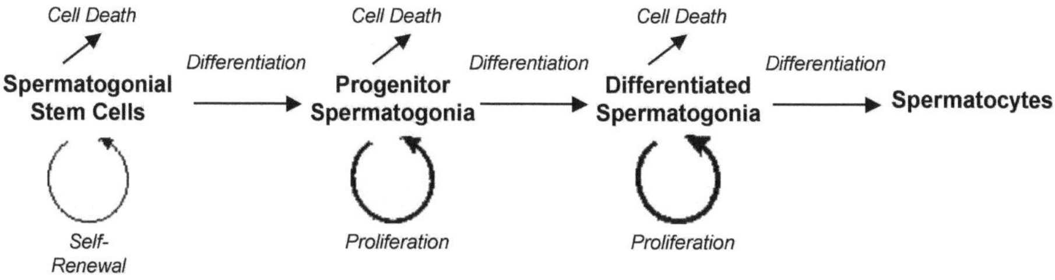

Fig. 4. A schematic representation of the cascade of spermatogonial differentiation. Spermatogenesis is a one-way differentiation event from stem cells to sperm. Therefore, a blockade in one step of differentiation may result in the accumulation of cells at prior differentiation stages, and ultimately stem cells. The amplification of stem cells can be achieved also by encouraging stem cell self-renewal and inhibiting stem cell death.

mulate in their testes *(54)*. In addition, transfection of GDNF in Sertoli cells leads to the expansion of the SSC population in vivo *(61)*. Likewise, GDNF may exert a similar function to block spermatogonial differentiation in vitro. A blockade of a differentiation process in unidirectional spermatogenesis could ultimately result in the accumulation of SSCs, thereby supporting the maintenance of SSCs in culture (Fig. 4).

The same study also suggested a similarity in regulatory mechanisms of SSCs and HSCs (59). Although bone morphogenetic protein 4 (BMP4) is known to play a critical role in germ cell specification during embryonic development in mice (14), BMP4 was found to decrease SSC numbers to 40% of control levels in vitro *(59)*. In this context, it has recently been shown that the number of HSCs significantly increases in transgenic mice that lack functional BMP signaling machinery *(62)*. Thus the BMP signaling might be involved in negatively regulating the number of stem cells in both the male germ line and the hematopoietic lineages.

The interpretation of these results described previously is based on the hypothesis that the regulation of spermatogonial/SSC differentiation alters the maintenance of SSCs in vitro. As illustrated in Fig. 4, however, the number of SSCs can also differ depending on the status of their death or proliferation. If the death of SSCs is inhibited or their proliferation stimulated, more SSCs should remain in culture. Thus further studies are required to better understand the mechanism of SSC fate decision (self-renewal, differentiation, or death), and the in vitro culture of SSCs is expected to provide an effective experimental system for such studies.

Recently, a culture system has been reported by which SSCs are dramatically amplified *(63)*. In this study, when testis cells derived from newborn mice were cultured with GDNF, bFGF, LIF, and epidermal growth factor, groups of aggregated germ cells emerged. Importantly, when digested using trypsin and replated into culture, these aggregated cells emerged again, indicating that the cells can be passaged. Repeated passaging of these cells resulted not only in a long-term maintenance of SSCs over 5 months, but also resulted in their remarkable amplification, estimated to be more than 10^{14}-fold. Such an extremely high degree of stem cell amplification has not been achieved with any other stem cell system, which may be related to intrinsic proliferation potential of different types of stem cells. For example, whereas mouse HSCs regenerate complete hematopoiesis after transplantation, their proliferation activity could cease even when the stem cell number reaches at only 5% of normal value *(64,65)*. Such an inhibition of repopulation activity has not been observed for mouse SSCs *(49)*. Thus SSCs may have a highly robust proliferation potential that can be induced in vitro using growth factors.

However, it should be noted that this remarkable proliferation was observed with neonatal SSCs and it remains to be addressed if adult SSCs retain a similar degree of proliferation potential. Furthermore, the robust proliferation activity of mouse SSCs was found to be strain-dependent *(63)*. Although neonatal SSCs derived from the DBA, DBA × C57BL/6 (B6) F_1, or ICR strain actively proliferate in vitro, those derived from the B6 or 129 strain do not. Therefore, there appear to be genetic mechanisms specific to mouse strains that predispose the proliferation potential of SSCs.

6. THE STEM CELL NICHE

The activity of stem cells and their fate decision are believed to be regulated intrinsically by stem cells and also extrinsically by supporting cells in the microenvironment where stem cells reside *(66)*. This microenvironment is called the stem cell niche. Although the mechanism of stem cell regulation by their niches is largely unknown for most of mammalian stem cell systems *(66)*, some information has begun to emerge recently. For HSCs, osteoblasts are now known to be a crucial element of their niches *(62,67)*. When osteoblasts are stimulated in vivo by parathyroid hormone/parathyroid hormone-related protein, they produce high levels of jagged 1, a ligand to Notch, and thereby stimulate HSC self-renewal, resulting in approximately twofold increase in the HSC population *(67)*. In addition, a twofold increase in the number of HSCs has been observed in mutant mice depleted of a BMP receptor, coinciding the doubling of osteoblast population in the HSC niches *(62)*. Similarly, with SSCs, it is known that when more vacant niches are available, more SSCs colonize recipient testes after transplantation *(41,68)*. Thus the availability of niches determines the number of stem cells in hematopoietic and germ cell lineages in vivo.

It is believed that SSC niches are composed of Sertoli cells, the basement membrane, and peritubular myoid cells, because all spermatogonia, including

SSCs, are contained in a space formed by these cellular and extracellular elements (*see* Fig. 2). However, how these niche components cross-talk with SSCs and regulate the SSC activity remains elusive. A study using a gene trap strategy in Sertoli cells has shown that these cells rapidly change their gene expression profiles in response to the contact with germ cells in vitro *(69)*. Such an in vitro approach may shed some light on the mechanism of intercellular communications involved in the niche functions.

7. SSC IDENTIFICATION MARKERS

Probably the most significant impedance in the study of stem cells is that the detection of stem cells relies on their function, rendering their assay retrospective and time-consuming with a low sensitivity. To prospectively study stem cells, identification markers need to be determined. A general strategy to determine stem cell markers is as follows. First, a molecule that could be a stem cell marker is chosen. Second, a population of cells is selected that express this molecule. Third, these selected cells are assayed for stem cell activity. If the molecule is expressed selectively or preferentially by stem cells, the selected cells should contain more stem cells and exhibit a higher level of stem cell activity than unselected cells.

Consequently, stem cell markers need to be cell-surface molecules, because the selected cells must be alive and functionally intact. Although an intracellular molecule, such as a transcription factor, could be expressed exclusively in stem cells, such a molecule cannot be used as a stem cell marker because it does not allow the selection of target cells without damaging or killing them. (An intracellular molecule can be used as a stem cell marker if donor animals are transgenic or donor cells are transfected with a marker gene (such as green fluorescent protein) and its expression is driven by the promoter of the molecule. *See* ref. *70*.) More specifically, in the search of SSC markers, testis cells are first selected based on the expression of a particular cell-surface molecule and then transplanted into recipient testes. If transplantation of selected cells gives rise to more spermatogenic colonies than that of unselected cells, the molecule is identified as a positive marker for SSCs. Conversely, if selected cells show a reduced stem cell activity, the molecule is identified as a negative marker for SSCs.

Based on the fact that SSCs reside on the basement membrane, Shinohara et al. investigated the enrichment efficiency of adult mouse SSCs by panning testis cells using tissue culture dishes that were coated with extracellular matrix *(71)*. Among the major components of seminiferous epithelium basement membrane, namely, laminin, collagen IV, and fibronectin, only the cells panned out using laminin showed a higher SSC activity (fourfold) than unselected cells, indicating that SSCs preferentially attach laminin in the basement membrane. Next, when testis cells were selected using antibodies against integrin (Int)-β1, a laminin receptor subunit, by magnet-assisted cell sorting, SSCs were enriched approximately fourfold *(71)*. Another laminin receptor subunit, Int-α6, was found to be more effective, allowing an eightfold enrichment for SSCs *(71)*. Although c-kit (Kit) has been known to be a marker for PGCs, HSCs, and ES cells, it was not expressed on SSCs, confirming previous results that Kit is expressed in advanced spermatogonia *(72)*.

An even higher SSC enrichment was achieved using fluorescent-activated cell sorting (FACS) technique *(73)*. It should be noted, however, that SSCs cannot be enriched by FACS from *intact* adult testis cells, probably because FACS is so sensitive that its cell separation ability is obscured by a high noise level resulting from the rare presence of SSCs in highly heterogeneous testis cells *(73)*. To circumvent this problem, adult testis cells were enriched for SSCs in vivo before FACS by suturing the testes of donor mice on the abdominal wall. A high body core temperature destroys heat-sensitive spermatogenesis, eliminating differentiating germ cells. Because 95% of testis cells are germ cells, this procedure (experimental cryptorchidism) results in an approximately 25-fold enrichment for SSCs *(74)*. The cells derived from cryptorchid testes were found to be more amenable for FACS. When transplanted into recipient testes, the Int-$\alpha6^{hi}$ Int-αv^{-} Side Scatter^{lo} (which reflects cell complexity) fraction of FACS-selected cells exhibited up to 7.2-fold higher stem cell activity than unselected cryptorchid testis cells *(73)*. Therefore, this two-step enrichment strategy (cryptorchidism + FACS) resulted in a total of 166-fold enrichment of intact adult testis cells for SSCs [(23 by cryptorchidism) ×(7.2 by FACS)] *(73)*.

Recent studies have identified more SSC markers and demonstrated a higher SSC enrichment efficiency. Kubota et al. have shown that SSCs do not express major histocompatibility complex (MHC)-I molecules but do express Thy-1, which is a known antigen for lymphocytes and HSCs *(75)*. After cryptorchidism and FACS, SSCs can be enriched approximately 700-fold in the Thy-1^{+} MHC-I^{-} Kit^{-} fraction. The cells in the Thy-1^{+} MHC-I^{-} Kit^{-} fraction also show an antigenic phenotype of Int-$\alpha6^{+}$ $CD24^{+}$ Int-αv^{-} Sca-1^{-} $CD34^{-}$. Kanatsu-Shinohara et al. have shown that SSCs also express CD9, which is associated with integrins and other cell-surface receptors *(76)*. Taken together, five molecules each are known to be expressed on SSCs (positive markers) and not expressed on SSCs (negative markers; Table 1).

Male germ line stem cells can also be selected based on their morphology *(77)*. Gonocytes (neonatal spermatogonia) derived from rat testes can readily be identified in a single cell suspension because of their large size. Some of the large cells have a round shape, but others have a more irregular shape with pseudopods. When rat gonocytes with or without pseudopods were individually picked up, pooled, and transplanted, stem cell activity was almost exclusively found in the

Table 1
Cell-Surface Marker Molecules for SSCs

Positive markers[a]	*Negative markers*[a]
Integrin α6	Integrin αv
Integrin β1	MHC-I
Thy-1	Sca-1
CD24	CD34
CD9	c-Kit

[a]Positive markers are the molecules expressed SSCs and negative markers are those not expressed by SSCs. (Based on refs. *71,74–76*.)

pseudopod cell population, demonstrating that rat neonatal stem cells can be morphologically selected *(77)*. However, this procedure is labor-intensive, and spermatogonia with pseudopods are not readily found in a single-cell suspension derived from adult rat testes or from mouse testes.

These studies show that the determination of SSC markers is in a rapid progress. Notably, however, even the highest enrichment of SSCs achieved to date (700-fold; ref. *75*) does not allow the purification of stem cells. Because SSCs represent only 0.01% of total testis cell population *(46)*, the 700-fold enrichment gives only 7% of stem cells in selected cells (700 × 0.01, 1 of 14 testis cells). Therefore, further investigations are required to determine SSC markers and prospectively identify stem cells.

Among different types of stem cells, the highest enrichment has been achieved with HSCs. Mouse HSCs have been enriched up to 2000-fold in the Lineage$^-$ Kit$^+$ Sca-1$^+$ Thy-1$^+$ fraction of bone marrow cells *(1)*. Because definitive HSCs represent 0.007% of bone marrow cells, 14% of selected marrow cells are stem cells (one of seven marrow cells). These studies of SSCs and HSCs raise three characteristics of stem cell markers. First, both SSCs and HSCs cannot be identified by the expression of a single molecule. In this context, it should be noted that none of the individual marker molecules are specific to stem cells. For instance, Thy-1 is also expressed in lymphocytes. Second, some, but not all, marker molecules are expressed in both stem cell populations *(75)*. Third, although a high degree of enrichment for HSCs and SSCs is possible by a multiparameter cell selection, purification and definitive identification of these stem cells have not been achieved. In addition, another difficulty in the determination of stem cell markers is that they could be species-specific. For example, HSC markers are different in mice and humans *(3)*. Thus, although SSC markers have been investigated only in mice, the markers determined in this species could be inappropriate to select/identify SSCs in another.

It has been an intensive focus of investigations for some time whether or not a set of molecules are expressed by all types of stem cells. Such molecules that could define "stemness" have been investigated using the DNA microarray technology *(78–80)*. Two studies explored the stemness genes expressed commonly in HSCs, ES cells, and neural stem cells and identified approximately 300 genes that were expressed in the three stem cell populations *(78,79)*. However, although these studies used virtually identical cell populations for microarray analyses, only six genes were commonly detected in both studies (1.2% overlap, ref. *81*). A similar study using microarrays identified nearly 400 genes shared by ES cells, neural stem cells, and retinal stem cells *(80)*. The comparison of these data demonstrated that there was only one gene detected in all the three studies (thus in HSCs, ES cells, neural stem cells, and retinal stem cells), namely, integrin-α6 *(80)*. Although this molecule is also expressed in SSCs (*see* Table 1), it can be found in a number of nonstem cells and its function on stem cell populations is unknown.

Several causes of this discrepancy can be raised. Technical difficulties could be one of them. As described previously, no stem cells have been purified. Thus the power of microarray technology could be clouded by the impurity of cell sources *(82,83)*. In addition, it is possible that stemness genes are differentially expressed depending on in vivo status of the cells (e.g., cell cycle, development) or differentially affected by experimental procedures (e.g., physical stresses during cell separation or culture, exposure to enzymes and growth factors, temperature). It is also possible that stemness genes are not present on microarrays currently available *(82,83)*. On the other hand, the simplest explanation could be that there are no universal stemness genes. Furthermore, even if such genes exist, they may not be regulated at the transcription level. The microarray-based studies of stem cell gene profiling collectively suggest at least that the stemness genes may not be expressed at a high level, which is detectable and distinguishable in microarray analyses *(82,83)*.

9. SSCs, MALE MUTATION BIAS, AND GENETIC DISEASES

SSCs are the foundation for the life-long production of sperm that transmit genes to the next generation. Therefore, any abnormality that occurs in the SSC genome can result in germ line mutations and cause inherited diseases in offspring. In this regard, recent clinical studies, including those of endocrine cancers, have shown that a strong sex-dependent bias exists in germ line mutations *(84)*, which, as described in the following sections, suggests the involvement of the regulation of stem cell fate decision in pathogenesis of inherited diseases.

It has been described that point mutations (base substitutions) occur primarily in the male germ line and are age-dependent, whereas small chromosomal changes (mainly intragenic deletions) occur more frequently in the female germ line and are not age-dependent *(84)*. A particularly strong male mutation bias has been demonstrated in point mutations of FGF receptor 2 (FGFR2), FGFR3, and Ret, which have been suggested to occur in spermatogonia and possibly in SSCs *(85–88)*.

Point mutations in FGFR1–3 are the cause of Apert, Crouzon, and Pfeiffer syndromes *(86–89)*. Apert syndrome (achondroplasia) is associated with short-limbed dwarfism, Crouzon syndrome with craniosynostosis and dysmorphic facial features, and Pfeiffer syndrome with premature fusion and deformity of the sutures of the skull. Ret is a signal-transducing component of GDNF receptor. Point mutations in Ret cause three familial cancer syndromes *(90–92)*: multiple endocrine neoplasia 2A (MEN2), which is associated with medullary thyroid carcinoma, pheochromocytoma, and parathyroid hyperplasia; MEN2B, medullary thyroid carcinoma associated with pheochromocytoma, enteric ganglioneuroma, and skeletal and ocular abnormalities; and familial medullary thyroid carcinoma. In all of these cases, point mutations that occur in corresponding genes (i.e., FGFRs and Ret) are gain-of-function mutations *(84,85)*. Furthermore, virtually all cases of these diseases are of paternal origin. In other words, mutations occur nearly exclusively in the male germ line and are transmitted to offspring through sperm *(84,85)*.

The incidence of these diseases has long been known to increase with paternal age *(84,85)*. The widely accepted cause of this age-dependent male mutation bias was the difference in the number of chromosomal replications that take place during male and female gametogenesis in humans. In the female, there are a total of 23 chromosomal replications regardless of age. In the male, the number of total chromosomal replications increases with age: 161 at age 20 and 610 at age 40 *(84)*. Thus it was believed that the male germ line has a greater chance for mutations.

However, an increase in mutation rate was not sufficient to explain the near-exclusive paternal origin of the diseases *(86–88)*. Only a slight increase in mutant sperm with paternal age was observed, which was much less than predicted by the clinical data *(84)*. In a recent study of Apert syndrome (caused by point mutations in FGFR2), Goriely et al. have suggested that the FGFR2 mutations are enriched with age because spermatogonia/SSCs with the mutant FGFR2 have a selective advantage that leads to their clonal expansion over time, in much the same way as the clonal expansion of some tumors *(86)*. Furthermore, a similar observation has also been reported with FGFR3 *(87)*, and it has been proposed that this may also be true for mutations in Ret, a GDNF receptor *(84,85)*.

It is intriguing to compare the observations made in these genetic diseases with those made in animal studies described earlier. Primitive spermatogonia accumulate in the testes of mutant mice that overexpress GDNF, which should result in the activation of its receptor *(54,61)*. In addition, GDNF augments the maintenance of SSCs in vitro *(59)*, and the combination of GDNF and bFGF highly stimulates the proliferation of cultured SSCs *(63)*. Based on the results of clinical and animal studies, therefore, it is likely that the stimulation of signaling pathways involving FGF and GDNF confers to spermatogonia/SSCs the selective advantage that results in their accumulation. This would result in a clonal expansion of mutant SSCs or their descendants over time, leading to age-dependent male mutation bias observed in human genetic diseases. Further investigations into the roles of FGFs and GDNF on the actions of SSCs and spermatogonia may be important to better understand the origin of male mutation bias and the mechanism of SSC fate decision.

10. SUMMARY

The development of spermatogonial transplantation in 1994 allowed, for the first time, investigations into SSCs based on their function. Since then, studies of SSCs have progressed rapidly and these cells can even be used for transgenesis *(93,94)*. However, some critical SSC properties still remain to be addressed and will be an important focus for future studies. Further investigations into the SSC identification markers are essential to better understand the biology of SSCs and to carry out prospective studies of SSCs. The mechanism of SSC fate decision is another important issue in SSC biology. The fate of SSCs should be regulated by the intrinsic potential of SSCs and by the extrinsic stimuli exerted by their niches. Investigations into the function of SSC niches could be facilitated by in vitro experiments, whereas those into the intrinsic potential of SSCs may require the determination of SSC markers or genetic manipulations of SSCs. Recent progress in clinical studies of sex-dependent mutation bias has provided important insights into the SSC biology. Because SSCs may contribute to the pathogenesis of paternally transmitted genetic diseases, our ability to understand the biology of SSCs will be critical for the development of potential therapeutic strategies for those diseases.

ACKNOWLEDGMENTS

The author thanks Kyle Orwig and Frances Clerk for their critical reading of this manuscript. The studies conducted at author's laboratory were supported by the Canadian Institutes of Health Research (MOP49444) and the Canada Foundation for Innovation (4177).

REFERENCES

1. Lagasse E, Shizuru JA, Uchida N, Tsukamoto A, Weissman IL Toward regenerative medicine. Immunity 2001;14:425–436.

2. Loeffler M, Potten CS. Stem cells and cellular pedigrees—a conceptual introduction. In: Potten CS, ed. Stem Cells. San Diego, Academic Press, 1997, pp. 1–27.
3. Weissman IL. Translating stem and progenitor cell biology to the clinic: barriers and opportunities. Science 2000;287:1442–1446.
4. Rudnicki MA. Marrow to muscle, fission versus fusion. Nature Med 2003;12:1461–1462.
5. Nagano MC. A surgical strategy using spermatogonial stem cells for restoring male fertility. In: Gosden RG, Tulandi T, eds. Preservation of Fertility. Lancaster, UK, The Parthenon Publishing Group, 2004, pp. 125–139.
6. Meistrich ML, Van Beek MEAB Spermatogonial stem cells. In: Desjardins C, Ewing LL, eds. Cell and Molecular Biology of the Testis. New York, Oxford University Press, 1993, pp. 266–295.
7. Kiger AA, Fuller MT. Male germ-line stem cells. In: Marshak DR, Gardner RL, Gottlieb D. eds. Stem Cell Biology. Cold Spring Harbor, Cold Spring Harbor Laboratory Press, 2001, pp. 149–187.
8. Hogan B. Primordial germ cells as stem cells. In: Marshak DR, Garnder RL, Gottlieb D, eds. Stem Cell Biology. Cold Spring Harbor, Cold Spring Harbor Laboratory Press, 2001, pp. 189–204.
9. Lawson KA, Hage WJ. Clonal analysis of the origin of primordial germ cells in the mouse. Ciba Found Symp 1994;182:68–91.
10. Tam PPL, Snow MHL. Proliferation and migration of primordial germ cells during compensatory growth in the mouse embryo. J Embryol Exp Morph 1981;64:133–147.
11. Russell LD, Ettlin RA, Shinha Hikim AP, Clegg ED, eds. Mammalian spermatogenesis. In: Histological and Histopathological Evaluation of the Testis. Clearwater, FL, Cache River Press, 1990, pp. 1–40.
12. Bellve AR, Cavicchia JC, Millette CF, O'Brien DA, Bhatnagar YM, Dym M. Spermatogenic cells of the prepuberal mouse. Isolation and morphological characterization. J Cell Biol 1977;741:68–85.
13. McCarrey JR. Development of the germ cell. In: Desjardins C, Ewing LL, eds. Cell and Molecular Biology of the Testis. New York, Oxford University Press, 1993, pp. 58–89.
14. Lawson KA, Dunn NR, Roelen BA, et al. Bmp4 is required for the generation of primordial germ cells in the mouse embryo. Genes Dev 1999;13:424–436.
15. Saitou M, Barton SC, Surani MA. A molecular programme for the specification of germ cell fate in mice. Nature 2002;418:293–300.
16. Godin I, Wylie CC. TGF beta 1 inhibits proliferation and has a chemotropic effect on mouse primordial germ cells in culture. Development 1991;113:1451–1457.
17. Zhao G-Q, Garbers DL. Male Germ cell specification and differentiation. Dev Cell 2002;2:537–547.
18. Brinster RL. Germline stem cell transplantation and transgenesis. Science 2002;296:2174–2176.
19. Illmensee K, Stevens LC. Teratomas and chimeras. Sci Am 1979;240:120–133.
20. Stevens LC. Origin of testicular teratomas from primordial germ cells in mice. J Natl Cancer Inst 1967;38:549–552.
21. Pierce GB. Teratocarcinoma: model for a developmental concept of cancer. Curr Top Dev Biol 1967;2:223–246.
22. Brinster RL. The effect of cells transferred into the mouse blastocyst on subsequent development. J Exp Med 1974;104:1049–1056.
23. Matsui JY, Zsebo K, Hogan BLM. Derivation of pluripotential embryonic stem cells from murine primordial germ cells in culture. Cell 1992;70:841–847.
24. Resnick JL, Bixler LS, Cheng L, Donovan PJ Long-term proliferation of mouse primordial germ cells in culture. Nature 1992;359:550–551.

25. Shim H, Gutierrez-Adan A, Chen LR, BonDurant RH, Behboodi E, Anderson GB. Isolation of pluripotent stem cells from cultured porcine primordial germ cells. Biol Reprod 1997;57:1089–1095.
26. Shamblott MJ, Axelman J, Wang S, et al. Derivation of pluripotent stem cells from cultured human primordial germ cells. Proc Natl Acad Sci USA 1998;95:13726–13731.
27. Stewart CL, Gadi I, Bhatt H. Stem cells from primordial germ cells can reenter the germ line. Dev Biol 1994;161:626–628.
28. Labosky PA, Barlow DP, Hogan BL. Mouse embryonic germ (EG) cell lines: transmission through the germline and differences in the methylation imprint of insulin-like growth factor 2 receptor (Igf2r) gene compared with embryonic stem (ES) cell lines. Development 1994;120:3197–3204.
29. Smith A 2001 Embryoinc stem cells. In: Marshak DR, Garnder RL, Gottlieb D, eds. Stem Cell Biology. Cold Spring Harbor, Cold Spring Harbor Laboratory Press, 2001, pp. 205–230.
30. Brook FA, Gardner RL. The origin and efficient derivation of embryonic stem cells in the mouse. Proc Natl Acad Sci USA 1997;94:5709–5712.
31. Tsunoda Y, Tokunaga T, Imai H, Uchida T. Nuclear transplantation of male primordial germ cells in the mouse. Development 1989;107:407–411.
32. Yamazaki, Y, Mann RW, Lee SS, et al. 2003 Reprogramming of primordial germ cells begins before migration into the gential ridge, making these cells inadequate donors for reproductive cloning. Proc Natl Acad Sci USA 2003;100:12207–12212.
33. Wakayama T, Yanagimachi R1 Mouse cloning with nucleus donor cells of different age and type. Mol Reprod Dev 2001;58:376–383.
34. Constancia M, Pickard B, Kelsey G, Reik W Imprinting mechanisms. Genome Res 1998;8:881–900.
35. Monk M. Epigenetic programming of differential gene expression in development and evolution. Dev Genet 1995;17:188–197.
36. Gage FH. Mammalian neural stem cells. Science 2000;287:1433–1438.
37. Brinster RL, Zimmermann JW. Spermatogenesis following male germ-cell transplantation. Proc Natl Acad Sci USA 1994;91:11298–11302.
38. Brinster RL, Avarbock MR. Germline transmission of donor haplotype following spermatogonial transplantation. Proc Natl Acad Sci USA 1994;9124:11303–11307.
39. Ogawa T, Arechaga JM, Avarbock MR, Brinster RL. Transplantation of testis germinal cells into mouse seminiferous tubules. Int J Dev Biol 1997;41:111–122.
40. Nagano MC. Spermatogonial transplantation. In: Gardner DK, Lane M, Watson A, eds. A Laboratory Guide to the Mammalian Embryo. Oxford, UK, Oxford University Press, 2004, pp. 334–351.
41. Ryu BY, Orwig KE, Avarbock MR, Brinster RL. Stem cell and niche development in the postnatal rat testis. Dev Biol 2003;263:253–263.
42. Johnston DS, Russell LD, Friel PJ, Griswold MD. Murine germ cells do not require functional androgen receptors to complete spermatogenesis following spermatogonial stem cell transplantation. Endocrinology 2001;142:2405–2408.
43. Mahato D, Goulding EH, Korach KS, Eddy EM. Spermatogenic cells do not require estrogen receptor-α for development or function. Endocrinology 2000;141:1273–1276.
44. Zhang X, Ebata KT, Nagano MC. Genetic analysis of the clonal origin of regenerating mouse spermatogenesis following transplantation. Biol Reprod 2003;69:1872–1878.
45. Dobrinski I, Ogawa T, Avarbock MR, Brinster RL. Computer assisted image analysis to assess colonization of recipient seminiferous tubules by spermatogonial stem cell from transgenic donor mice. Mol Reprod Dev 1999;53:142–148.

46. Nagano MC. Homing efficiency and proliferation kinetics of male germ line stem cells following transplantation in mice. Biol Reprod 2003;69:701–707.
47. Shinohara T, Orwig KE, Avarbock MR, Brinster RL. Remodeling of the postnatal mouse testis is accompanied by dramatic changes in stem cell number and niche accessibility. Proc Natl Acad Sci USA 2001;98:6186–6191.
48. Orwig KE, Shinohara T, Avarbock MR, Brinster RL. Functional analysis of stem cells in the adult rat testis. Biol Reprod 2002;66:944–949.
49. Ogawa T, Ohmura M, Yumura Y, Sawada H, Kubota Y. Expansion of murine spermatogonial stem cells through serial transplantation. Biol Reprod 2003;68:316–322.
50. Franca LR, Ogawa T, Avarbock MR, Brinster RL, Russell LD. Germ cell genotype controls cell cycle during spermatogenesis in the rat. Biol Reprod 1998;59:1371–1377.
51. Ogawa T, Dobrinski I, Avarbock MR, Brinster RL. Transplantation of male germ line stem cells restores fertility in infertile mice. Nat Med 2000;6:29–34.
52. de Rooij DG, Okabe M, Nishimune Y. Arrest of spermatogonial differentiation in jsd/jsd, Sl17H/Sl17H, and cryptorchid mice. Biol Reprod 1999;61:842–847.
53. Boettger-Tong HL, Johnston DS, Russell LD, Griswold MD, Bishop CE. Juvenile spermatogonial depletion (jsd) mutant seminiferous tubules are capable of supporting transplanted spermatogenesis. Biol Reprod 2000;63:1185–1191.
54. Meng X, Lindahl M, Hyvonen ME, et al. Regulation of cell fate decision of undifferentiated spermatogonia by GDNF. Science 2000;287:1489–1493.
55. Furuchi T, Masuko K, Nishimune Y, Obinata M, Matsui Y Inhibition of testicular germ cell apoptosis and differentiation in mice misexpressing Bcl-2 in spermatogonia. Development 1996;122:1703–1709.
56. Matzuk MM, Lamb DJ. Genetic dissection of mammalian fertility pathways. Nat Cell Biol 2002;4(Suppl.):s41–s49.
57. Nagano M, Shinohara T, Avarbock MR, Brinster RL. Retrovirus-mediated gene delivery into male germ line stem cells. FEBS Lett 2000;475:7–10.
58. Nagano M, Watson DJ, Ryu BY, Wolfe JH, Brinster RL. Lentiviral vector transduction of male germ line stem cells in mice. FEBS Lett 2002;524:111–115.
59. Nagano M, Ryu BY, Brinster CJ, Avarbock MR, Brinster RL. Maintenance of mouse male germ line stem cells in vitro. Biol Reprod 2003;68:2207–2214.
60. Mather JP, Attie KM, Woodruff TK, Rice GC, Phillips DM. Activin stimulates spermatogonial proliferation in germ-Sertoli cell cocultures from immature rat testis. Endocrinology 1990;127:3206–3214.
61. Yomogida K, Yagura Y, Tadokoro Y, Nishimune Y. Dramatic expansion of germinal stem cells by ectopically expressed human glial cell line-derived neurotrophic factor in mouse Sertoli cells. Biol Reprod 2003;69:1303–1307.
62. Zhang J, Niu C, Ye L, et al. Identification of the haematopoietic stem cell niche and control of the niche size. Nature 2003;425:836–841.
63. Kanatsu-Shinohara M, Ogonuki N, Inoue K, et al. Long-term proliferation in culture and germline transmission of mouse male germline stem cells. Biol Reprod 2003;69:612–616.
64. Pawliuk R, Eaves C, Humphries RK. Evidence of both ontogeny and transplant dose-regulated expansion of hematopoietic stem cells in vivo. Blood 1996;88:2852–2858.
65. Iscove NN, Nawa K. Hematopoietic stem cells expand during serial transplantation in vivo without apparent exhaustion. Curr Biol 1997;7:805–808.
66. Watt FM, Hogan BLM. Out of Eden: stem cells and their niches. Science 2000;287:1427–1430.
67. Calvi LM, Adams GB, Weibrecht KW, et al. Osteoblastic cells regulate the haematopoietic stem cell niche. Nature 2003;425:841–846.

68. Ohta H, Yomogida K, Dohmae K, Nishimune Y. Regulation of proliferation and differentiation in spermatogonial stem cells: the role of c-kit and its ligand SCF. Development 2000;127:2125–2131.
69. Vidal F, Lopez P, Lopez-Fernandez LA, et al. Gene trap analysis of germ cell signaling to Sertoli cells: NGF-TrkA mediated induction of Fra1 and Fos by post-meiotic germ cells. J Cell Sci 2001;114:435–443.
70. Giuili G, Tomljenovic A, Labrecque N, Oulad-Abdelghani M, Rassoulzadegan M, Cuzin F. Murine spermatogonial stem cells: targeted transgene expression and purification in an active state. EMBO Rep 2002;3:753–759.
71. Shinohara T, Avarbock MR, Brinster RL. β1- and α6-integrin are surface markers on mouse spermatogonial stem cells. Proc Natl Acad Sci USA 1999;96:5504–5509.
72. Yoshinaga K, Nishikawa S, Ogawa M, et al. Role of c-kit in mouse spermatogenesis: identification of spermatogonia as a specific site of c-kit expression and function. Development 1991;113:689–699.
73. Shinohara T, Orwig KE, Avarbock MR, Brinster RL. Spermatogonial stem cell enrichment by multiparameter selection of mouse testis cells. Proc Natl Acad Sci USA 2000;97:8346–8351.
74. Shinohara T, Avarbock MR, Brinster RL. Functional analysis of spermatogonial stem cells in Steel and cryptorchid infertile mouse models. Dev Biol 2000;220:401–411.
75. Kubota H, Avarbock MR, Brinster RL. Spermatogonial stem cells share some, but not all, phenotypic and functional characteristics with other stem cells. Proc Natl Acad Sci USA 2003;100:6487–6492.
76. Kanatsu-Shinohara M, Toyokuni S, Shinohara T. CD9 is a surface marker on mouse and rat male germline stem cells. Biol Reprod 2004;70:70–75.
77. Orwig KE, Ryu BY, Avarbock MR, Brinster RL. Male germ-line stem cell potential is predicted by morphology of cells in neonatal rat testes. Proc Natl Acad Sci USA 2002;99:11706–11711.
78. Ramalho-Santos M, Yoon S, Matsuzaki Y, Mulligan RC, Melton DA. "Stemness:" transcriptional profiling of embryonic and adult stem cells. Science 20002;298: 97–600.
79. Ivanova NB, Dimos JT, Schaniel C, Hackney JA, Moore KA, Lemischka IR. A stem cell molecular signature. Science 2002;298:601–604.
80. Fortunel NO, Otu HH, Ng HH, et al. Comment on " 'Stemness': transcriptional profiling of embryonic and adult stem cells" and "a stem cell molecular signature." Science 2003;302:393.
81. Evsikov AV, Solter D. Comment on " 'Stemness': transcriptional profiling of embryonic and adult stem cells" and "a stem cell molecular signature." Science 2003;302:393.
82. Vogel G. 'Stemness' genes still elusive. Science 2003;302:371.
83. Ivanova NB, Dimos JT, Schaniel C, et al. Response to comments on " 'stemness': transcriptional profiling of embryonic and adult stem cells" and "a stem cell molecular signature" Science 2003;302:393.
84. Crow JF. The origins, patterns and implications of human spontaneous mutation. Nat Rev Genet 2000;1:40–47.
85. Crow JF. There's something curious about paternal-age effects. Science 2003;301:606–607.
86. Goriely A, McVean GA, Rojmyr M, Ingemarsson B, Wilkie AO. Evidence for selective advantage of pathogenic FGFR2 mutations in the male germ line. Science 2003;301:643–646.
87. Tiemann-Boege I, Navidi W, Grewal R, et al. The observed human sperm mutation frequency cannot explain the achondroplasia paternal age effect. Proc Natl Acad Sci USA 2002;99: 14952–14957.
88. Oldridge M, Lunt PW, Zackai EH, et al. Genotype-phenotype correlation for nucleotide substitutions in the IgII-IgIII linker of FGFR2. Hum Mol Genet 1997;6:137–143.

89. Vajo Z, Francomano CA, Wilkin DJ. The molecular and genetic basis of fibroblast growth factor receptor 3 disorders: the achondroplasia family of skeletal dysplasias, Muenke craniosynostosis, and Crouzon syndrome with acanthosis nigricans. Endocr Rev 2000;21:23–39.
90. Santoro M, Carlomagno F, Romano A, et al. Activation of RET as a dominant transforming gene by germline mutations of MEN2A and MEN2B. Science 1995;267:381–383.
91. Santoro M, Melillo RM, Carlomagno F, Fusco A, Vecchio G. Molecular mechanisms of RET activation in human cancer. Ann N Y Acad Sci 2002;963:116–121.
92. Takahashi M. The GDNF/RET signaling pathway and human diseases. Cytokine Growth Factor Rev 2001;12:361–373.
93. Nagano M, Brinster CJ, Orwig KE, Ryu BY, Avarbock MR, Brinster RL. Transgenic mice produced by retroviral transduction of male germ-line stem cells. Proc Natl Acad Sci USA 2001;98:13090–13095.
94. Hamra FK, Gatlin J, Chapman KM, Grellhesl DM, Garcia JV, Hammer RE, Garbers DL. Production of transgenic rats by lentiviral transduction of male germ-line stem cells. Proc Natl Acad Sci USA 2002;99:14931–14936.
95. Donovan PJ. Growth factor regulation of mouse primordial germ cell development. Curr Top Dev Biol 1994;19:189–225.
96. Nagano M, Avarbock MR, Brinster RL. Pattern and kinetics of mouse donor spermatogonial stem cell colonization in recipient testes. Biol Reprod 1999;60:1429–1436.

3 Umbilical Cord Stem Cells

Kathy E. Mitchell

Contents

1. INTRODUCTION

The two most basic properties of stem cells are the capacities to self-renew and to differentiate into multiple cell or tissue types *(1–3)*. Generally, stem cells are categorized as one of three types: embryonic stem cells (ES), embryonic germ cells (EG), or adult stem cells. ES cells are derived from the inner cell mass of the blastula (Fig. 1). They proliferate indefinitely and can differentiate spontaneously into all three tissue layers of the embryo *(4)* and into germ cells as well *(5–7)*. EG cells are derived from primordial germ cells (*see* Fig. 1), a small set of stem cells that reside in the protected environment of the yolk stalk, so that they remain undifferentiated during embryogenesis. As with ES cells, EG cells have the capacity to differentiate into all three tissue layers *(8)*. Adult stem cells are found in most tissues and in the circulation. They may have less replicative capacity than ES or EG cells and, until recently, were thought to have restricted developmental fates *(9)*. This classification system omits a significant source of stem cells derived from the extraembryonic tissues (umbilical cord, placenta and amniotic tissues/fluids), which are derived from neither the adult organism nor the embryo proper. This review will describe studies of stem cells derived from

From: *Contemporary Endocrinology: Stem Cells in Endocrinology*
Edited by: L. B. Lester © Humana Press Inc., Totowa, NJ

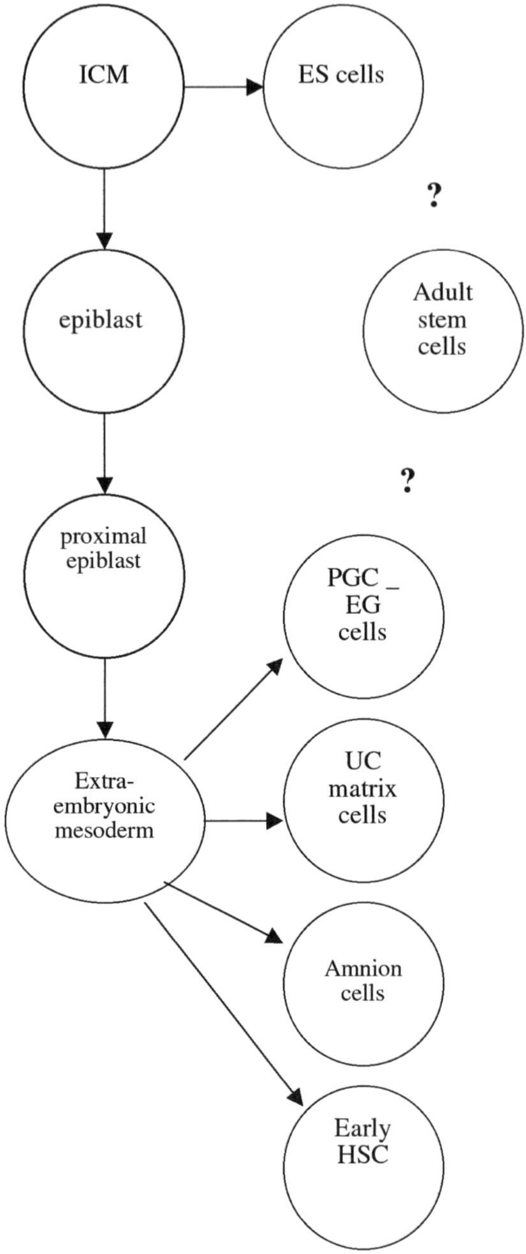

Fig. 1. Stem cells and origins from inner cell mass (ICM) and extraembryonic mesoderm. ES cells arise from cells derived from the ICM. EG cells, umbilical cord matrix cells, cells from amniotic tissues, and early hematopoietic stem cells (HSC) arise from extraembryonic mesoderm.

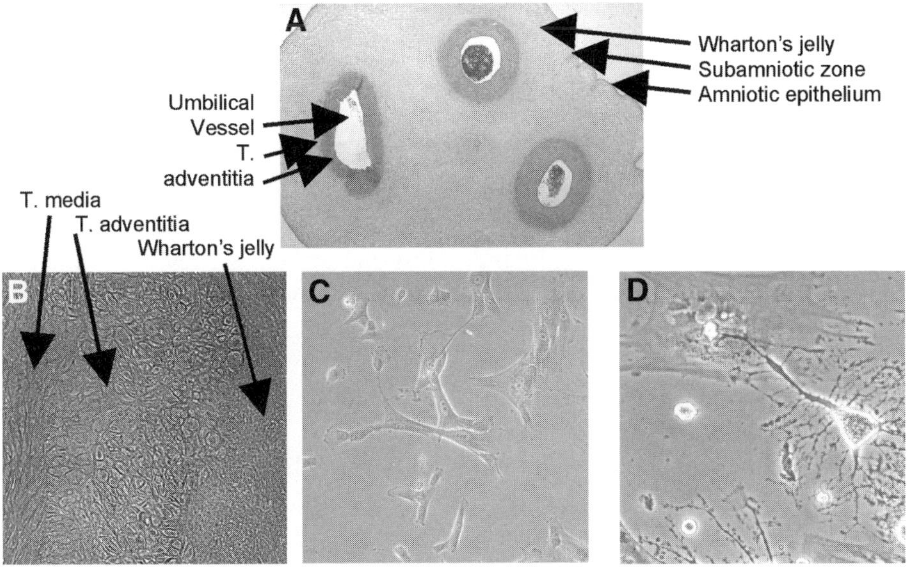

Fig. 2. Human umbilical cord matrix cells. **(A)** Umbilical cords have two arteries and one vein surrounded by Wharton's jelly. **(B)** Pockets of cobblestone-appearing cells between the adventitia and Wharton's jelly. **(C)** Umbilical cord matrix cells in culture. **(D)** Human umbilical cord cells treated by neural induction method of Woodbury et al. *(33)*.

extraembryonic tissues with an emphasis on cells derived from umbilical cord, their developmental origins, and relationships to other types of stem cells and potential in regenerative medicine.

2. STRUCTURE AND DEVELOPMENT OF THE UMBILICAL CORD

The fully developed umbilical cord has one vein and two arteries surrounded by mucous or gelatinous connective tissue also known as Wharton's jelly and is covered with amnion (Fig. 2). There are three distinct zones of stromal cells and matrix that can be identified: subamniotic layer, Wharton's jelly, and media and adventitia surrounding the vessels but no differences along the longitudinal axis *(10)*. The Wharton's jelly region, the most abundant, has cleft-like spaces of stroma matrix molecules of collagens type I, III, and VI, with collagen type VI, laminin, and heparin sulphate proteoglycan around the clefts. The jelly-filled, cleft-like spaces are surrounded by stromal cells that are slender and spindle-shaped myofibroblasts that express vimentin and smooth muscle actin as well as desmin *(11)*. Earlier cords have only vimentin and desmin. The structure and composition of the umbilical cord, rich in highly resilient matrix and myofibroblasts, protects the vessels from compression and may also facilitate an exchange between cord blood and amniotic fluid.

The umbilical cord is derived from extraembryonic mesoderm (*see* Fig. 1). After the blastula develops, cells from the inner cell mass (from which ES cells are derived) form the epiblast *(12)*. Cells destined to become the extraembryonic mesoderm arise from the proximal epiblast and are the earliest mesoderm to migrate through the primitive streak *(13)*. Extraembryonic mesoderm increases over the next few stages of embryogenesis to line the trophectoderm shell, the amniotic ectoderm, and the yolk sac endoderm and form the connecting stalk as well. Thus extraembryonic mesoderm contributes to the chorion, amnion, yolk sac, and, eventually, the umbilical cord *(14)*.

Primordial germ cells (from which EG stem cells are derived) and early hematopoietic stem cells arise from extraembryonic mesoderm (*see* Fig. 1). Hematopoiesis occurs in the yolk sac blood islands 8–8.5 days postconception in the mouse *(15,16)*. These yolk sac hematopoietic stem cells provide early, local hematopoiesis during development and circulate through the embryo to provide oxygen and nutrients. Primordial germ cells arise from the extraembryonic mesoderm and appear in the yolk sac as distinguishable entities at about 7 days postconception in the mouse *(17)*. They migrate to the genital ridges of the developing fetus by about 11.5–12.5 days postconception. Primordial germ cells retrieved from the genital ridges and cultured in vitro are multipotential *(8)*. The migration of primordial germ cells is controlled by a number of factors, including c-Kit and members of the nanos family *(18)*. Primordial germ cells, which do not home correctly to the genital ridges, undergo apoptosis. If apoptosis does not occur, these cells can form pediatric germ cell tumors *(19)*.

Recent work has shown that the umbilical cord is a rich source of stem cells. Ende coined the term *Berashis cells,* meaning "beginning cells," to describe the primitive multipotential cells found in human umbilical cord blood and suggested that they may be related to fetal stem cells *(20,21)*. Three types of stem cells have been identified in umbilical cord: myofibroblast-like cells from the umbilical cord matrix, and hematopoietic and mesenchymal stem cells from cord blood. Stem cells obtained from umbilical cord and placental blood express low levels of human leukocyte antigens (HLA) and have a universal donor potential *(22)*. This is an important source of stem cells for bone marrow replacement when HLA-matched donors cannot be found. The properties of umbilical cord stem cells, their relationship to other types of stem cells, and their immunogenic properties are areas of much interest in the emerging fields of stem cell biology and regenerative medicine.

3. STEM CELLS DERIVED FROM EXTRAEMBRYONIC TISSUES

3.1. Umbilical Cord Matrix Cells

Umbilical cord matrix may be the remnants of the yolk stalk, the protected environment where early hematopoietic stem cells and primordial germ cells arise. As such, it may be a reservoir of cells with stem cell-like characteristics that can migrate into the developing fetus at appropriate times during development. Umbilical cord matrix cells express markers for stem cells, including many that are expressed in ES, EG, and neural precursor or stem cells (Table 1). In addition, umbilical cord matrix cells can be easily expanded and maintained in culture for more than 80 population doublings. They express low levels of telomerase. They also form structures reminiscent of embryoid bodies when cultured past confluence. They express smooth muscle actin and vimentin, markers for myofibroblasts; nestin, neuron-specific enolase (NSE), and glial fibrillary acidic protein (GFAP), markers for neural stem cells; and c-Kit, Oct-4, Tra-1-60, markers expressed in ES and EG cells. Importantly, umbilical cord matrix cells do not form teratomas in nude mice *(23)* or when injected into rat brain or muscle *(24)*.

Pluripotency of ES cells has been linked to expression of Oct-4, a Pit-Oct-Unc transcription factor *(25)*. Until recently, it was believed that Oct-4 expression in mature animals was confined exclusively to germ cells *(26)*. Initially expressed in all cells in the morula, Oct-4 becomes restricted to the inner cell mass at the blastula stage. Oct-4 is expressed by nearly 100% of isolated umbilical cord matrix cells after 10 passages and is localized to the nucleus. The full-length transcript was cloned from umbilical cord matrix cells and has 100% homology to the reported human embryonic form of Oct-4 *(23)*. The role of Oct-4 in umbilical cord matrix cells is not known. In ES cells, the precise level of Oct-4 expression seems to determine cell fate with high levels of Oct-4 expression pushing ES cells toward extraembryonic mesoderm or endodermal lineages and low Oct-4 expression resulting in cells that become trophectoderm *(27)*. Only ES cells expressing normal Oct-4 levels remained pluripotent. Recently, a population of bone marrow stromal cells was isolated after serum deprivation that expressed Oct-4 *(28)*. Oct-4 expression was also found in amniotic fluid cells *(29)*. Taken together, these findings suggest that Oct-4 may play a role in nonembryonic stem cells. This is being investigated for umbilical cord matrix cells in our laboratory.

Umbilical cord matrix cell express many of the markers Shamblott et al. *(30)* identified in derivatives of cultured EG cells including NSE, vimentin, and nestin—markers for neural precursors—and glial markers, 2',3'-cyclic nucleotide 3'-phosphodiesterase, and GFAP, also expressed in early neural precursors (*see* Table 1). In addition, umbilical cord matrix cells express c-Kit, which is important for proper migration of primordial germ cells. Expression of these

Table 1
Comparison of Markers for Stem Cells Expressed in ES, EG, UCM, Amniotic, and NS Cells

	ES cells	*EG cells*	*UCM cells*	*Amniotic*	*NS cells*
Oct-4	+	+	+	+	NA
Telomerase	+	+	+	+	–
Vimentin	NA	+	+	+	+
Nestin	NA	+	+	+	+
NSE	NA	+	+	+	+
GFAP	NA	+	+	+	+

ES, embronic stem; EG, embryonic germ; UCM, umbilical cord matrix; NS, neural stem; NSE, neuron-specific enolase; GFAP, glial fibrillary acidic protein; NA, not applicable.

proteins, including Oct-4, by both umbilical cord matrix cells and EG cells suggests a possible relationship between the two cell types, particularly in light of their residing in the same region of the developing fetus and common origin from extraembryonic mesoderm.

Umbilical cord matrix cells can be differentiated to form neuron-like cells based on morphology, expression of neuron-specific proteins, and development of voltage-gated potassium channels found in early neurons that are important for development of electrical excitability *(31,32)*. Some cells differentiate spontaneously to express neuronal markers. Induction by the method of Woodbury et al. *(33)* greatly enhances the number of cells that differentiate into a neuron-like cell (approximately 80%) *(31)*. Umbilical cord matrix cells induced by this method form primitive networks between the cells with long axon-like processes, refractile cell bodies and dendrite-like processes, highly reminiscent of primary neurons in culture (Fig. 2D). The induced umbilical cord matrix cells express neurofilament M, Tuj1, growth cone-associated protein (GAP43), and tyrosine hydroxylase, which are markers for more mature neurons. Thus, as with many stem cells, umbilical cord matrix stem cells appear to differentiate along a neuronal fate readily, with some differentiation occurring spontaneously.

Umbilical cord matrix cells have also been used in in vivo xenotransplantation. Studies by Weiss et al. *(24)* suggest that porcine umbilical cord matrix cells survive, migrate, and begin to express markers for mature neurons when transplanted into rat brain. Umbilical cord matrix cells loaded with the fluorescent dye, PKH26, were transplanted into rat brains and detectable at periods from 2 to 6 weeks after transplantation. After 4 weeks, the umbilical cord matrix cells were detected primarily along the injection tract and were small and spherical, with very few processes. However, the transplanted umbilical cord cells did express neuronal filament 70 (NF70) based on detection with an antibody specific for porcine but not rodent NF70. In contrast, 6 weeks after injection, about 10% of the detectable umbilical cord matrix cells had migrated away from the injection site and into the region just ventral to the corpus callosum. These umbilical cord matrix cells also expressed NF70. Taken together, these studies suggest that umbilical cord matrix cells may have the capacity to differentiate into neurons in vitro and in vivo. More work needs to be done to establish that the umbilical cord matrix cells can generate action potentials in vitro and form new neuronal connections in vivo. Studies are under way to address these issues and to establish whether umbilical cord matrix cells can ameliorate neural deficits after oxygen deprivation of the brain or in a Parkinson's disease model in rat.

3.2. Umbilical Cord Blood Cells

Umbilical cord blood is a rich source of hematopoietic stem/progenitor cells and has been used successfully as an important source of cells for hematopoietic stem cell (HSC) transplantation *(34)*. Although somewhat controversial, umbilical cord blood is also thought to be a source of mesenchymal stem cells (MSC). MSC can be differentiated into cells other than blood, but may also be important for long-term engraftment in bone marrow transplants with umbilical cord blood *(35)*. There is much interest in the potential of umbilical cord blood as a source of multipotential stem cells; umbilical cord blood is often banked and cryogenically stored for use by the individual from whom the cord blood was taken or as a source for donation to other individuals in need of bone marrow transplants or other cell-based therapies.

Umbilical cord blood is an important source of HSC for bone marrow transplants for which HLA-matched donors cannot be found. Umbilical cord blood stem cell progenitors are used now routinely as an alternative to bone marrow transplant *(36)*. There are many potential advantages in using the HSC from cord blood as compared with HSC derived from bone marrow. First, HSC in umbilical cord blood occur at higher frequency than in peripheral blood *(37)* and at comparable levels to their occurrence in bone marrow, making up about 2% of the total mononuclear cell population *(38)*. Importantly, umbilical cord HSC have a greater ability to replicate than bone marrow-derived HSC and can be manipulated genetically as well *(39)*. They can be collected noninvasively with no risk to mother or child. Because of their increased proliferative rate, HSC can be expanded ex vivo, unlike adult hematopoietic stem cells *(40,41)*. This potential for expansion can be augmented by treatment with a cocktail of growth factors (thrombo poetin, stem cell factor, interleukin-3, flt3-ligand, and basic fibroblastic growth factor) allowing for a 500-fold expansion of $CD34^+$ HSC from umbilical cord blood *(42)*. $CD34^+$ umbilical cord cells may also have potentials beyond the hematopoietic lineages. Pesce et al. *(43)* showed that $CD34^+$ umbilical cord cells can differentiate into muscle fibers in immune-suppressed mice and can also form myotubes when cocultured with muscle cells in vivo. The abilities to expand ex vivo, genetically manipulate, and cryogenically store umbilical cord blood HSC in addition to their potential to contribute to repair of other tissues holds great promise for future stem cell-based therapies.

Although umbilical cord blood is known to be a rich source of HSC *(44,45)*, the existence of MSC in umbilical cord blood has been somewhat controversial *(46)*. However, in recent studies, MSC have been isolated from cord blood through methods used for isolation of MSC from bone marrow *(47)*. The umbilical cord-derived MSC displayed a fibroblast-like morphology and were smooth muscle actin and fibronectin positive. This suggests that they may be related to the cells isolated from umbilical cord matrix, which may migrate into the cord blood circulation. Other groups have isolated MSC from umbilical cord blood that could be expanded in culture and induced to differentiate into osteocytes, chondrocytes, and adipocytes as well as hepatocytes of mesenchymal origin *(48)*. They were also able to induce the cells to express markers for neurons and glia. Hou et al. isolated MSC from umbilical cord blood by negative selection. These cells do not express CD34, CD11a, or CD11b, but do express CD29 and CD71, which is identical to markers of MSC derived from bone marrow *(49)*. Hou et al. also isolated clonal populations of MSC that could differentiate into adipocytes, chondrocytes, osteocytes, hepatocytes, neuronal, and glial cells based on expression of specific markers.

Cells that resemble neural stem cells have been isolated from umbilical cord blood *(50)*. Nestin, an intermediate filament expressed in neural precursors, is expressed by a large percentage of human cord blood monocytes that also coexpress CD133. However, nestin expression was not detected in adult monocytes *(50)*. Buzanska et al. *(51)* showed that nestin-expressing cells from umbilical cord blood could be directed to differentiate into early neurons that expressed TUJ1 (a neuron-specific class III β-tubulin), astrocytes expressing GFAP, and galactocerebrosidase expressing oligodendrocytes by treatment with brain-derived neurotrophic factor and retinoic acid. Similarly, other studies have shown that CD45-negative cells from umbilical cord blood could be expanded in culture and then be induced to form cells that express neuronal and glial markers TUJ1 and GFAP *(52)*. Many other studies have shown the potential for cells from cord blood to differentiate into cells that express neuronal or glial proteins using a number of different induction protocols *(53)*. Interestingly, many of the proteins are expressed in umbilical cord cells without any treatment to induce them. For example, GFAP was expressed in about one-third of the isolated cells. This was increased by treatment with retinoic acid. Similar results were found for expression of NeuN. These studies show that a population of cells within umbilical cord blood express markers and have properties very similar to those of umbilical cord matrix cells and neural precursor cells (*see* Table 1).

3.3. Other Extraembryonic Stem Cells

Other cells with stem cell-like properties have been identified in the extraembryonic tissues. Oct-4-expressing cells have been identified in human amniotic fluid *(29)*. Amniotic fluid cells express stem cell factor, smooth muscle actin, and vimentin and are rapidly proliferating compared with adult cells *(54)*. They may also express telomerase as telomerase activity has been detected in amniotic fluid *(55)*. Amniotic cells also express a number of glial and neuronal proteins, including neurofilament proteins, microtubule-associated protein 2, GFAP, 2',3'-cyclic nucleotide 3'-phosphodiesterase, myelin basic protein, and galactocerebroside *(56,57)*. These properties are similar to those of cells isolated from umbilical cord matrix, suggesting that they may have a common origin.

An interesting observation made by several investigators is that many neuronal and glial proteins are expressed in extraembryonic tissues. Initially, expression of some neuronal and glial proteins, NSE and S100, in cord blood and amniotic fluid was thought to be indicative of neonatal neuronal damage *(58–61)*. But recent studies have shown that high levels of NSE and S-100 are expressed in umbilical cord blood after normal delivery. They are expressed at higher levels in the artery than venous blood, suggesting fetal origin *(62)*. Wijnberger et al. did a more extensive analysis of neuronal and glial protein expression in the placenta and umbilical cord, looking for expression of S-100, NSE, GFAP, and GAP43 *(63)*. They found that many cell types, including myofibroblasts of Wharton's jelly, are positive for NSE and S-100, as are cells of the vascular wall, amnion epithelium, and macrophages and monocytes in umbilical cord blood. GFAP and GAP43 were not detected, however. S-100 is also expressed in placental tissues *(64)*. These results suggest that extraembryonic tissues are possibly a rich source of stem cells with neural precursor type properties.

4. RELATIONSHIP TO ES, EG, AND ADULT STEM CELLS

ES cells are derived from the inner cell mass of the blastula. EG cells are derived proximal to the epiblast, residing temporarily in a protected environment of the yolk stalk so that they remain undifferentiated. Adult stem cells are found in most tissues, as well as in circulation. Adult stem cells are usually quiescent but become activated under conditions of stress or injury. What are the origins of adult stem cells and how do they keep from differentiating? These are some of the most critical questions in stem cell biology. It has been suggested that stem cells may not be the first cells to show up in a tissue, but rather may appear later in development when they can populate adult niches. Adult stem cells may be differentiated appropriately for their tissue, but also have other potentials if in a different microenvironment.

Are multipotential adult stem cells related to the primitive stem cells of the umbilical cord? Most multipotential adult stem cells share common characteristics with the myofibroblast-like cells isolated from umbilical cord matrix *(31)*. Postnatal stem cells in the adult, from a wide variety of sources, appear to be capable of differentiation into multiple tissue types. Cells derived from bone marrow *(65)*, skin *(66)*, astrocytes *(67)*, synoviocytes *(68)*, adipose *(69)*, and dental pulp *(70)* have recently been shown to be multipotential. Many of these multipotential stem cells may have a common precursor in that they are tissue-specific myofibroblasts. Myofibroblasts are found throughout the body and include bone marrow stromal cells, astrocytes, synoviocytes, and pericytes *(71)*. Myofibroblasts in the adult take part in growth, development, and repair of normal tissue. They can also be the cause of organ fibrosis, scar formation, and tumors. Myofibroblasts have some tissue-specific functions but are similar in morphology, function, and biochemistry regardless of their location *(71)*. Perhaps myofibroblasts or their precursors exist as a pool of pluripotent stem cells that exist in equilibrium between stem cells that are buried in the diverse organs and those that circulate from the bone marrow, similar to monocytes and macrophages as suggested by Labat for adult stem cells *(72)*. There are intrinsic differences in fetal versus adult myofibroblasts that regulate their responses to cytokines, which in turn may account for the ability for scarless repair by fetal myofibroblasts *(73)*. This may be a critical characteristic that favors younger myofibroblasts, such as those isolated from umbilical cord matrix for therapeutic applications.

5. UMBILICAL CORD STEM CELLS AND THE IMMUNE SYSTEM

Although much of the enthusiasm about the potentials for therapeutic applications of ES cells is based on the hope that they will evade the immune system, very little work has been done to investigate this potential. Immunological rejection may be an important barrier for ES cell-based therapies if MHC molecules responsible for immune-mediated graft rejection are expressed by ES cells after they differentiate. Human ES cells express HLA class I but not class II molecules. Expression of both classes of molecules increases with differentiation in vitro or in vivo *(74)*. As with ES cells, mesenchymal stem cells express low levels of HLA class I molecules but not class II *(75)*. Importantly, they were able to suppress mixed lymphocytic cultures and retained this capability even after differentiation.

Tumor formation (teratomas) by ES cells is a major hurdle that needs to be overcome before this source of cells can be used in therapeutic applications. Preliminary findings show that, unlike ES cells, human umbilical cord matrix cells do not form tumors in immune compromised mice *(23)*. Porcine umbilical cord matrix cells do not illicit an immune response when injected into rat brain or muscle, nor are they rejected at 4 weeks *(24)*. The mechanism of this immune evasion is not known but may involve the low expression of HLA class I molecules and expression of HLA-G *(23)*, a nonclassical HLA that suppresses immune response at the maternal–fetal interface *(76)* and in muscle *(77)*.

Umbilical cord blood HSC have low immunogenicity with a lower incidence of graft-vs-host disease when used for transplantation in cancer patients, even when the number of HLA markers that are matched are lower *(78)*. The mechanism of this potential to evade the immune system is not understood. However, β2-microglobulin is expressed constitutively in cord blood cells *(79)* and is known to be an integral part of MHC expression in killer T cells and, thus, may play a role in immune evasion of umbilical cord blood HSC *(80)*. Stem cells from umbilical cord appear to have the unique ability to evade the immune system, which makes their use therapeutically particularly exciting. More research on the mechanisms by which umbilical cord stem cells suppress immune response and how long after differentiation this is maintained is essential.

6. POTENTIAL FOR CELL-BASED THERAPIES

Umbilical cord blood is commonly used in cell-based therapies today for reconstitution of the bone marrow after bone marrow ablation for cancers of the blood *(36)*. There are some new experimental therapies using bone marrow transplant with cord blood cells being developed for other diseases. Umbilical cord blood transplantation in Wiskott Aldrich syndrome, which results in severe immune deficiency and early death if not treated, was found to result in rapid and reliable recovery of immune function, with low risk of graft-vs-host disease *(81)*. Using umbilical cord blood stem cells taken from unrelated donors, Staba et al. *(82)* treated children with Hurler's syndrome, who lack of a functional enzyme, alpha-L-iduronidase. These researchers were able to treat these patients without bone marrow ablation and to have improvement in survival and less neuronal degeneration than Hurler's patients who received bone marrow transplants. The researchers speculate that stem cells from cord blood may transport α-L-iduronidase across the blood–brain barrier more effectively. In addition, they are younger cells and do not have to be matched as closely. Research is under way to expand the use of umbilical cord blood cells to treat other disorders such as β-thalassemia *(83)*.

Animal models suggest that umbilical cord blood cells may be useful in treatment of amyotrophic lateral sclerosis by slowing motor neuron degeneration when injected intravenously *(84)*. Ende and coworkers found that intravenous injection of umbilical cord blood cells could extend the survival of several mouse knockout models of human disease, including amyotrophic lateral sclerosis *(85)*, Alzheimer's *(85)*, Huntington's *(86)*, Parkinson's *(87)*, and type 1 diabetes *(88)*. Human umbilical cord blood cells also improve the mobility of rats with spinal cord injuries when injected intravenously. Cord blood cells were observed in the areas of injury of spinal cord but not others and never seen in the control, uninjured animals *(89)*. Similarly, umbilical cord blood cells were able to improve function in a stroke model in the rat when injected intravenously. The human umbilical cord blood cells differentiated into cells that expressed glial or neuronal markers *(90)*. This suggests that umbilical cord blood cells have the ability to target to and heal neurologic defects.

Cells from umbilical cord matrix may also be a source of cells for treatment of neurodegenerative disease. Medicetty et al. *(91)* treated rats with a unilateral 6-hydroxydopamine (6-OHDA) lesion that caused parkinsonian-like symptoms. Four weeks after the 6-OHDA lesion, rats were injected with umbilical cord matrix cells or sham transplants. Four weeks after transplantation, there was a significant decrease in apomorphine-induced rotatory behavior in the parkinsonian rats that received umbilical cord matrix cell transplants as compared with parkinsonian rats that received a sham transplant. Normal rats, without 6-OHDA lesions, were transplanted with umbilical cord matrix cells but showed no changes in behavior. This work suggests that umbilical cord matrix cells can target areas of neurodegeneration and play a role in healing of neural tissue. Amniotic cells may have a similar potential *(92)*. Labeled amniotic epithelial cells were injected into monkeys with spinal cord injuries. Some labeled neurons were subsequently found in the spinal cord. Glial scar formation was decreased compared with animals that did not receive amniotic epithelial cells. More importantly, the function of the animals improved suggesting that amniotic epithelial cells help in axon regrowth. These studies suggest that cells from umbilical cord blood and other cells from extraembryonic tissues may be an important source of stem cells for a variety of therapeutic applications.

7. SUMMARY

There is much hope today for the many potential benefits that can be achieved through stem cell research, including a better understanding of the basic biology of stem cells that may provide insights into cancer when proper control of proliferation and differentiation have gone awry, for developmental processes, and for drug discovery. There is significant potential to discover new drugs through stem cell research that will increase the proliferative capacity of specific populations of cells in the brain to ameliorate Parkinson's disease or in the islets to produce new insulin-producing cells or discover new chemotherapeutic agents that target the cancer stem cell and thus improve long-term survival of cancer patients. What is clear is that there is much yet to be learned; stem cell biology and regenerative medicine are in their infancy. We need to study cells from many sources to be able to harness these potentials. The cells from the umbilical cord and other extraembryonic tissues are a particularly exciting and promising source of primitive stem cells based on their ready availability, low immunogenicity, and lack of tumorigenicity. The study of extraembryonic stem cells may also reveal the origins of the adult stem cell. Extraembryonic stem cells may also be a particularly useful tool in drug development because of their ready availability, making it possible to harvest cells that represent a genetically diverse population or stem cells that carry specific genetic defects.

ACKNOWLEDGMENTS

Supported by P20 RR 15563-02 COBRE-NIH and RO1-NS/HL36124. Jeremy Traas is also acknowledged for his research contributions.

REFERENCES

1. McKay R. Stem cells in the central nervous system. Science 1997;276:66–71.
2. Gordon MY, Blackett NM. Reconstruction of the hematopoietic system after stem cell transplantation. Cell Transplant 1998;7:339–344.
3. Scheffler B, Horn M, Blumcke I, et al. Marrow-mindedness: a perspective on neuropoiesis. Trends Neurosci 1999;22:348–357.
4. Smith A. Embryo-derived stem cells: of mice and men. Annu Rev Cell Dev Biol 2001;17:435–462.
5. Hubner K, Fuhrmann G, Christenson LK, et al. Derivation of oocytes from mouse embryonic stem cells. Science 2003;300:1251–1256.
6. Toyooka Y, Tsunekawa N, Akasu R, Noce T. Embryonic stem cells can form germ cells in vitro. PNAS 2003;100:11457–11462.
7. Clark AT, Bodnar MS, Fox M, et al. Spontaneous differentiation of germ cells from human embryonic stem cells in vitro. Hum Mol Genet 2004;13:727–739.
8. Shamblott MJ, Axelman J, Wang S, et al. Derivation of pluripotent stem cells from cultured human primordial germ cells. PNAS 1998;95:13726–13731.
9. Paul G, Li JY, Brundin P. Stem cells: hype or hope? Drug Discov Today 2002;7:295–302.
10. Nanaev AK, Kohnen G, Milovanov AP, Domogatsky SP, Kaufmann P. Stromal differentiation and architecture of the human umbilical cord. Placenta 1997;18:53–64.
11. Takechi K, Kuwabara Y, Mizuno M. Ultrastructural and immunohistochemical studies of Wharton's jelly umbilical cord cells. Placenta 1993;14:235–245.
12. Gardner RL. Cell lineage and cell commitment in the early mammalian embryo. Mead Johnson Symp Perinat Dev Med 1979;16:18–24.
13. Lawson KA, Meneses JJ, Pedersen RA. Clonal analysis of epiblast fate during germ layer formation in the mouse embryo. Development 1991;113:891–911.

14. Vogler H. Human Blastogenesis. Formation of the Extraembryonic Cavities. Bibliotheca Anatomica 30. Karger, Basel, 1987.
15. Moore MA, Metcalf D. Ontogeny of the haemopoietic system: yolk sac origin of in vivo and in vitro colony forming cells in the developing mouse embryo. Br J Haematol 1970;18:279–296.
16. Weissman IL, Warnke R, Butcher EC, Rouse R, Levy R. The lymphoid system. Its normal architecture and the potential for understanding the system through the study of lymphoproliferative diseases. Hum Pathol 1978;9:25–45.
17. Mintz B, Russell ES. Gene-induced embryological modifications of primordial germ cells in the mouse. J Exp Zool 1957;134:207–237.
18. Tres, LL, Rosselot C, Kierszenbaum AL Primordial germ cells: what does it take to be alive? Mol Reprod Dev 2004;68:1–4.
19. Schneider DT, Schuster AE, Fritsch MK, et al. Multipoint imprinting analysis indicates a common precursor cell for gonadal and nongonadal pediatric germ cell tumors. Cancer Res 2001;61:7268–7276.
20. Ende, N. History of umbilical cord blood transplantation. Lancet 1995;346:1161.
21. Ende N. Berashis cells in human umbilical cord blood vs. embryonic stem cells. J Med 2002;33:167–171.
22. von Drygalski A, Adamson J. Placental/umbilical cord blood (PCB) stem cells for transplantation: early clinical outcomes and the status of ex vivo expansion strategies. Keio J Med 2000;49:141–151.
23. Traas J, Kaptur R, Schermerhorn T, Chun R, Mitchell KE Stem cell gene array analysis of Oct-4 positive human umbilical cord matrix cells. Mol Cell Biol 2003;14:115a.
24. Weiss ML, Mitchell KE, Hix JE, et al. Transplantation of porcine umbilical cord matrix cells into the rat brain. Exp Neurol 2003;182:288–299.
25. Suzuki N, Rohdewohld H, Neuman T, Gruss P, Scholer HR. Oct-6: a POU transcription factor expressed in embryonal stem cells and in the developing brain. EMBO J 1990;9:3723–3732.
26. Pesce M, Scholer HR. Oct-4: control of totipotency and germline determination. Mol Reprod Dev 2000;55:452–457.
27. Niwa H, Miyazaki J, Smith AG. Quantitative expression of Oct-3/4 defines differentiation, dedifferentiation or self-renewal of ES cells. Nat Genet 2000;24:372–376.
28. Pochampally RR, Smith JR, Ylostalo J, Prockop DJ. Serum deprivation of human marrow stromal cells (hMSCs) selects for a subpopulation of early progenitor cells with enhanced expression of OCT-4 and other embryonic genes. Blood 2004;103:1647–1652.
29. Prusa AR, Marton E, Rosner M, Bernaschek G, Hengstschlager M. Oct-4-expressing cells in human amniotic fluid: a new source for stem cell research? Hum Reprod 2003;18:1489–1493.
30. Shamblott MJ, Axelman J, Littlefield JW, et al. Human embryonic germ cell derivatives express a broad range of developmentally distinct markers and proliferate extensively in vitro. Proc Natl Acad Sci USA 2001;98:113–118.
31. Mitchell KE, Weiss ML, Mitchell BM, et al. Matrix cells from Wharton's jelly form neurons and glia. Stem Cells 2003;21:50–60.
32. Helwig B, Van Wye T, Hoynowski S, Mitchell KE. Defining key proteins in stem cell based neuronal development using proteomics. Mol Cell Biol 2003;14:115a.
33. Woodbury D, Schwarz EJ, Prockop DJ, Black IB. Adult rat and human bone marrow stromal cells differentiate into neurons. J Neurosci Res 2000;61:364–370.
34. Broxmeyer HE, Douglas GW, Hangoc G, et al. Human umbilical cord blood as a potential source of transplantable hematopoietic stem/progenitor cells. Proc Natl Acad Sci USA 1989;86:3828–3832.
35. Sirchia G, Rebulla P. Placental/umbilical cord blood transplantation. Haematologica 1999;84:738–747.

36. Gluckman E, Rocha V, Boyer-Chammard A, et al. Outcome of cord-blood transplantation from related and unrelated donors. Eurocord Transplant Group and the European Blood and Marrow Transplantation Group. N Engl J Med 1997;337:373–381.
37. Murohara T, Ikeda H, Duan J, et al. Transplanted cord blood-derived endothelial precursor cells augment postnatal neovascularization. J Clin Invest 2000;105:1527–1536.
38. Wu AG, Michejda M, Mazumder A, et al. Analysis and characterization of hematopoietic progenitor cells from fetal bone marrow, adult bone marrow, peripheral blood, and cord blood. Pediatr Res 1999;46:163–169.
39. Mayani H, Lansdorp PM. Biology of human umbilical cord blood-derived hematopoietic stem/progenitor cells. Stem Cells 1998;16:153–165.
40. Lansdorp PM, Poon S, Chavez E, et al. Telomeres in the haemopoietic system. Ciba Found Symp 1997;211:209–218; discussion 219–222.
41. Globerson A. Hematopoietic stem cells and aging. Exp Gerontol 1999;34:137–146.
42. Kashiwakura I, Takahashi TA. Basic fibroblast growth factor-stimulated ex vivo expansion of haematopoietic progenitor cells from human placental and umbilical cord blood. Br J Haematol 2003;122:479–488.
43. Pesce M, Orlandi A, Iachininoto MG, et al. Myoendothelial differentiation of human umbilical cord blood-derived stem cells in ischemic limb tissues. Circ Res 2003;93:e51–e62.
44. Hows JM. Status of umbilical cord blood transplantation in the year 2001. J Clin Pathol 2001;54:428–434.
45. Benito AI, Diaz MA, Gonzalez-Vicent M, Sevilla J, Madero L. Hematopoietic stem cell transplantation using umbilical cord blood progenitors: review of current clinical results. Bone Marrow Transplant 2004;33:675–690.
46. Mareschi K, Biasin E, Piacibello W, Aglietta M, Madon E, Fagioli F. Isolation of human mesenchymal stem cells: bone marrow versus umbilical cord blood. Haematologica 2001;86:1099–1100.
47. Romanov YA, Svintsitskaya VA, Smirnov VN. Searching for alternative sources of postnatal human mesenchymal stem cells: candidate MSC-like cells from umbilical cord. 2003;Stem Cells 21:105–110.
48. Lee OK, Kuo TK, Chen WM, Lee KD, Hsieh SL, Chen TH. Isolation of multipotent mesenchymal stem cells from umbilical cord blood. Blood 2004;103:1669–1675.
49. Hou L, Cao H, Wang D, et al. Induction of umbilical cord blood mesenchymal stem cells into neuron-like cells in vitro. Int J Hematol 2003;78:256–261.
50. Ha Y, Lee JE, Kim KN, Cho YE, Yoon DH. Intermediate filament nestin expressions in human cord blood monocytes (HCMNCs). Acta Neurochir (Wien) 2003;145:483–487.
51. Buzanska L, Machaj EK, Zablocka B, Pojda Z, Domanska-Janik K. Human cord blood-derived cells attain neuronal and glial features in vitro. J Cell Sci 2002;115:2131–2138.
52. Bicknese AR, Goodwin HS, Quinn CO, Henderson VC, Chien SN, Wall DA. Human umbilical cord blood cells can be induced to express markers for neurons and glia. Cell Transplant 2002;11:261–264.
53. Sanchez-Ramos JR, Song S, Kamath SG, et al. Expression of neural markers in human umbilical cord blood. Exp Neurol 2001;171:109–115.
54. Kaviani A, Perry TE, Dzakovic A, Jennings RW, Ziegler MM, Fauza DO. The amniotic fluid as a source of cells for fetal tissue engineering. J Pediatr Surg 2001;36:1662–1665.
55. Mosquera A, Fernandez JL, Campos A, Goyanes VJ, Ramiro-Diaz J, Gosalvez J. Simultaneous decrease of telomere length and telomerase activity with ageing of human amniotic fluid cells. J Med Genet 1999;36:494–496.
56. Sakuragawa N, Thangavel R, Mizuguchi M, Hirasawa M, Kamo I. Expression of markers for both neuronal and glial cells in human amniotic epithelial cells. Neurosci Lett 1996;209:9–12.

57. Uchida S, Inanaga Y, Kobayashi M, Hurukawa S, Araie M, Sakuragawa N. Neurotrophic function of conditioned medium from human amniotic epithelial cells. J Neurosci Res 2000;62:585–590.
58. Zinsmeyer J, Marangos PJ, Issel EP, Gross J. Neuron specific enolase in amniotic fluid—a possible indicator for fetal distress and brain implication. J Perinat Med 1987;15:199–202.
59. Elimian A, Figueroa R, Verma U, Visintainer P, Sehgal PB, Tejani N. Amniotic fluid neuron-specific enolase: a role in predicting neonatal neurologic injury? Obstet Gynecol 1998;92:546–550.
60. Kintzel K, Sonntag J, Strauss E, Obladen M. Neuron-specific enolase: reference values in cord blood. Clin Chem Lab Med 1998;36:245–247.
61. Gazzolo D, Vinesi P, Marinoni E, et al. S100B protein concentrations in cord blood: correlations with gestational age in term and preterm deliveries. Clin Chem 2000;46:998–1000.
62. Amer-Wahlin I, Herbst A, Lindoff C, Thorngren-Jerneck K, Marsal K, Alling C. Brain-specific NSE and S-100 proteins in umbilical blood after normal delivery. Clin Chim Acta 2001;304:57–63.
63. Wijnberger LD, Nikkels PG, van Dongen AJ, et al. Expression in the placenta of neuronal markers for perinatal brain damage. Pediatr Res 2002;51:492–496.
64. Marinoni E, Di Iorio R, Gazzolo D, et al. Ontogenetic localization and distribution of S-100beta protein in human placental tissues. Obstet Gynecol 2002;99:1093–1099.
65. Jiang Y, Jahagirdar BN, Reinhardt RL, et al. Pluripotency of mesenchymal stem cells derived from adult marrow. Nature 2002;418:41–49.
66. Toma JG, Akhavan M, Fernandes KJ, et al. Isolation of multipotent adult stem cells from the dermis of mammalian skin. Nat Cell Biol 2001;3:778–784.
67. Laywell ED, Rakic P, Kukekov VG, Holland EC, Steindler DA. Identification of a multipotent astrocytic stem cell in the immature and adult mouse brain. Proc Natl Acad Sci USA 2000;97:13883–13888.
68. De Bari C, Dell'Accio F, Tylzanowski P, Luyten FP. Multipotent mesenchymal stem cells from adult human synovial membrane. Arthritis Rheum 2001;44:1928–1942.
69. Zuk PA, Zhu M, Ashjian P, et al. Human adipose tissue is a source of multipotent stem cells. Mol Biol Cell 2002;13:4279–4295.
70. Miura M, Gronthos S, Zhao M, et al. SHED: stem cells from human exfoliated deciduous teeth. Proc Natl Acad Sci USA 2003;100:5807–5812.
71. Powell, DW, Mifflin RC, Valentich JD, Crowe SE, Saada JI, West AB. Myofibroblasts. I. Paracrine cells important in health and disease. Am J Physiol 1999;277:C1–C9.
72. Labat ML. Stem cells and the promise of eternal youth: embryonic versus adult stem cells. Biomed Pharmacother 2001;55:179–185.
73. Moulin V, Tam BY, Castilloux G, et al. Fetal and adult human skin fibroblasts display intrinsic differences in contractile capacity. J Cell Physiol 2001;188:211–222.
74. Bradley JA, Bolton EM, Pedersen RA. Stem cell medicine encounters the immune system. Nat Rev Immunol 2002;2:859–871.
75. Le Blanc K, Tammik C, Rosendahl K, Zetterberg E, Ringden O. HLA expression and immunologic properties of differentiated and undifferentiated mesenchymal stem cells. Exp Hematol 2003;31:890–896.
76. Rouas-Freiss N, Kirszenbaum M, Dausset J, Carosella ED. Fetomaternal tolerance: role of HLA-G molecule in the protection of the fetus against maternal natural killer activity). C R Acad Sci III 1997;320:385–392.
77. Wiendl H, Mitsdoerffer M, Hofmeister V, et al. The non-classical MHC molecule HLA-G protects human muscle cells from immune-mediated lysis: implications for myoblast transplantation and gene therapy. Brain 2003;126:176–185.

78. Barker JN, Wagner JE. Umbilical cord blood transplantation: current practice and future innovations. Crit Rev Oncol Hematol 2003;48:35–43.
79. Beerheide W, von Mach MA, Ringel M, et al. Downregulation of beta2-microglobulin in human cord blood somatic stem cells after transplantation into livers of SCID-mice: an escape mechanism of stem cells? Biochem Biophys Res Commun 2002;294:1052–1063.
80. Hoglund P, Glas R, Menard C, et al. Beta2-microglobulin-deficient NK cells show increased sensitivity to MHC class I-mediated inhibition, but self tolerance does not depend upon target cell expression of H-2Kb and Db heavy chains. Eur J Immunol 1998;28:370–378.
81. Knutsen AP, Steffen M, Wassmer K, Wall DA. Umbilical cord blood transplantation in Wiskott Aldrich syndrome. J Pediatr 2003;142:519–523.
82. Staba SL, Escolar ML, Poe M, et al. Cord-blood transplants from unrelated donors in patients with Hurler's syndrome. N Engl J Med 2004;350:1960–1969.
83. Hall JG, Martin PL, Wood S, Kurtzberg J. Unrelated umbilical cord blood transplantation for an infant with beta-thalassemia major. J Pediatr Hematol Oncol 2004;26:382–385.
84. Garbuzova-Davis S, Willing AE, Zigova T, et al. Intravenous administration of human umbilical cord blood cells in a mouse model of amyotrophic lateral sclerosis: distribution, migration, and differentiation. J Hematother Stem Cell Res 2003;12:255–270.
85. Ende N, Weinstein F, Chen R, Ende M. Human umbilical cord blood effect on sod mice (amyotrophic lateral sclerosis). Life Sci 2000;67:53–59.
86. Ende N, Chen R. Human umbilical cord blood cells ameliorate Huntington's disease in transgenic mice. J Med 2001;32:231–240.
87. Ende N, Chen R. Parkinson's disease mice and human umbilical cord blood. J Med 2002;33:173–180.
88. Ende N, Chen R, Mack R. NOD/LtJ type I diabetes in mice and the effect of stem cells (Berashis) derived from human umbilical cord blood. J Med 2002;33:181–187.
89. Saporta S, Kim JJ, Willing AE, Fu ES, Davis CD, Sanberg PR. Human umbilical cord blood stem cells infusion in spinal cord injury: engraftment and beneficial influence on behavior. J Hematother Stem Cell Res 2003;12:271–278.
90. Chen J, Sanberg PR, Li Y, et al. Intravenous administration of human umbilical cord blood reduces behavioral deficits after stroke in rats. Stroke 2001;32:2682–2688.
91. Medicetty S, Bledsoe AR, Mitchell KE, Troyer D, Weiss ML. Transplantation of human umbilical cord matrix stem cells alleviates apomorphine-induced rotations in Parkinsonian rats. Neuroscience Meeting Abstract, 2003.
92. Sankar V, Muthusamy R. Role of human amniotic epithelial cell transplantation in spinal cord injury repair research. Neuroscience 2003;118:11–17.

4 Differentiation Potential of Adult Stem Cells

Henry E. Young and Asa C. Black, Jr.

CONTENTS

1. ADULT PRECURSOR CELLS

Stem cells are a subcategory of cells designated as "precursor" cells. Precursor cells provide the cellular building blocks to maintain the tissues and organs of the body throughout the life-span of an individual. Precursor cells also provide the cellular building blocks for tissue replacement and repair following injury. There are three basic categories of precursor cells: lineage-uncommitted pluripotent stem cells; germ layer lineage-committed ectodermal, mesodermal, and endodermal stem cells; and lineage-committed progenitor cells. These three categories of precursor cells are based on their life-span, the nature of their lineage commitment, their ability to form various differentiated cell types, and their programmed developmental lineage pattern (Fig. 1).

1.1. Life Span

Differentiated cells and lineage-committed cells have a finite life span. These tissue-specific cells have a "mitotic clock" of 50–70 population doublings before programmed replicative cell senescence and cell death occurs. The mitotic clock for these tissue-specific cells begins at birth. From birth to approximately 20 years of age, about the time an individual attains full stature, there is an exponential increase in the mitotic clock of these cells to about 30 population doublings. From this point, there is an inverse relationship between the increasing age of

From: *Contemporary Endocrinology: Stem Cells in Endocrinology*
Edited by: L. B. Lester © Humana Press Inc., Totowa, NJ

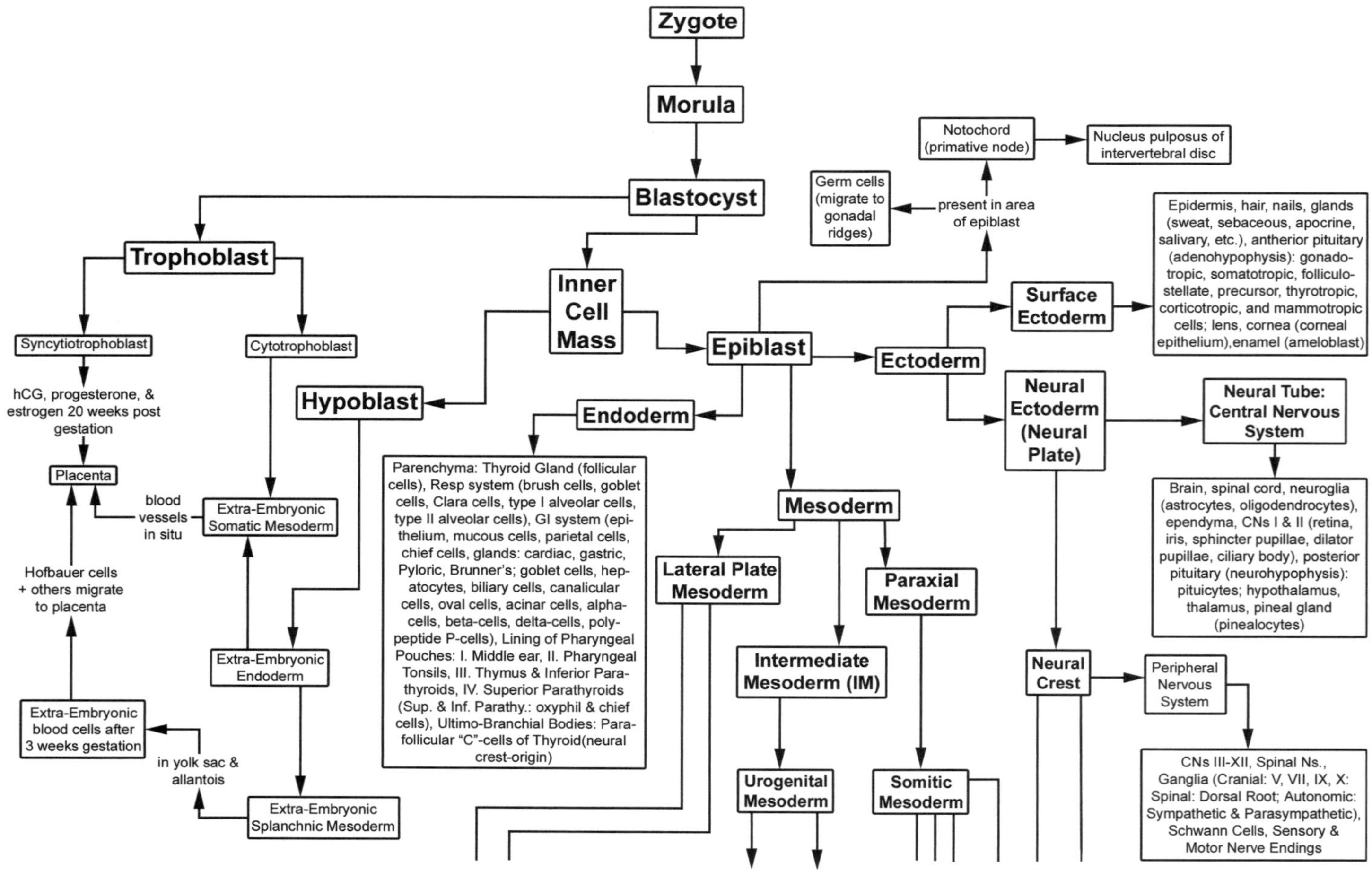
Zygote
Morula
Blastocyst
Trophoblast
Syncytiotrophoblast
Cytotrophoblast
hCG, progesterone, & estrogen 20 weeks post gestation
Placenta
blood vessels in situ
Extra-Embryonic Somatic Mesoderm
Hofbauer cells + others migrate to placenta
Extra-Embryonic Endoderm
Extra-Embryonic blood cells after 3 weeks gestation
in yolk sac & allantois
Extra-Embryonic Splanchnic Mesoderm
Inner Cell Mass
Hypoblast
Epiblast
Endoderm
Parenchyma: Thyroid Gland (follicular cells), Resp system (brush cells, goblet cells, Clara cells, type I alveolar cells, type II alveolar cells), GI system (epithelium, mucous cells, parietal cells, chief cells, glands: cardiac, gastric, Pyloric, Brunner's; goblet cells, hepatocytes, biliary cells, canalicular cells, oval cells, acinar cells, alpha-cells, beta-cells, delta-cells, polypeptide P-cells), Lining of Pharyngeal Pouches: I. Middle ear, II. Pharyngeal Tonsils, III. Thymus & Inferior Parathyroids, IV. Superior Parathyroids (Sup. & Inf. Parathy.: oxyphil & chief cells), Ultimo-Branchial Bodies: Parafollicular "C"-cells of Thyroid(neural crest-origin)
Mesoderm
Lateral Plate Mesoderm
Intermediate Mesoderm (IM)
Urogenital Mesoderm
Paraxial Mesoderm
Somitic Mesoderm
Germ cells (migrate to gonadal ridges)
present in area of epiblast
Notochord (primative node)
Nucleus pulposus of intervertebral disc
Ectoderm
Surface Ectoderm
Epidermis, hair, nails, glands (sweat, sebaceous, apocrine, salivary, etc.), antherior pituitary (adenohypophysis): gonadotropic, somatotropic, folliculo-stellate, precursor, thyrotropic, corticotropic, and mammotropic cells; lens, cornea (corneal epithelium),enamel (ameloblast)
Neural Ectoderm (Neural Plate)
Neural Tube: Central Nervous System
Brain, spinal cord, neuroglia (astrocytes, oligodendrocytes), ependyma, CNs I & II (retina, iris, sphincter pupillae, dilator pupillae, ciliary body), posterior pituitary (neurohypophysis): pituicytes; hypothalamus, thalamus, pineal gland (pinealocytes)
Neural Crest
Peripheral Nervous System
CNs III-XII, Spinal Ns., Ganglia (Cranial: V, VII, IX, X: Spinal: Dorsal Root; Autonomic: Sympathetic & Parasympathetic), Schwann Cells, Sensory & Motor Nerve Endings

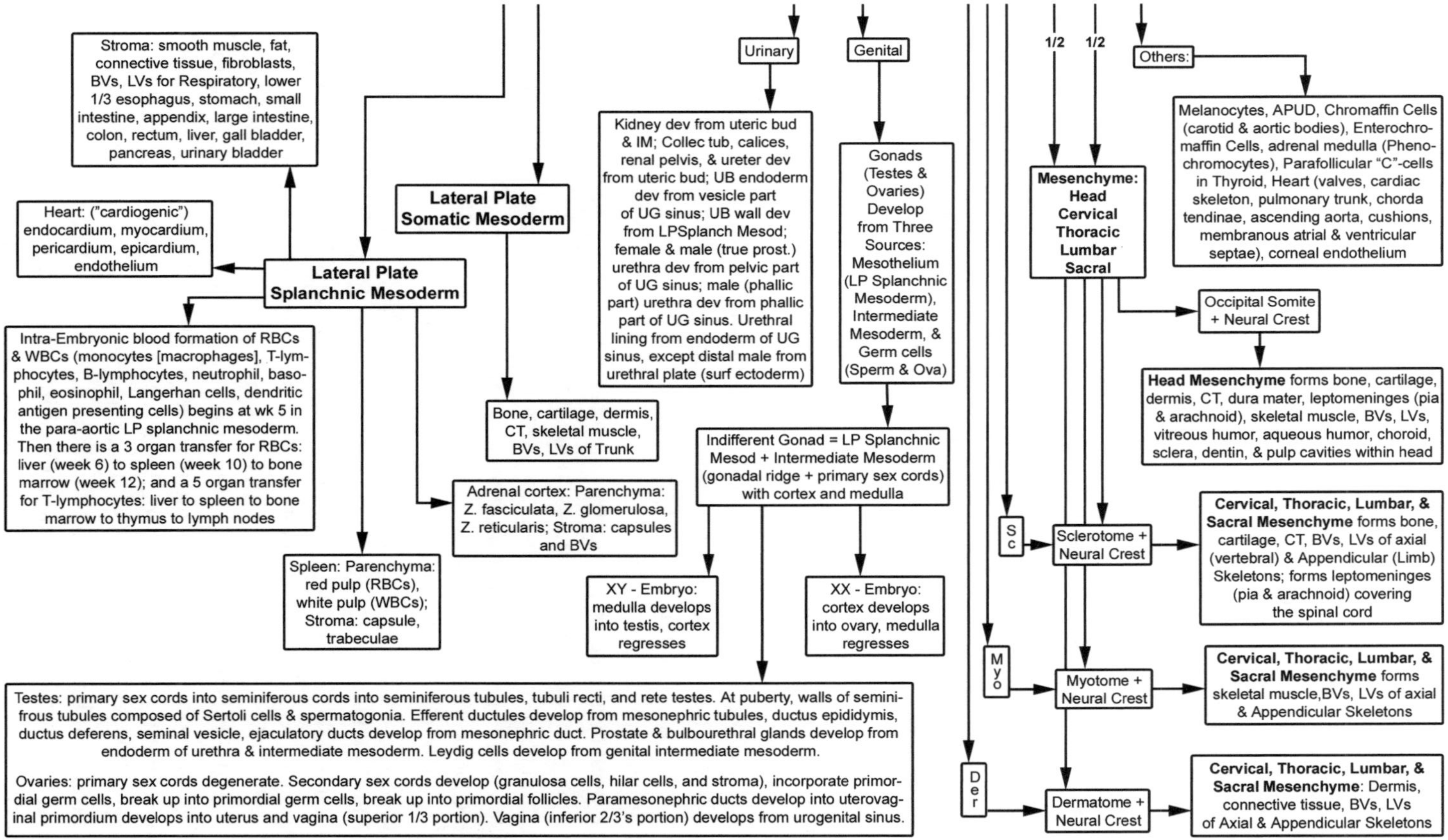

Fig. 1. Lineage flow chart for mammalian embryogenetic development. (Reproduced with permission from Young and Black. Adult stem cells. Anat Rec 2004;276A:75–102, Copyright 2004, Wiley-Liss, Inc.)

individuals and the decreasing population doublings on their respective mitotic clocks. However, if individuals do not succumb to excessive replacement and repair, diseases, or acute trauma leading to death, their remaining population doublings from age 20 would equate to a total life expectancy of approximately 120 years of age.

1.2. Pluripotent Stem Cells

The pluripotent stem cell forms the first category of adult precursor cells. These cells are lineage-uncommitted. They are the most undifferentiated of the precursor cells. They have extensive capabilities for self-renewal that far exceed the mitotic clock of 50–70 population doublings characteristic of differentiated cells and progenitor cells that are committed to specific tissue lineages. They are telomerase-positive, which is consistent with their extensive capabilities for self-renewal. Pluripotent stem cells can commit to a particular germ layer lineage, a process that will eventually result in their becoming lineage-committed progenitor cells. After this happens, they will exhibit a mitotic clock of 50–70 population doublings before programmed cellular senescence and death occurs *(1)*.

Because of its developmental lineage (*see* Fig. 1), the pluripotent stem cell has the potential to form cells belonging to any of the three primary germ layer lineages. Thus it has the capacity to form any cell of the body. Young and coworkers have induced pluripotent ("epiblastic-like") stem cells derived from rats and humans to form more than 80 cell types. The identity of 46 of these cell types have been confirmed by objective assays *(1,2)*.

Pluripotent stem cells demonstrate a unique profile of cell surface cluster of differentiation (CD) markers. Young and coworkers found that pluripotent epiblastic-like stem cells derived from human adult and geriatric donors exhibit CD10 and CD66e markers. They do not exhibit CD1a, CD2, CD3, CD4, CD5, CD7, CD8, CD9, CD11b, CD11c, CD13, CD14, CD15, CD16, CD18, CD19, CD20, CD22, CD23, CD24, CD25, CD31, CD33, CD34, CD36, CD38, CD41, CD42b, CD45, CD49d, CD55, CD56, CD57, CD59, CD61, CD62E, CD65, CD66e, CD68, CD69, CD71, CD79, CD83, CD90, CD95, CD105, CD117, CD123, CD135, CD166, Glycophorin-A, MHC-I, human leukocyte antigen (HLA)-DRII, FMC-7, Annexin-V, or LIN cell-surface markers. Other investigators have found similar results for pluripotent stem cells with some variations *(3)*. In the lineage-uncommitted state, adult-derived pluripotent epiblastic-like stem cells express various embryonic stem cell markers, such as stage-specific embryonic antigen (SSEA)-1, SSEA-3, SSEA-4, CD66e, human carcinoembryonic antigen, carcinoembryonic antigen, carcinoembryonic antigen cell adhesion molecule-1, and Oct-4 gene expression. Once induced to differentiate, pluripotent stem cells demonstrate tissue-specific phenotypic differentiation expression markers for somatic cells of the body (Table 1 *[1–31]*).

Pluripotent stem cells are responsive to proliferation agents such as platelet-derived growth factors. They do not exhibit contact inhibition at confluence, but continue to proliferate to form multiple confluent layers in vitro. This characteristic sets them apart from germ layer lineage stem cells and progenitor cells. Pluripotent stem cells are responsive to any lineage-induction agent (e.g., brain-derived neurotrophic factor, bone morphogenetic protein-2, hepatocyte growth factor) across all three primary germ layer lineages. As long as pluripotent stem cells remain lineage-uncommitted, they are unresponsive to progression agents (e.g., insulin, insulin-like growth factor-I, insulin-like growth factor-II) that accelerate the time frame of expression for tissue-specific phenotypic differentiation expression markers. Pluripotent stem cells remain quiescent in a serum-free environment lacking proliferation agents, lineage-induction agents, progression agents, or inhibitory factors (e.g., recombinant human leukemia inhibitory factor, recombinant murine leukemia inhibitory factor, antidifferentiation factor *[1–5]*). Pluripotent stem cells comprise approximately 1% of the adult precursor cell population. These stem cells are located in all tissues of the body throughout the life-span of an individual. The preferred harvest sites for pluripotent stem cells are skeletal muscle, dermis, or bone marrow *(2,3)*.

1.3. Germ Layer Lineage Stem Cells

A second category of adult precursor cells consists of the germ layer lineage ectodermal, mesodermal, and endodermal stem cells. These stem cells demonstrate extensive capabilities for self-renewal, far exceeding the mitotic clock of 50–70 population doublings for differentiated cells and lineage-committed tissue-specific cells. Germ layer lineage stem cells are telomerase-positive. This characteristic is consistent with their extensive capabilities for self-renewal. They retain this capacity as long as they remain uncommitted to particular tissue and cell types. However, after germ layer lineage stem cells commit to a particular tissue type, they become tissue-specific progenitor cells. As with all progenitor cells, they then exhibit a mitotic clock of 50–70 population doublings before programmed cellular senescence and death occurs *(2,6–10)*.

Because of its developmental lineage (*see* Fig. 1), the germ layer lineage ectodermal stem cell (EctoSC) has the potential to form gonadotrophs, somatotrophs, thyrotrophs, corticotrophs, mammanotrophs, amine precursor uptake decarboxylase (APUD) cells, chromaffin cells, enterochromaffin cells, pheochromocytes, adrenal medulla, parafollicular-C-cells, neurons, astrocytes, oligodendrocytes, dorsal root ganglion cells, sympathetic ganglion cells, parasympathetic ganglion cells, ependyma, keratinocytes, hair, nails, sweat glands, sebaceous glands, apocrine glands, salivary gland mucous cells, salivary gland serous cells, lens, corneal epithelium, enamel, olfactory epithelium, retina, iris, smooth muscle (sphincter & dilator pupillae), ciliary body, pituicytes, hypothalamus, thalamus, pinealocytes, spinal nerves, Schwann cells, motor nerve endings, Meissner's touch corpuscles, Merkel's disks, Krause's end bulbs, free nerve endings, Pacinian touch corpuscles, melanocytes, odontocytes, cementocytes, heart valves, cardiac skeleton, pulmonary trunk, chordae tendinae, ascending aorta, cardiac cushions, membranous atrial septum, membranous ventricular septum, and corneal endothelium *(3,5,11)*. Thus far we have induced over 20 of these differentiated cell types. We have developed assay procedures to verify the identity of 10 of these cell types within populations of germ layer lineage ectodermal stem cells derived from humans and rats (*see* Table 1).

Because of its developmental lineage (*see* Fig. 1), the germ layer lineage mesodermal stem cell has the potential to form cells of the adrenal cortex, Sertoli cells, interstitial cells of Leydig, ovarian stroma, follicular cells/granulosa cells, thecal cells, skeletal muscle, smooth muscle, cardiac muscle, unilocular adipocytes, multilocular adipocytes, fibrous connective tissues, dermis, tendons, ligaments, dura mater, arachnoid mater, pia mater, organ capsules, organ stroma, tunica adventitia, tunica serosa, fibrous scar tissue, hyaline cartilage, articular cartilage, elastic cartilage, growth plate cartilage, fibrocartilage, endochondral bone, intramembranous bone, arterial endothelial cells, venous endothelial cells, capillary endothelial cells, lymphoidal endothelial cells, sinusoidal endothelial cells, erythrocytes, monocytes, macrophages, T-lymphocytes, B-lymphocytes, plasma cells, eosinophils, basophils, Langerhans cells, dendritic cells, natural killer cells, bone marrow stroma, proximal convoluted tubule, distal convoluted tubule, loop of Henle, podocytes, juxtaglomerular cells, mesangial cells, transitional epithelium, seminiferous tubules, tubuli recti, rete testis, efferent ductules, ductus epididymis, ductus deferens, seminal vesicle, ejaculatory ducts, fallopian tubes, uterine endometrium, uterine glands, and upper two-thirds of the vagina *(3,6–8,11)*. Thus far we have induced more than 40 of these cell types and have developed assay procedures to objectively verify 25 of them within populations of germ layer lineage mesodermal stem cells derived from humans and rats (*see* Table 1).

Because of its developmental lineage (*see* Fig. 1), the germ layer lineage endodermal stem cell has the potential to form thyroid follicular cells, parathyroid oxyphil cells, parathyroid chief cells, pancreatic α cells, pancreatic β cells, pancreatic δ cells, pancreatic poly peptide-P cells, brush cells, goblet cells, Clara cells, type I alveolar cells, type II alveolar cells, epithelium of esophagus, gastric mucous cells, gastric parietal cells, gastric chief cells, cardiac glands, gastric glands, pyloric glands, Brunner's glands, epithelium of small intestine, epithelium of large intestine, epithelium of appendix, epithelium of rectum, epithelium of gall bladder, goblet cells, hepatocytes, biliary cells, canalicular cells, oval cells, acinar cells, lining epithelium of pharyngeal pouches, lining of middle ear, pharyngeal tonsils, and thymus *(1–3,11)*. We have induced more than 20 of these cell types and have developed assay procedures to objectively verify 11 of them within rodent and human germ layer lineage endodermal stem cell lines (*see* Table 1).

Young et al. *(6,8)* studied the expression of CD markers in germ layer lineage stem cells generated from human fetal, neonatal, adult, and geriatric donors. They found that the mesodermal stem cell exhibited CD10, CD13, CD34, CD56, CD90, and MHC-I CD markers. They did not find expression of CD1a, CD2, CD3, CD4, CD5, CD7, CD8, CD9, CD11b, CD11c, CD14, CD15, CD16, CD18, CD19, CD20, CD22, CD23, CD24, CD25, CD31, CD33, CD36, CD38, CD41, CD42b, CD45, CD49d, CD55, CD57, CD59, CD61, CD62E, CD65, CD66e, CD68, CD69, CD71, CD79, CD83, CD95, CD105, CD117, CD123, CD135, CD166, Glycophorin-A, HLA-DRII, FMC-7, Annexin-V, or LIN cell surface markers. Other investigators have observed some variations on this pattern *(3)*. Once induced to differentiate, germ layer lineage stem cells demonstrate phenotypic differentiation expression markers specific for their tissues and characteristic of the germ layer from which the cell was derived (*see* Table 1) *(2,3)*.

Germ layer lineage stem cells are responsive to proliferation agents such as platelet-derived growth factors. They exhibit contact inhibition at confluence in vitro. These stem cells are unresponsive to lineage-induction agents that have actions outside their germ layer tissue lineage. For example, germ layer lineage mesodermal stem cells are unresponsive to brain-derived neurotrophic factor (which acts on ectodermal lineage cells) and hepatocyte growth factor (which acts on endodermal lineage cells), but are responsive to bone morphogenetic protein-2 (which acts on mesodermal lineage cells). They are unresponsive to progression agents that accelerate the time frame of expression for tissue-specific phenotypic differentiation expression markers. Germ layer lineage stem cells remain quiescent in a serum-free environment lacking proliferation agents, lineage-induction agents, progression agents, and inhibitory factors *(2–4,9,10)*. Ectodermal, mesodermal, and endodermal germ layer lineage stem cells compose approximately 9% of the precursor cell population. These stem cells are located in all tissues of the body throughout the life-span of an individual. The preferred harvest sites for germ layer lineage stem cells are skeletal muscle, dermis, bone marrow, or an organ of the respective germ layer lineage *(2,3)*.

1.4. Progenitor Cells

A third category of adult precursor cells are the tissue-specific, lineage-committed progenitor cells. Progenitor cells have a finite life-span that begins at birth. Progenitor cells have a "mitotic clock" of 50–70 population doublings before programmed replicative cell senescence and cell death occurs.

A second characteristic of tissue-specific progenitor cells is that they are the immediate precursor cells for adult differentiated cells. They are preprogrammed to commit to particular cell lineages and are unidirectional in their ability to form differentiated cell types. There are four subcategories of tissue-specific progeni-

Table 1
Induction of Phenotypic Expression in Postnatal Precursor Cell Lines

Phenotypic markers	*ELSC (1–3,10)*	*EctoSC (1–3,5,10)*	*MSC (6–10)*	*EndoSC (1–3,10)*	*PanPC (1)*	*DIC (1)*	*ILS (1)*
Embryonic	+	–	–	–	–	ND	–
SSEA-1 *(46)*[c]	+	–	–	–	–	ND	–
SSEA-3 *(47)*	+	–	–	–	–	ND	–
SSEA-a4 *(48)*	+	–	–	–	–	ND	–
CD66e *(13)*[b]	+	–	–	–	–	ND	–
HCEA *(2)*	+	–	–	–	–	ND	–
CEA *(49)*	+	–	–	–	–	ND	–
CEA-CAM-1 *(49)*[d]	+	–	–	–	–	ND	–
Oct-4 *(50)*	+	ND	ND	ND	ND	ND	ND
Telomerase	+	ND	+	ND	ND	ND	ND
Ectoderm							
Neuronal progenitor cells[e]	+	+	–	–	–	ND	–
Neurons[f]	+	+	–	–	–	ND	–
Ganglia[g]	+	+	–	–	–	ND	–
Astrocytes[h]	+	+	–	–	–	ND	–
Oligodendrocytes[i]	+	+	–	–	–	ND	–
Radial glial cells[j]	+	+	–	–	–	ND	–
Synaptic vesicles[k]	+	+	–	–	–	ND	–
Keratinocytes	+	+	–	–	–	ND	–
Mesoderm							
Skeletal muscle[m]	+	–	+	–	–	ND	–
Smooth Muscle[n]	+	–	+	–	–	ND	–
Cardiac Muscle[o]	+	–	+	–	–	ND	–
White fat[p]	+	–	+	–	–	ND	–
Brown fat[q]	+	–	+	–	–	ND	–
Hyaline cartilage[r]	+	–	+	–	–	ND	–
Articular cartilage[r]	+	–	+	–	–	ND	–
Elastic cartilage[r]	+	–	+	–	–	ND	–
Growth plate Cartilage[r]	+	–	+	–	–	ND	–
Fibrocartilage[r]	+	–	+	–	–	ND	–
Intramembranous Bone[s]	+	–	+	–	–	ND	–
Endochondral bone[t]	+	–	+	–	–	ND	–
Tendon ligament[u]	+	–	+	–	–	ND	–
Dermis[v]	+	–	+	–	–	ND	–
Scar tissue[w]	+	–	+	–	–	ND	–
Endothelial cells[x]	+	–	+	–	–	ND	–
Hematopoietic cells[y]	+	–	+	–	–	ND	–

Table 1 (Continued)

Endodermal progenitor cells[z]	+	–	–	+	–	ND	–
GI epithelium[aa]	+	–	–	+	–	ND	–
Liver biliary cells[bb]	+	–	–	+	–	ND	–
Liver canalicular cells[cc]	+	–	–	+	–	ND	–
Liver hepatocytes[dd]	+	–	–	+	–	ND	–
Liver oval cells[ee]	+	–	–	+	–	ND	–
Pancreatic progenitor cells[ff]	+	–	–	+	+	ND	–
Pancreas ductal cells[gg]	+	–	–	+	+	ND	+
Pancreatic α-cells[hh]	+	–	–	+	+	+	+
Pancreatic β-cells[ii]	+	–	–	+	+	+	+
Pancreatic δ-cells[jj]	+	–	–	+	+	+	+

[a]MC480, Developmental Studies Hybridoma Bank (DSHB), Iowa City, IA.

[b]Vector, Burlingame, CA.

[c]Sigma.

[d]Hixson, Providence, RI.

[e]Neuronal progenitor cells werre identified using FORSE-1 (DSHB) for neural precursor cells *(51,52)*, RAT-401 (DSHB) for nestin *(53)*, HNES (Chemicon, Temecula, CA) for nestin *(2)*, and MAB353 (Chemicon) for nestin *(54)*.

[f]Neurons were identified using 8A2 (DSHB) for neurons *(55)*, S-100 (Sigma) for neurons *(56)*, T8660 (Sigma) for β-tubulin III *(57–59)*, RT-97 (DSHB) for neurofilaments *(60)*, N-200 (Sigma) for neurofilament-200 *(61,62)*, and SV2 (DSHB) for synaptic vesicles *(63)*.

[g]Ganglia were identified using TuAg1 (Hixson) for ganglion cells *(64,65)*.

[h]Astrocytes were identified using CNPase (Sigma) for astroglia and oligodendrocytes *(66–68)*.

[i]Oligodendrocytes were identified using Rip (DSHB) for oligodendrocytes *(69)* and CNPase (Sigma) for oligodendrocytes and astroglia *(66–68)*.

[j]Radial glial cells were identified using 40E-C (DSHB) for radial glial cells *(70)*.

[k]Synaptic vesicles were identified using SV2 (DSHB) for synaptic vesicles *(63)*.

[l]Keratinocytes were identified using VM-1(DSHB) to keratinocyte cell surface protein *(71,72)*.

[m]Skeletal muscle was identifed as mononucleated myoblasts staining with OP137 (Calbiochem, San Diego, CA) for MyoD *(73)*, F5D (DSHB) for myogenin *(74)*, and DEU-10 (Sigma) for desmin *(75)*, and as multinucleated spontaneously contracting structures staining with MF-20 (DSHB) for sarcomeric myosin *(76)*, MY-32 (Sigma) for skeletal muscle fast myosin *(77)*, ALD-58 (DSHB) for myosin heavy chain *(78)*, and A4.74 (DSHB) for myosin fast chain *(79)*.

[n]Smooth muscle was identified as mononucleated cells staining with antibodies IA4 (Sigma) for smooth muscle α-actin *(80)* and Calp (Sigma) for calponin *(81,82)*.

[o]Cardiac muscle was identified as binucleated cells co-staining with MF-20 (DSHB) + IA4 (Sigma) for sarcomeric myosin and smooth muscle α- actin *(83,84)*, MAB3252 (Chemicaon) for cardiotin *(85)* and MAB1548 for cardiac muscle (Chemicon).

[p]White fat, also denoted as unilocular adipose tissue, was identified as a mononucleated cell with peripherally located nucleus and containing a large central intracellular vacuole filled with refractile lipid and stained histochemically for saturated neutral lipid using Oil Red-O (Sigma) and Sudan Black-B (Chroma-Gesellschaft, Roboz Surgical Co, Washington, DC) *(7)*.

Table 1 (Continued)

[q]Brown fat, also denoted as multilocular adipose tissue, was identified as a mononucleated cell with a centrally located nucleus containing multiple small intracellular vacuoles filled with refractile lipid and stained histochemically for saturated neutral lipid using Oil Red-O (Sigma) and Sudan Black-B (Chroma-Gesellschaft) *(8,9)*.

[r]Cartilage: structures thought to be cartilage nodules were tentatively identified as aggregates of rounded cells containing pericellular matrix halos. Cartilage nodules were confirmed by both histochemical and immunochemical staining. Histochemically, cartilage nodules were visualized by staining the pericellular matrix halos for proteoglycans containing glycosaminoglycan side chains with chondroitin sulfate and keratan sulfate moieties. This was accomplished using Alcian Blue (Alcian Blau 8GS, Chroma-Gesellschaft), Safranin-O (Chroma-Gesellschaft) at pH 1.0, and Perfix/Alcec Blue. Verification of glycosaminoglycans specific for cartilage was confirmed by loss of extracellular matrix staining following digestion of the material with chondroitinase-AC (ICN Biomedicals, Cleveland, OH) and keratanase (ICN Biomedicals) *(7,8,86,87)* before staining (negative staining control). Immunochemically, the chondrogenic phenotype was confirmed by initial intracellular staining followed by subsequent staining of the periculluar and extracellular matrices with CIIC1 (DSHB) for type II collagen *(88)*, HC-II ((ICN Biomedicals, Aurora, OH) for type II collagen *(89,90)*, D1-9 (DSHB) for type IX collagen *(91)*, 9/30/8A4 (DSHB) for link protien *(92)*, and 12C5 (DSHB) for versican *(94)*. Types of cartilage were segregated based on additional attributes. *Hyaline cartilage* was identified by a perichondrial-like connective tissue surrounding the prevously stained cartilage nodule and histochemical costaining for type I collagen *(95)*. *Articular cartilage* was identified as the above stained cartilage nodule without a perichondrial-like connective tissue covering *(96)*. *Elastic cartilage* was identified by nodular staining for elastin fibers and a perichondrial-like connective tissue surrounding the above stained cartilage nodule and histochemical co-staining for type I collagen *(95)*. Growth plate cartilage was identified by nodular staining for cartilage phenotypic markers and co-staining for calcium phosphate using the von Kossa procedure *(6–8)*. Fibrocartilage was identified as three-dimensional nodules demonstrating extracellualr histochemical staining for type I collagen *(95)* and co-staining for pericellular matrices rich in chondroitin sulfates A and C. The latter were assessed by Alcian Blue pH1.0 staining. Negative staining controls were digested prior to staining with chondroitinase-ABC or chondroitinase-AC *(7,8,86,87)*.

[s]Intramembranous bone was identified as a direct transition from stellate-shaped stem cells to three-dimensional nodules displaying only osteogenic phenotypic markers WV1D1(9C5) (DSHB) for bone sialoprotein II *(97)*, MPIII (DSHB) for osteopontine *(98)*, and the von Kossa procedure, (Silber Protein, Chroma-Gesellschaft) for calcium phosphate. In the von Kossa procedure, negative staining controls were preincubated in EGTA, a specific chelator for calcium (Sigma) *(6–8,96)*.

[t]Endochondral bone was identified as the formation of a three-dimensional structure with progressional staining from one displaying chondrogenic phenotypic markers i.e., pericellular type II collagen, type IX collage, chondroitin sulfate/keratan sulfate glycosaminoglycans (see previous) to three-dimensional nodules displaying osteogenic phenotypic markers; that is, WV1D1(9C5) (DSHB) for bone sialoprotein II *(97)*, MPIII (DSHB) for osteopontine *(98)*, and the von Kossa procedure (Silber Protein, Chroma-Gesellschaft) for calcium phosphate. In the von Kossa procedure, negative staining controls were preincubated in EGTA, a specific chelator for calcium (Sigma) *(6–8,96)*.

[u]Tendon/ligament was identified as linear structures with cellualr staining for fibroblast-specific protein IB10 (Sigma) *(99)* and displaying extracellular histochemical staining for type I collagen *(95)*.

[v]Dermis was identified by the presence of interwoven type I collagen fibers *(95)* interspersed with spindle-shaped cells staining for fibroblast-specific protein IB10 (Sigma) *(99)* with an extracellular matrix rich in chondroitin sulfate and dermatan sulfate glycosaminoglycans as assessed by Alcian Blue pH 1.0 staining. In the latter procedure, negative staining controls were digested with chondroitinase-ABC or chondroitinase-AC prior to staining *(6,7,86,87)*.

Table 1 (Continued)

[w]Scar tissue was identified as interwoven type I collagen fibers *(95)* interspersed with spindle-shaped cells staining for fibroblast specific protien IB10 (Sigma) *(99)* with an extracellular matrix rich in chondroitin sulfate glycosaminoglycans as assessed by Alcian Blue pH 1.0 staining. In the latter procedure, negative staining controls were digested with chondroitinase-ABC or chondroitinase-AC prior to staining *(6,7,86,87)*.

[x]Endothelial cells were identified by staining with antibodies P2B1 (DSHB) for CD31-PECAM *(8)*, H-Endo (Chemicon)f or CD146 *(100,101)*, P8B1 (DSHB) for VCAM *(8,102)*, and P2H3 (DSHB) for CD62e selectin-E *(8)*.

[y]Hematopoietic cells were identified using H-CD34 (Vector) for sialomucin-containing hematopoietic cells *(8,13)*; Hermes-1 (DSHB) for CD44—hyaluronate receptor *(103–105)*; and H5A4 (DSHB) for DC11b-granulocytes, monocytes; and natural killer cells, H5H5 (DSHB) for CD43—leukocytes, H4C4 (DSHB) for CD44—hyaluronate receptor, H5A5 (DSHB) for CD45—all leukocytes, and H5C6 (DSHB) for CD63—macrophages, monocytes, and platelets *(106,107)*.

[z]Endodermal progenitor cells were identified with H-AFP (Vector) and R-AFP (Nordic Immunological Laboratories, Tilburg, The Netherlands) for α-fetoprotein *(108)*.

[aa]GI Epithelium was identified with HESA (Sigma) for GI-epithelium *(2,3,10)*.

[bb]Liver biliary cells were identified with OC2, OC3, OC4, OC5, OC10, DPP-IV, and OV6 (Hixson) for biliary epithelial cells, liver progenitor cells, oval cells, and canalicular cells *(65, 109–113)*.

[cc]Liver canalicular cells were identified with antibodies H4Ac19 (DSHB), DPP-IV, OV6, and LAP (Hisxon) for bile canalicular cells, liver progenitor cells, biliary epithelial cells, and canalicular cell surface protein *(64,65,109, 110,111,113,114)*.

[dd]Liver hepatocytes were identified with H-1 and H-4 (Hixson) for hepatocyte cell surface marker and hepatocyte cytoplasm, respectively *(111,112)*, and 151-IgG for liver progenitor cells, and biliary epithelial cells *(112,113)*.

[ee]Liver oval cells were identified with OC2 and OV6 (Hixson) for oval cells, liver progenitor cells, and biliary epithelial cells *(112,113)*.

[ff]Pancreatic progenitor cells were tentatively identified as three-dimensional structures void of chondrogenic or osteogenic phenotypic markers. This identity was confirmed by the presence phenotypic markers for pancreatic ductal cells, β-cells, α-cells, and δ-cells *(1–3,10)*.

[gg]Pancreatic ductal cells were identified with cytokeratin-19 (Chemicon) to pancreatic ductal cells *(1–3,10)*.

[hh]Pancreatic α-cells were identified with YM-PS087 (Accurate, Westbury, NY) an antibody to glucagon *(1–3,10)*.

[ii]Pancreatic b-cells were identified with YM-PS088 (Accurate) an antibody to insulin *(1–3,10)*.

[jj]Pancreatic d-cells were identified with 11180 (ICN) an antibody to somatostatin *(1–3,10)*.

ELSC, pluripotent epiblastic-like stem cells (isolated and cloned); EctoSC, germ layer lineage ectodermal stem cells (induced); MSC, germ layer lineage mesodermal (pluripotent mesenchymal) stem cells (isolated and cloned); EndoSC, germ layer lineage endodermal stem cells (induced); Pan PC, pancreatic progenitor cells induced from germ layer lineage endodermal stem cells; DIC, diffuse population of islet cells induced from GLL endodermal stem cells; ILS, islet-like structures induced from pancreatic progenitor stem cells; SSEA-1, stage-specific embroyonic antigen-1 antibody MC480 (DSHB); SSEA-3, stage-specific embryonic antigen-3, antibody MC631 (DSHB); SSEA-4, stage-specific embryonic antighen-4, antibody MC-813-70 (DHSB); CD66e, carcinoembryonic antigen; HCEA, human carcinoembryonic antigen; CEA, carcinoembryonic antigen;CEA-CAM1, carcino-embryonic antigen-cell adhesion molecule; Oct-4, a gene directly involved in the capacity for self-renewal and pluripotency of mammalian embryonic stem cells; ND, not determined.

tor cells: unipotent, bipotent, tripotent, and multipotent. Progenitor cells may be unipotent, having the ability to form only a single differentiated cell type. A precursor cell of endodermal origin residing in the thyroid gland, designated the thyroid progenitor cell, is an example of a unipotent progenitor cell. This cell will form thyroid follicular cells *(11)*. A progenitor cell may be bipotent, having the ability to form two differentiated cell types. A precursor cell of intermediate mesodermal origin located within the ovary, designated the ovarian stromal cell, is an example of a bipotent progenitor cell. This cell will form granulosa cells and thecal cells *(11)*. A progenitor cell may be tripotent, having the ability to form three differentiated cell types. A precursor cell of mesodermal origin, the chondro-osteo-adipoblast, is an example of a tripotent progenitor cell. This cell will only form chondrocytes (cartilage), osteocytes (bone), or adipocytes (fat cells) *(12)*. A progenitor cell may be multipotent, having the ability to form multiple cell types. A precursor cell of ectodermal origin residing in the adenohypophysis, designated the adenohypophyseal progenitor cell, is an example of a multipotent progenitor cell. This cell will form gonadotrophs, somatotrophs, thyrotrophs, corticotrophs, and mammotrophs *(11)*.

Progenitor cells for particular cell lineages have unique profiles of cell surface CD markers *(13)* and unique profiles of phenotypic differentiation expression markers (*see* Table 1). They are responsive to proliferation agents such as platelet-derived growth factors and exhibit contact inhibition at confluence in vitro. They are unresponsive to lineage-induction agents that have actions outside their respective tissue lineage. However, they are responsive to progression agents that accelerate the time frame of expression for tissue-specific phenotypic differentiation expression markers. Progenitor cells remain quiescent in a serum-free environment lacking lineage induction agents, progression agents, proliferation agents, and inhibitory factors *(2–4)*. Progenitor cells compose approximately 90% of the precursor cell population. They are located in all tissues of the body throughout the life-span of an individual. However, progenitor cells have a rather unique distribution. Fifty percent of the precursor cells within a tissue or organ are its own respective lineage-committed progenitor cells. Approximately 40% of the remaining precursor cells are progenitor cells specific for other tissues. For example, although myogenic, fibrogenic, and hematopoietic progenitor cells are the predominant precursor cells in skeletal muscle, dermis, and bone marrow, respectively, lesser quantities of other progenitor cells including neuronal progenitor cells and hepatic progenitor cells have also been found in these tissues *(2,3)*.

2. USE OF ADULT PRECURSOR CELLS FOR THERAPEUTIC MODALITIES

Based on our current knowledge, we propose that various therapeutic modalities could be performed using adult autologous, syngeneic, or allogeneic pluripotent stem cells, germ layer lineage stem cells, or progenitor cells. However, use of the adult-derived pluripotent stem cells or germ layer lineage stem cells would require that they be made to undergo lineage/tissue induction to form specific tissue types. We have begun to study the potential advantages for using syngeneic, allogeneic, and autologous adult stem cells in transplantation and replacement therapies. The model systems used in these experiments include gene therapy and therapies for neuronal diseases, hematopoietic diseases, diabetes mellitus, and myocardial infarction. Studies involving the repair of articular cartilage, bone, and skeletal muscle have also been undertaken *(1,2)*. As an example of this approach, the use of adult pluripotent stem cells as donor tissue for generating pancreatic islets as a potential therapy for diabetes mellitus is discussed.

2.1. Therapy for Diabetes Mellitus

Diabetes mellitus is a metabolic syndrome with a diversity of etiologies, clinical presentations, and outcomes. It is characterized by insulinopenia, fasting or postprandial hyperglycemia, and insulin resistance. Type 1 diabetes mellitus, referred to as juvenile or insulin-dependent diabetes mellitus is typically characterized by insulinopenia, hyperglycemia, and secondary insulin resistance *(14)*. Type 2 diabetes mellitus, referred to as adult onset or non-insulin-dependent diabetes mellitus, is characterized by hyperglycemia and varying degrees of primary insulin resistance with elevated plasma insulin concentrations, but a decreased insulin response to challenge by a secretagogue *(15)*. Diabetes mellitus need not be overt and grossly hyperglycemic to induce detrimental metabolic changes. A growing body of evidence suggests that there are detrimental consequences to normal physical challenges such as aging, which may be inherently linked to alterations in body composition. Such challenges may result in subclinical diabetogenic changes. It is becoming increasingly clear that loss of physical strength, functional status, and immune competence are related to decreases in lean body mass observed in diabetogenic states *(16–18)*.

In 1933, Walsh and colleagues showed that protein wasting in type 1 diabetes mellitus could be eliminated by administration of insulin *(19)*. Later studies suggested that the degree of protein wasting may be related to the degree of pancreatic function and insulin availability *(20)*. A single mechanism of action, which describes the effect of insulin on proteolysis or proteogenesis, remains to be clearly elucidated. Decreased lean body mass in diabetes mellitus may be due to decreased number and translational efficiency of ribosomes *(21,22)* and to alterations in peptide chain elongation and termination *(23)*. Several studies additionally suggest that these effects may be modulated in part by modifications in insulin-like growth factor I (IGF-I). Streptozotocin diabetic rats that are insulin-deficient lack IGF-I. Growth retardation in diabetic infants has been ascribed to a lack of proper insulinization *(24)*. More recent studies suggest that protein nutrition, insulin, and growth may be modulated via IGF-I *(25,26)*. Tobin et al. *(27–29)* demonstrated that transplantation with normal islets of Langerhans completely restores normal body protein levels in rats.

Islet transplantation, rather than whole organ transplantation, has been investigated as a possible treatment for type 1 diabetes mellitus in selected patients unresponsive to exogenous insulin therapy *(30)*. Recently, the Edmonton group *(31–35)* reported that sufficient islet mass from as few as two pancreases, in combination with a new regimen involving a glucocorticoid-free immunosuppressive protocol, engendered sustained freedom (>1 year) of insulin independence in 8 of 8 *(32)* and 12 of 12 *(34,35)* patients with type 1 diabetes mellitus. Their findings indicated that islet transplantation alone was associated with minimal risk and resulted in good metabolic control *(32,33)*. However, because of the paucity of cadaveric organ donors, less than 0.5% of patients with type 1 diabetes mellitus could receive an islet transplant at this time. Thus alternative sources of insulin-secreting tissue are urgently needed *(31)*.

Recent reports *(36–38)* suggest that reversal of insulin-dependent diabetes mellitus can be accomplished using chemically induced islets generated in vitro from pancreatic ductal endodermal stem cells. In addition, Lumelsky et al. *(39)* reported the formation of three-dimensional insulin-secreting pancreatic islets that spontaneously differentiated from embryonic stem cells. Based on these reports, we began preliminary in vitro studies to ascertain the ability of adult pluripotent epiblastic-like stem cells to form insulin-secreting pancreatic islet-like structures. A clone of adult rat pluripotent epiblastic-like stem cells *(1)* was used for these studies.

One of the major differences we noted between reports of embryonic stem cells and the adult pluripotent epiblastic-like stem cells is their respective activities in serum-free defined media in the absence of lineage-induction or differentiation inhibitory agents. In serum-free medium in the absence of differentiation inhibitory agents (i.e., leukemia inhibitory factor or a fibroblast feeder layer), embryonic stem cells will spontaneously differentiate into all the somatic cells present in the body *(40,41)*. Indeed, Soria et al. *(42,43)*, Assady et al. *(44)*, and Lumelsky et al. *(39)* used spontaneous differentiation directly or in combination with directed differentiation to generate pancreatic islets from embryonic stem cells. In contrast, adult-derived pluripotent epiblastic-like stem cells remain quiescent in serum-free defined media in the absence of differentiation inhibitory agents (i.e., leukemia inhibitory factor or antidifferentiation factor) *(1,2)*. In other words, these adult pluripotent epiblastic-like stem cells are not preprogrammed to form any type of cell. Furthermore, pluripotent epiblastic-like stem cells remain quiescent unless a specific lineage-, tissue-, or cell-inductive agent is present in the medium *(1,3,4,7–10)*. Because pluripotent epiblastic-like stem cells do not exhibit spontaneous differentiation, we attempted to use direct lineage-induction to generate pancreatic islet-like structures. The initial population of stem cells consisted of a clone of pluripotent epiblastic-like stem cells derived from an adult rat by single-cell repetitive clonogenic analysis *(1)*. In a sequential fashion, we induced these undifferentiated pluripotent stem cells to commit to and form germ layer lineage endodermal stem cells and then to form pancreatic progenitor cells. As the stem cells became increasingly lineage-committed, there was a concomitant loss of pluripotentiality within the induced cell line (Table 1).

Next, we used the islet-inductive mixture of Bonner-Weir et al. *(38)* in an attempt to induce pancreatic islet-like structures in the three stem cell populations: pluripotent epiblastic-like stem cells, germ layer lineage endodermal stem cells, and pancreatic progenitor cells. For each cell line, 10^3 stem cells were plated per well ($n = 96$) and treated with serum-free defined medium containing the islet-inductive mixture *(1,38)*. The mean number of induced islet-like structures formed per well (± standard error of the mean) was 0.364 ± 0.066 for the pluripotent epiblastic-like stem cells, 1.177 ± 0.117 for the germ layer lineage endodermal stem cells, and 10.104 ± 0.480 for the pancreatic progenitor cells. The increase in the number of constructs formed by the pancreatic progenitor cells was statistically significant compared with that induced in the pluripotent epiblastic-like stem cells or the germ layer lineage endodermal stem cells ($p < 0.05$, analysis of variance). After treatment with the islet-inductive cocktail, the cultures were stained with antibodies to insulin, glucagon, and somatostatin. Induced pluripotent epiblastic-like stem cells showed minimal intracellular staining for any of the antibodies used (Fig. 2A–C). Induced germ layer lineage endodermal stem cells showed a diffuse population of individual cells stained for insulin, glucagon, and somatostatin (Fig. 2D–F). Induced pancreatic progenitor cells demonstrated nodular islet-like structures that exhibited intracellular staining for insulin, glucagon, and somatostatin (Fig. 2G–I).

We then examined the biological activity of the two cell populations induced to form islet cells (i.e., the diffuse population of islet cells) (Fig. 2D–F), induced from endodermal stem cells, and the nodular islet-like structures (Figs. 2G–I, 3A,B) induced from pancreatic progenitor cells. The biological activity examined was the ability of these cells to secrete insulin in response to a glucose challenge. This was compared with the biological activity of native pancreatic islet tissue. For native pancreatic islet tissue, 200 × 150 mm pancreatic islet equivalent units (Fig. 3C,D) were isolated from pancreases taken from adult male Wistar Furth rats *(27–29)* for each trial ($n = 8$). Diffuse islet cells were derived from a starting population of 5×10^3 adult pluripotent stem cells induced to form endodermal stem cells by cultivation through two passages in endodermal inductive medium (*1*). Twenty-four hours after replating, the endodermal stem cell cultures were switched to islet-inductive medium (*1,38*). Cultures were

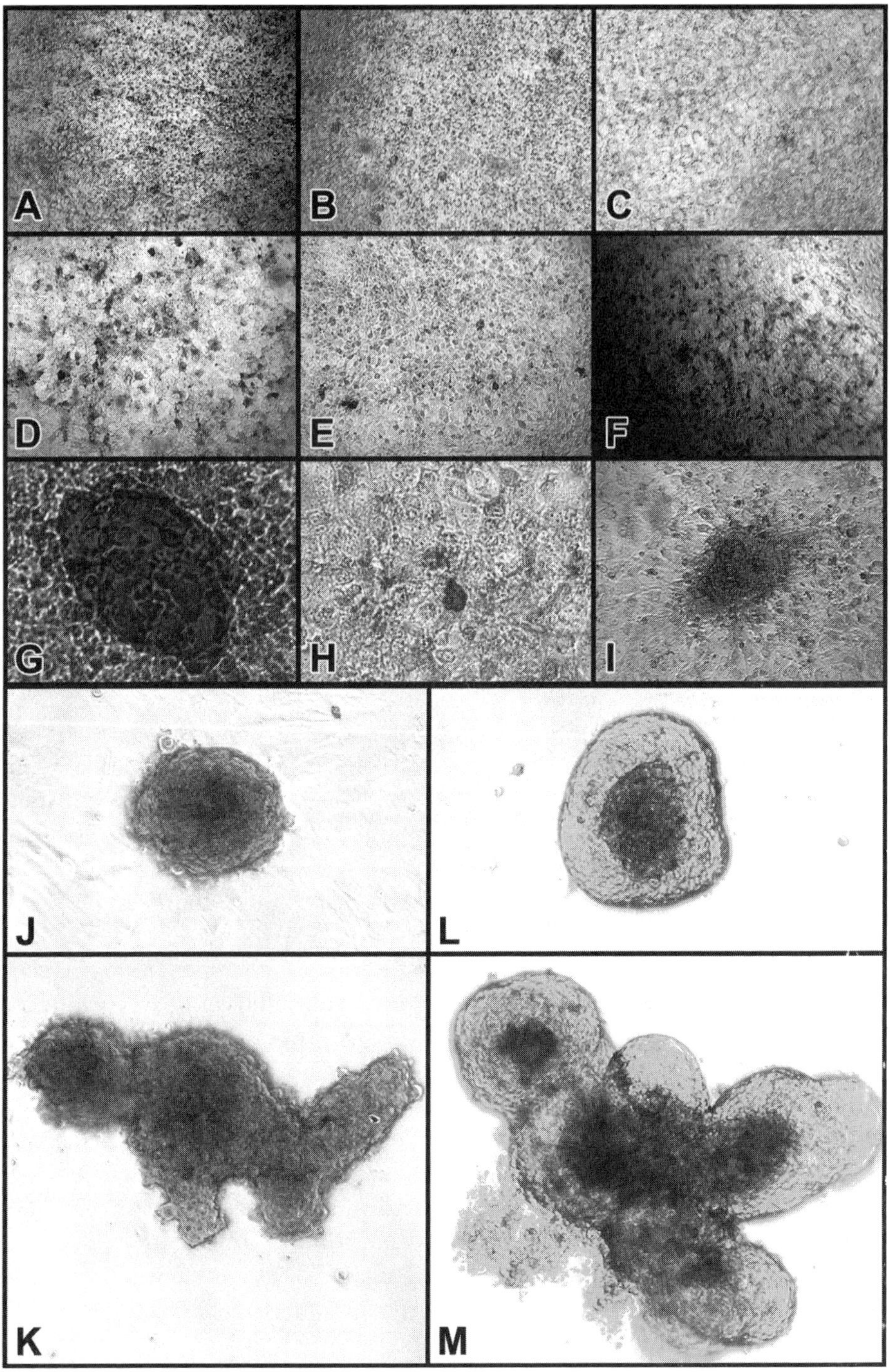
A
B
C
D
E
F
G
H
I
J
L
K
M

Fig. 2. (*opposite page*) Expression of insulin, glucagon, and somatostatin in adult rat pluripotent epiblastic-like stem cells, pluripotent epiblastic-like stem cells induced to form germ layer lineage endodermal stem cells, germ layer lineage endodermal stem cells induced to form pancreatic progenitor cells, and native pancreatic islets isolated from adult Wistar-Furth rats. (Reproduced with permission from Young et al. Clonogenic analysis reveals reserve stem cells in postnatal mammals. II. Pluripotent epiblastic-like stem cells. Anat Rec 277A:178–203, 2004, Copyright 2004, Wiley-Liss, Inc.). **(A–C)** Pluripotent epiblastic-like stem cells were expanded in medium containing proliferative activity (like that of PDGF) and inductive-inhibitory activity (like that of antidifferentiation factor). Twenty-four hours after plating the cultures were switched to islet-inductive medium (*38*), containing serum with endodermal inductive activity (*1*). Cultures were incubated for 2 weeks and processed for enzyme-linked immunoculture assay (ELICA) using primary antibodies to insulin, glucagon, and somatostatin. Visualization of bound antibody occurred with 3,3′-diaminobenzidine (DAB). Original magnifications, ×100. **(A)** Minimal intracellular staining for insulin. **(B)** Minimal intracellular staining for glucagon. **(C)** Minimal intracellular staining for somatostatin. **(D–F)** Germ layer lineage endodermal stem cells were generated from pluripotent epiblastic-like stem cells by directed lineage induction. Pluripotent epiblastic-like stem cells were expanded in medium containing proliferative activity and inhibitory activity with respect to induction. Twenty-four hours after plating, pluripotent epiblastic-like stem cells were switched to medium containing endodermal inductive activity (*1*) for two passages. By the end of the second passage in endodermal inductive medium, the cells increased to a uniform size and shape and assumed contact inhibition, forming a single confluent layer of cells. Twenty-four hours after replating germ layer lineage endodermal stem cells, the cultures were switched to islet-inductive medium (*1,38*). Cultures were incubated for 2 weeks and processed for ELICA using primary antibodies to insulin, glucagon, and somatostatin. Visualization of bound antibody occurred with DAB. Original magnifications, ×100. **(D)** Diffuse distribution of individual cells stained intracellularly for insulin. **(E)** Diffuse distribution of individual cells stained intracellularly for glucagon. **(F)** Diffuse distribution of individual cells stained intracellularly for somatostatin. **(G–I)** Pancreatic progenitor cells were generated from germ layer lineage endodermal stem cells by directed lineage induction. Germ layer lineage endodermal stem cells were expanded in endodermal inductive medium. Twenty-four hours after replating germ layer lineage endodermal stem cells were switched to pancreatic progenitor cell induction medium (*1*). A minimum of two passages were required for the induction process. Twenty-four hours after replating, the cultures were switched to islet-inductive medium (*1,38*). Cultures were incubated for 2 weeks and processed for ELICA using primary antibodies to insulin, glucagon, and somatostatin. Visualization of bound antibody occurred with DAB. Original magnifications: ×400 **(G)**, ×300 **(H)**, ×200 **(I)**. G. Three-dimensional nodular islet-like structure and surrounding mononucleated cells showing moderate to heavy intracellular staining for insulin. **(H)** Three-dimensional nodular islet-like structure with a few centrally located cells showing heavy intracellular staining for glucagon. **(I)** Three-dimensional nodular islet-like structure and some surrounding mononucleated cells showing moderate to heavy intracellular staining for somatostatin. **(J–M)** Nodular islet-like structures **(A,B)** induced from an adult rat pluripotent epiblastic-like stem cell clone via directed lineage induction. Cultures were photographed with phase contrast incubated for 2 weeks before testing each trial (*n* = 12). Nodular islet-like structures were derived from a starting population of 5×10^3 adult pluripotent stem cells induced sequentially by directed lineage induction to first form endodermal stem cells by cultivation with endodermal induction medium *(1)*. The endodermal stem cells were induced to form pancreatic progenitor cells by cultivation with pancreatic progenitor cell induction medium *(1)*. And pancreatic progenitor cells were induced to form islet-like structures by cultivation with islet-inductive medium *(1,38)*. Cultures were incubated for 2 weeks before testing each trial (*n* = 12). The progression of adult pluripotent stem cells to endodermal stem cells, endodermal stem cells to diffuse islet cells, endodermal stem cells to pancreatic progenitor cells, and pancreatic progenitor cells to nodular islet-like structures was monitored by successive loss of pluripotency within the induced cell lines (*see* Table 1) and the resultant morphology of the cultures.

Each well of the native islets, induced diffuse islet cells, and induced islet-like structures were incubated sequentially with testing medium (TM) only, followed by TM containing 5 m*M* glucose for 24 hours, followed by TM containing 5 m*M* glucose for 1 hour, followed by TM containing 25 m*M* glucose for 1 hour. The media were removed and the amount of secreted insulin was determined by double antibody competitive binding radioimmunoassay (RIA) using rat insulin standards and antibodies raised against rat-specific insulin (Linco, St. Louis, MO) according to the manufacturer's directions. The mean value for insulin secretion from native islets was determined and designated as 100%. The mean values for insulin secretion from diffuse islet cells and islet-like structures were also determined and expressed as percent mean of native islets.

Fig 2 (*continued*) microscopy, original magnifications ×100. **(J,K)** Islet-like structures were induced from pluripotent epiblastic-like stem cell clone derived from an adult rat by sequential directed lineage induction. In this process, pluripotent epiblastic-like stem cells were induced to form germ layer lineage endodermal stem cells, which were induced to form pancreatic progenitor stem cells, which were induced to form islet-like structures (*1*). The induced transition from pluripotent epiblastic-like stem cells to germ layer lineage endodermal stem cells, germ layer lineage endodermal stem cells to pancreatic progenitor cells, and pancreatic progenitor cells to islet-like structures was monitored by changes in phenotypic lineage expression markers (*see* Table 1). Cultures were photographed with phase contrast microscopy, original magnifications ×100. **(J)** Induced single islet-like structure. **(K)** Induced group of islet-like structures. **(L,M)** Pancreatic islets from 9- to 10-week-old male Wistar Furth rats (approximately 220 g) were isolated as described (*1*). Cultures were incubated for 24 hours and photographed with phase contrast microscopy, original magnifications ×100. **(L)** Native Wistar-Furth pancreatic islet. **(M)** Native Wistar-Furth islet grouping.

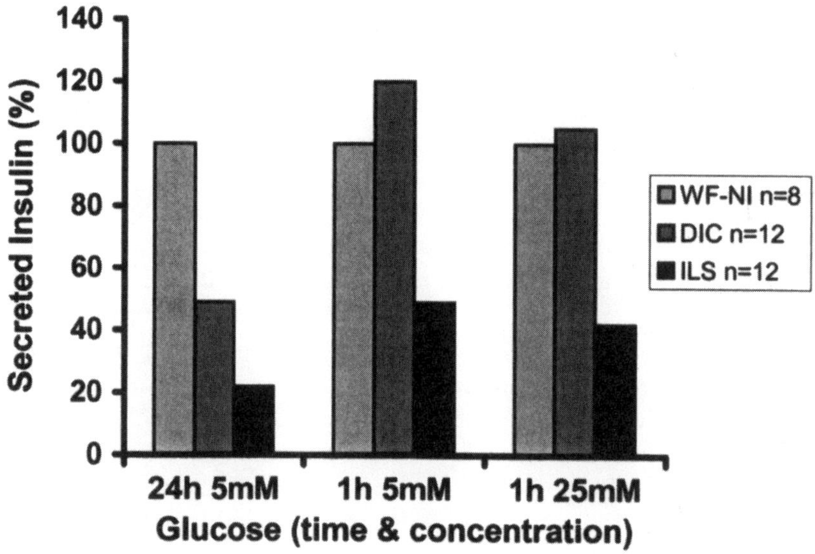

Fig. 3. Glucose-mediated insulin secretion. The efficacy of insulin secretion in vitro by native Wistar-Furth islets, diffuse islet cells, and nodular islet-like structures were compared at basal (5 m*M*) and elevated (25 m*M*) glucose concentrations.

A series of positive and negative controls was performed to ensure that the RIA measured only rat insulin secreted into the media and not bovine insulin taken up and subsequently released by the cells *(1,45)*. The positive controls consisted of a concentration range of rat insulin standards included with the rat-specific RIA kit. The negative controls consisted of serum-free defined medium with and without the insulin secretagogues in a cell-free system. Because our testing medium also contained a small amount of bovine insulin, its presence was monitored using the same concentration range (0.1 to 10 ng/mL bovine insulin) as rat insulin standards in the RIA kit. No insulin was detected in any of the negative controls analyzed.

Pancreatic β cells induced from adult pluripotent stem cells as either diffuse islet cells or islet-like structures demonstrated a positive response to the glucose challenge, secreting 50% and 22%, respectively, the amount of insulin secreted by native islets during incubation with 5 m*M* glucose for 24 hours. When this was followed in each well by incubation in 5 m*M* glucose for 1 hour, the diffuse islet cells secreted 120% and the nodular islet-like structures secreted 49% of the amount secreted by the native islets. A subsequent incubation with 25 m*M* glucose for 1 hour resulted in secretion by the diffuse islet cells of 105% and the nodular islet-like structures of 42% of the amount of insulin secreted by the native islets (*see* Fig. 3).

3. CONCLUSION

There are potential advantages for using adult precursor cells in transplantation and replacement therapies. Precursor cells can be directly isolated from newborn to geriatric individuals, including patients awaiting treatment. Use of autologous precursor cells circumvents the inherent morbidity and mortality associated with human leukocyte antigen mismatches that require the use of immunosuppressant drugs to prevent rejection of allogeneic or syngeneic tissues and organs. Based on the presence of telomerase and their inherent capabilities for extensive self-renewal, a small number of pluripotent stem cells or germ layer lineage stem cells obtained at harvest can be stimulated to form vast quantities of cells. Once induced to commit to a particular cell type, these stem cells assume all the characteristics of lineage-committed progenitor cells, including a mitotic clock of 50–70 population doublings before programmed cellular senescence and cell death occurs. Pluripotent stem cells and germ layer lineage stem cells can be stored for long periods with minimal loss of cell viability, pluripotentiality or function. Adult pluripotent stem cells can be induced to form cells from the three primary germ layer lineages (i.e., ectoderm, mesoderm, and endoderm). Adult germ layer lineage stem cells can subsequently form any somatic cell type within their respective germ layer lineages. These results suggest that adult-derived stem cells comprise a potential donor source for the production of endocrine cell types, as well as other somatic cells, for various therapeutic protocols.

ACKNOWLEDGMENTS

Supported by grants from Rubye Ryle Smith Charitable Trust, Lucille M. and Henry O. Young Estate Trust, MedCen Community Health Foundation, and MorphoGen Pharmaceuticals, Inc. We would like to thank Nicholas Henson, Julie Floyd, John Knight, technical assistants, volunteers, and collaborators for their insight and work ethic. The antibodies CEA-CAM-1, TuAG1, OC2, OC3, OC4, OC5, OC10, DPP-IV, OV6, LAP, H-1, and H-4 were generously provided by Douglas Hixson (Providence, RI). The following antibodies were obtained from the Developmental Studies Hybridoma Bank developed under the auspices of the NICHD and maintained by The University of Iowa, Department of Biological Sciences, Iowa City, IA: MC480, MC631, and MC813-70 developed by D. Solter; FORSE-1 developed by P. Patterson; RAT-401 and Rip developed by S. Hockfield; RT-97 developed by J. Wood; 8A2 developed by V. Lemmon; SV2 developed by K.M. Buckley; VM-1 developed by V.B. Morhenn; 151-Ig was developed by A. Hubbard; 40E-C developed by A. Alvarez-Buylla; F5D developed by W.E. Wright; MF-20 and ALD-58 developed by D.A. Fischman; A4.74 developed by H.M. Blau; CIIC1 developed by R. Holmdahl and K. Rubin; D1-9 developed by X.-J. Ye and K. Terato; 9/30/8A4 and 12/21/1C6 developed by

B. Caterson; 12C5 developed by R.A. Asher; WV1D1 (9C5) and MP111B10 developed by M. Solursh and A. Frazen; P2B1 and P2H3 developed by E.A. Wayner and G. Vercellotti; P8B1 developed by E.A. Wayner and T. LeBien; HA4c19 developed by A. Hubbard; Hermes-1 developed by E.C. Butcher; and H4C4, H5A5, H5C5, H5C6, and H5A4 developed by J.T. August and J.E.K. Hildreth.

REFERENCES

1. Young HE, Duplaa C, Yost MJ, et al. Clonogenic analysis reveals reserve stem cells in postnatal mammals. II. Pluripotent epiblastic-like stem cells. Anat Rec 2004;277A:178–203.
2. Young HE, Duplaa C, Romero-Ramos M, et al. Adult reserve stem cells and their potential for tissue engineering. Cell Biochem Biophys 2004;40:1–80.
3. Young HE, Black Jr AC. Adult stem cells. Anat Rec 2004;276A:75–102.
4. Young HE, Wright RP, Mancini ML, Lucas PA, Reagan CR, Black AC Jr. Bioactive factors affect proliferation and phenotypic expression in progenitor and pluripotent stem cells. Wound Repair Regen 1998;6:65–75.
5. Romero-Ramos M, Vourc'h P, Young HE, et al. Neuronal differentiation of stem cells isolated from adult muscle. J Neurosci Res 2002;69:894–907
6. Young HE, Steele TA, Bray RA, et al. Human pluripotent and progenitor cells display cell surface cluster differentiation markers CD10, CD13, CD56, and MHC Class-I. Proc Soc Exp Biol Med 1999;221:63–71.
7. Young HE, Duplaa C, Young TM, et al. Clonogenic analysis reveals reserve stem cells in postnatal mammals. I. Pluripotent mesenchymal stem cells. Anat Rec 2001;263:350–360.
8. Young HE, Steele TA, Bray RA, et al. Human reserve pluripotent mesenchymal stem cells are present in the connective tissues of skeletal muscle and dermis derived from fetal, adult, and geriatric donors. Anat Rec 2001;264:51–62.
9. Young HE. Stem cells and tissue engineering. In: Huard J, Fu FH, eds. Gene Therapy and Tissue Engineering in Orthopaedic and Sports Medicine. Boston, Birkhauser, 2000, pp. 143–173.
10. Young HE. Existence of reserve quiescent stem cells in adults, from amphibians to humans. Curr Top Microbiol Immunol 2004;280:71–109.
11. Kacsoh B. Endocrine Physiology. McGraw-Hill, New York, 2000.
12. Pittenger MF, Mackay AM, Beck SC, et al. Multilineage potential of adult human mesenchymal stem cells. Science 1999;284:143–147.
13. Kishimoto T, Kikutani H, von dem Borne AEGK, et al. Leucocyte Typing VI, White Cell Differentiation Antigens. Garland Publishing, Hamden, 1997.
14. Eisenbarth GS, Connelly J, Soeldner JS. The "natural" history of type I diabetes. Diabetes/ Metab Rev 1987;3:873–891.
15. Ward WK, Beard JC, Porte D Jr. Clinical aspects of islet B-cell function in non-insulin-dependent diabetes mellitus Diabetes Metab Rev 1986;2:297–313.
16. Chandra RK. Nutritional regulation of immunity and risk of infection in old age. Immunology 1989;67:141–147.
17. Fiatarone MA, Marks EC, Ryan ND, Meridith CN, Lipsitz LA, Evans WJ. High-intensity strength training in nonagenarians. Effects on skeletal muscle. JAMA 1990;263:3029–3034.
18. Frontera WR, Hughes VA, Lutz KJ, Evans WJ. A cross-sectional study of muscle strength and mass in 45- to 78-yr-old men and women. J Appl Physiol 1991;71:644–650.
19. Walsh CH, Soler NG, James H, et al. Studies in whole body potassium and whole body nitrogen in newly diagnosed diabetics. Q J Med 1976;45:295–301.

20. Nair KS, Garrow JS, Ford C, Mahler RF, Halliday D. Effect of poor diabetic control and obesity on whole body protein metabolism in man. Diabetologia 1983;25:400–403
21. Morgan HE, Jefferson LS, Wolpert EB, Rannels DE. Regulation of protein synthesis in heart muscle. II. Effect of amino acid levels and insulin on ribosomal aggregation. J Biol Chem 1971;246:2163–2170.
22. Jefferson LS, Li JB, Rannels SR. Regulation by insulin of amino acid release and protein turnover in the perfused rat hemicorpus. J Biol Chem 1977;252:1476–1483.
23. Peavy DE, Taylor JM, Jefferson LS. Correlation of albumin production rates and albumin mRNA levels in livers of normal, diabetic and insulin-treated diabetic rats. Proc Nat Acad Sci USA 1978;75:5879–5883.
24. Froesch ER, Guler HP, Schmid C, Ernst M, Zapf J. Insulin-like growth factors. In: Rifkin H, Porte D, eds. Ellenberg and Rifkin's Diabetes Mellitus: Theory and Practice. New York, Elsevier Press, 1990, pp. 154–169.
25. Lemozy S, Pucilowska JB, Underwood LE. Reduction of insulin-like growth factor-I (IGF-I) in protein-restricted rats is associated with differential regulation of IGF-binding protein messenger ribonucleic acids in liver and kidney, and peptides in liver and serum. Endocrinology 1994;135:617–623.
26. Straus DS. Nutritional regulation of hormones and growth factors that control mammalian growth. FASEB J 1994;8:6–12.
27. Tobin BW, Marchello MJ. Islet transplantation reverses carcass protein loss in diabetic rats without inducing disproportionate fat accumulation. Diabetologia 1995;38:881–888.
28. Tobin BW, Lewis JT, Tobin BL, Finegood DT. Insulin action in previously diabetic rats receiving graded numbers of islets of Langerhans. Transplantation 1995;59:1464–1469.
29. Tobin BW, Welch-Holland KR, Marchello MJ. Pancreatic islet transplantation improves body composition, decreases energy intake and normalizes energy efficiency in previously diabetic female rats. J Nutr 1997;127:1191–1197.
30. Weir GC, Bonner-Weir S. Islet transplantation as a treatment for diabetes. J Am Optom Assoc 1998;69:727–732.
31. Shapiro AM, Lakey JR. Future trends in islet transplantation. Diabetes Technol Therapeutics 2000;2:449–452.
32. Shapiro AM, Lakey JR, Ryan EA, et al. Islet transplantation in seven patients with type 1 diabetes mellitus using a glucocorticoid-free immunosuppressive regimen. N Engl J Med 2000;343:230–238.
33. Shapiro AM, Ryan EA, Lakey JR. Pancreatic islet transplantation in the treatment of diabetes mellitus. Best Pract Res Clin Endocrinol Metab 2001;15:241–264.
34. Ryan EA, Lakey JR, Shapiro AM. Clinical results after islet transplantation. J Investig Med 2001;49:559–562.
35. Ryan EA, Lakey JR, Rajotte RV, et al. Clinical outcomes and insulin secretion after islet transplantation with the Edmonton protocol. Diabetes 2001;50:710–719.
36. Cornelius JG, Tchernev V, Kao KJ, Peck AB. In vitro-generation of islets in long-term cultures of pluripotent stem cells from adult mouse pancreas. Horm Metab Res 1997;29:271–277.
37. Ramiya VK, Maraist M, Arfos KE, Schatz DA, Peck AB, Cornelius JG. Reversal of insulin-dependent diabetes using islets generated in vitro from pancreatic stem cells. Nat Med 2000;6:278–282.
38. Bonner-Weir S, Taneja M, Weir GC, Tatarkiewic, K, Song K-H, Sharma A, O'Neil JJ. In vitro cultivation of human islets from expanded ductal tissue. Proc Natl Acad Sci USA 2000;97:7999–8004.
39. Lumelsky N, Blondel O, Laeng P, Velasco I, Ravin R, McKay R. Differentiation of embryonic stem cells to insulin-secreting structures similar to pancreatic islets. Science 2001;292:1389–1393.

40. Thomson JA, Itskovitz-Eldor J, Shapiro SS, et al. Embryonic stem cell lines derived from human blastocysts. Science 1998;282:1145–1147.
41. Shamblott MJ, Axelman J, Wang S, et al. Derivation of pluripotent stem cells from cultured human primordial germ cells. Proc Natl Acad Sci USA 1998;95:13726–13731.
42. Soria B, Roche E, Berna G, Leon-Quinto T, Reig JA, Martin F. Insulin-secreting cells derived from embryonic stem cells normalize glycemia in streptozotocin-induced diabetic mice. Diabetes 2000;49:157–162.
43. Soria B, Skoudy A, Martin F. From stem cells to beta cells: new strategies in cell therapy of diabetes mellitus. Diabetologia 2001;4:407–415.
44. Assady S, Maor G, Amit M, Itskovitz-Eldor J, Skorecki, KL, Tzukerman M. Insulin production by human embryonic stem cells. Diabetes 2001;50:1691–1697.
45. Rajagopal J, Anderson WJ, Kume S, Martinez OI, Melton DA. Insulin staining of ES cell progeny from insulin uptake. Science 2003;299:363.
46. Solter D, Knowles BB. Monoclonal antibody defining a stage-specific mouse embryonic antigen (SSEA-1). Proc Natl Acad Sci USA 1978;75:5565–5569.
47. Damjanov I, Fox N, Knowles BB, Solter D, Lange PH, Fraley EE. Immunohistochemical localization of murine stage-specific embryonic antigens in human testicular germ cell tumors. Am J Pathol 1982;108:225–230.
48. Kannagi R, Cochran NA, Ishigami F, et al. Stage specific embryonic antigens (SSEA-3 and -4) are epitopes of a unique globo-series ganglioside isolated from human treatocarcinoma cells. EMBO J 1983;2:2355–2361.
49. Estrera VT, Luo W, Phan D, Earley K, Hixson DC, Lin SH. The cytoplasmic domain of C-CAM1 tumor suppressor is necessary and sufficient for suppressing the tumorigenicity of prostate cancer cells. Biochem Biophys Res Commun 1999;263:797–803.
50. Pesce M, Scholer HR. Oct-4: gatekeeper in the beginnings of mammalian development. Stem Cells 2001;19:271–278.
51. Tole S, Kaprielian Z, Ou SK, Patterson PH. FORSE-1: a positionally regulated epitope in the developing rat central nervous system. J Neurosci 1995;15:957–969.
52. Tole S, Patterson PH. Regionalization of the developing forebrain: a comparison of FORSE-1, Dlx-2, and BF-1. J Neurosci 1995;15:970–980.
53. Hockfield S, McKay RD. Identification of major cell classes in the developing mammalian nervous system. J Neurosci 1985;5:3310–3328.
54. Gritti A, Frolichsthal-Schoeller P, Galli R, et al. Epidermal and fibroblast growth factors behave as mitogenic regulators for a single multipotent stem cell-like population from the subventricular region of the adult mouse forebrain. J Neurosci 1999;19:3287–3297.
55. Drazba J, Pierce M, Lemmon V. Studies of the developing chick retina using monoclonal antibody 8A2 that recognizes a novel set of gangliosides. Dev Biol 1991;145:154–163.
56. Baudier J, Glasser N, Gerard D. Ions binding to S100 proteins. I. Calcium- and zinc-binding properties of bovine brain S100 alpha alpha, S100a (alpha beta), and S100b (beta beta) protein: Zn2+ regulates Ca2+ binding on S100b protein. J Biol Chem 1986;261:8192–8203.
57. Banerjee A, Roach MC, Wall KA, Lopata MA, Cleveland DW, Luduena RF. A monoclonal antibody against the type II isotype of beta-tubulin. Preparation of isotypically altered tubulin. J Biol Chem 1988;263:3029–3034.
58. Banerjee A, Roach MC, Trcka P, Luduena RF. Increased microtubule assembly in bovine brain tubulin lacking the type III isotype of beta-tubulin. J Biol Chem 1990;265:1794–1799.
59. Joshi HC, Cleveland DW. Diversity among tubulin subunits: toward what functional end? Cell Motil Cytoskeleton 1990;16:159–163.

60. Wood JN, Anderton BH. Monoclonal antibodies to mammalian neurofilaments. Biosci Rep 1981;1:263–268.
61. Debus E, Weber K, Osborn M. Monoclonal antibodies specific for glial fibrillary acidic (GFA) protein and for each of the neurofilament triplet polypeptides. Differentiation 1983;25:193–203.
62. Franke FE, Schachenmayr W, Osborn M, Altmannsberger M. Unexpected immunoreactivities of intermediate filament antibodies in human brain and brain tumors. Am J Pathol 1991;139:67–79.
63. Feany MB, Lee S, Edwards RH, Buckley KM. The synaptic vesicle protein SV2 is a novel type of transmembrane transporter. Cell 1992;70:861–867.
64. Faris RA, McEntire KD, Thompson NL, Hixson DC. Identification and characterization of a rat hepatic oncofetal membrane glycoprotein. Cancer Res 1990;50:4755–4763.
65. Hixson DC, Faris RA, Thompson NL. An antigenic portrait of the liver during carcinogenesis. Pathobiology 1990;58:65–77.
66. Sprinkle TJ, Agee JF, Tippins RB, Chamberlain CR, Faguet GB, De Vries GH. Monoclonal antibody production to human and bovine 2¢:3¢-cyclic nucleotide 3¢-phosphodiesterase (CNPase): high-specificity recognition in whole brain acetone powders and conservation of sequence between CNP1 and CNP2. Brain Res 1987;426:349–357.
67. Sprinkle TJ. 2¢,3¢-cyclic nucleotide 3¢-phosphodiesterase, an oligodendrocyte-Schwann cell and myelin-associated enzyme of the nervous system. Crit Rev Neurobiol 1989;4:235–301.
68. Reynolds R, Carey EM, Herschkowitz N. Immunohistochemical localization of myelin basic protein and 2¢,3¢-cyclicnucleotide 3¢-phosphohydrolase in flattened membrane expansions produced by cultured oligodendrocytes. Neuroscience 1989;28:181–188.
69. Friedman B, Hockfield S, Black JA, Woodruff KA, Waxman SG. In situ demonstration of mature oligodendrocytes and their processes: an immunocytochemical study with a new monoclonal antibody, rip. Glia 1989;2:380–390.
70. Alvarez-Buylla A, Buskirk DR, Nottebohm F. Monoclonal antibody reveals radial glia in adult avian brain. J Comp Neurol 1987;264:159–170.
71. Oseroff AR, Pfendt EA, DiCicco L, Morhenn VB. A murine monoclonal antibody (VM-1) against human basal cells inhibits the growth of human keratinocytes in culture. J Invest Dermatol 1985;84:257–261.
72. Morhenn VB. VM-1 for keratinocyte, basal, cell attachment antigen (human). In: Developmental Studies Hybridoma Bank Product Catalog. The University of Iowa, Iowa City, 2002, p. 24.
73. Thulasi R, Dias P, Houghton PJ, Houghton JA. Alpha 2a-interferon-induced differentiation of human alveolar rhabdomyosarcoma cells: correlation with down-regulation of the insulin-like growth factor type I receptor. Cell Growth Differ 1996;7:531–541.
74. Wright WE, Binder M, Funk W. Cyclic amplification and selection of targets (CASTing) for the myogenin consensus binding site. Mol Cell Biol 1991;11:4104–4110.
75. Debus E, Weber K, Osborn M. Monoclonal antibodies to desmin, the muscle-specific intermediate filament protein. EMBO J 1983b;2:2305–2312.
76. Bader D, Masaki T, Fischman DA. Immunochemical analysis of myosin heavy chain during avian myogenesis in vivo and in vitro. J Cell Biol 1982;95:763–770.
77. Naumann K, Pette D. Effects of chronic stimulation with different impulse patterns on the expression of myosin isoforms in rat myotube cultures. Differentiation 1994;55:203–211.
78. Shafiq SA, Shimizu T, Fischman DA. Heterogeneity of type 1 skeletal muscle fibers revealed by monoclonal antibody to slow myosin. Muscle Nerve 1984;7:380–387.
79. Webster C, Silberstein L, Hays AP, Blau HM. Fast muscle fibers are preferentially affected in Duchenne muscular dystrophy. Cell 1988;52:503–513.

80. Skalli O, Ropraz P, Trzeciak A, Benzonana G, Gillessen D, Gabbiani G. A monoclonal antibody against alpha-smooth muscle actin: a new probe for smooth muscle differentiation. J Cell Biol 1986;103:2787–2796.
81. Frid MG, Shekhonin BV, Koteliansky VE, Glukhova MA. Phenotypic changes of human smooth muscle cells during development: late expression of heavy caldesmon and calponin. Dev Biol 1992;153:185–193.
82. Lazard D, Sastre X, Frid MG, Glukhova MA, Thiery JP, Koteliansky VE. Expression of smooth muscle-specific proteins in myoepithelium and stromal myofibroblasts of normal and malignant human breast tissue. Proc Natl Acad Sci USA 1993;90:999–1003.
83. Eisenberg CA, Markwald RR. Mixed cultures of avian blastoderm cells and the quail mesoderm cell line QCE-6 provide evidence for the pluripotentiality of early mesoderm. Dev Biol 1997;191:167–181.
84. Eisenberg CA, Gourdie RG, Eisenberg LM. Wnt-11 is expressed in early avian mesoderm and required for the differentiation of the quail mesoderm cell line QCE-6. Development 1997;124:525–536.
85. Schaart G, Moens L, Endert JM. Ramaekers FC. Biochemical characterization of cardiotin, a sarcoplasmic reticulum associated protein. FEBS Lett 1997;403:168–172.
86. Young HE, Dalley BK, Markwald RR. Glycoconjugates in normal wound tissue matrices during the initiation phase of limb regeneration in adult Ambystoma. Anat Rec 1989;223:231–241.
87. Young HE, Dalley BK, Markwald RR. Effect of selected denervations on glycoconjugate composition and tissue morphology during the initiation phase of limb regeneration in adult Ambystoma. Anat Rec 1989;223:223–230.
88. Holmdahl R, Rubin K, Klareskog L, Larsson E, Wigzell H. Characterization of the antibody response in mice with type II collagen-induced arthritis, using monoclonal anti-type II collagen antibodies. Arthritis Rheum 1986;29:400–410.
89. Burgeson RE, Hollister DW. Collagen heterogeneity in human cartilage: identification of several new collagen chains. Biochem Biophys Res Commun 1979;87:1124- 1131.
90. Kumagai J, Sarkar K, Uhthoff HK, Okawara Y, Ooshima A. Immunohistochemical distribution of type I, II and III collagens in the rabbit supraspinatus tendon insertion. J Anat 1994;185:279–284.
91. Ye XJ, Terato K, Nakatani H, Cremer MA, Yoo TJ. Monoclonal antibodies against bovine type IX collagen (LMW fragment): production, characterization, and use for immunohistochemical localization studies. J Histochem Cytochem 1991;39:265–271.
92. Caterson B. 9/30/8-A-4 for link protein, 12/21/1-C-6 for proteoglycan hyaluronic acid binding region. In: Developmental Studies Hybridoma Bank Product Catalog. NICHHD. University of Iowa, Iowa City, 2001, p. 12.
93. Caterson B, Baker JR, Christner JE, Lee Y, Lentz M. Monoclonal antibodies as probes for determining the microheterogeneity of the link proteins of cartilage proteoglycan. J Biol Chem 1985;260:11348–11356.
94. Asher RA, Scheibe RJ, Keiser HD, Bignami A. On the existence of a cartilage-like proteoglycan and link proteins in the central nervous system. Glia 1995;13:294–308.
95. Young HE, Carrino DA, Caplan AI. Histochemical analysis of newly synthesized and accumulated sulfated glycosaminoglycans during musculogenesis in the embryonic chick leg. J Morphol 1989;201:85–103.
96. Young HE, Ceballos EM, Smith JC, et al. Pluripotent mesenchymal stem cells reside within avian connective tissue matrices. In Vitro Cell Dev Biol Anim 1993;29A:723–736.
97. Kasugai S, Nagata T, Sodek J. Temporal studies on the tissue compartmentalization of bone sialoprotein (BSP), osteopontin (OPN), and SPARC protein during bone formation in vitro. J Cell Physiol 1992;152:467–477.

98. Gorski JP, Griffin D, Dudley G, et al. Bone acidic glycoprotein-75 is a major synthetic product of osteoblastic cells and localized as 75- and/or 50-kDa forms in mineralized phases of bone and growth plate and in serum. J Biol Chem 1990;265:14956–14963.
99. Ronnov-Jessen L, Celis JE, Van Deurs B, Petersen OW. A fibroblast-associated antigen: characterization in fibroblasts and immunoreactivity in smooth muscle differentiated stromal cells. J Histochem Cytochem 1992;40:475–486.
100. Solovey A, Lin Y, Browne P, Choong S, Wayner E, Hebbel RP. Circulating activated endothelial cells in sickle cell anemia. N Eng J Med 1997;337:1584–1590.
101. St Croix B, Rago C, Velculescu V, et al. Genes expressed in human tumor endothelium. Science 2000;289:1197–1202.
102. Dittel BN, McCarthy JB, Wayner EA, LeBien TW. Regulation of human B-cell precursor adhesion to bone marrow stromal cells by cytokines that exert opposing effects on the expression of vascular cell adhesion molecule-1 (VCAM-1). Blood 1993;81:2272–2282.
103. Picker LJ, Nakache M, Butcher EC. Monoclonal antibodies to human lymphocyte homing receptors define a novel class of adhesion molecules on diverse cell types. J Cell Biol 1989;109:927–937.
104. Lewinsohn DM, Nagler A, Ginzton N, Greenberg P, Butcher EC. Hematopoietic progenitor cell expression of the H-CAM (CD44) homing-associated adhesion molecule. Blood 1990;75:589–595
105. Butcher EC. Hermes-1 for CD44. In: Developmental Studies Hybridoma Bank Product Catalog. The University of Iowa, Iowa City, 2002, p. 12.
106. Hildreth JE, August JT. The human lymphocyte function-associated (HLFA) antigen and a related macrophage differentiation antigen (HMac-1): functional effects of subunit-specific monoclonal antibodies. J Immunol 1985;134:3272–3280.
107. August JT, Hildreth JEK. H5A4 for CD11b (Mac-1, CR3), H5H5 for CD43 (human) sialophorin, H4C4 for CD44 human hyaluronate receptor, H5A5 for CD45 (lymphocyte common antigen) (human), H5C6 for CD63 (human) LIMP. In: Developmental Studies Hybridoma Bank Product Catalog. The University of Iowa, Iowa City, 2002, p. 11.
108. Mujoo K, Ali M, Sahib MK. Isolation, characterization, and synthesis of alpha-fetoprotein from neonatal rat brain. J Neurochem 1983;41:1223–1228.
109. Hixson DC, De Lourdes Ponce M, Allison JP, Walborg EF Jr. Cell surface expression by adult rat hepatocytes of a non-collagen glycoprotein present in rat liver biomatrix. Exp Cell Res 1984;152:402–414.
110. Hixson DC, Brown J, McBride AC, Affigne S. Differentiation status of rat ductal cells and ethionine-induced hepatic carcinomas defined with surface-reactive monoclonal antibodies. Exp Mol Pathol 2000;68:152–169.
111. Walborg EF Jr, Tsuchida S, Weeden DS, et al. Identification of dipeptidyl peptidase IV as a protein shared by the plasma membrane of hepatocytes and liver biomatrix. Exp Cell Res 1985;158:509–518.
112. Faris RA, Monfils BA, Dunsford HA, Hixson DC. Antigenic relationship between oval cells and a subpopulation of hepatic foci, nodules, and carcinomas induced by the "resistant hepatocyte" model system. Cancer Res 1991;51:1308–1317.
113. Gordon GJ, Coleman WB, Hixson DC, Grisham JW. Liver regeneration in rats with retrorsine-induced hepatocellular injury proceeds through a novel cellular response. Am J Pathol 2000;156:607–619.
114. Hubbard AL, Bartles JR, Braiterman LT. Identification of rat hepatocyte plasma membrane proteins using monoclonal antibodies. J Cell Biol 1985;100:1115–1125.

5 Growth Conditions for Primate vs Murine Embryonic Stem Cells

Gillian M. Beattie, Nathan Bucay, Rohan Humphrey, Ana D. Lopez, and Alberto Hayek

CONTENTS

1. INTRODUCTION

Cultured embryonic stem (ES) cells are continuous cell lines derived from 3- to 5-day-old embryonic blastocysts. Essentially an artifact of tissue culture, they can, under certain physiological conditions, sustain an undifferentiated state with the capacity to divide and renew themselves indefinitely while having the ability to differentiate into all cell types when so instructed by specific extracellular signals. An understanding of these fundamental properties and elucidation of the underlying mechanisms involved is important for implementation of potential stem cell-based therapies for human disease.

From: *Contemporary Endocrinology: Stem Cells in Endocrinology*
Edited by: L. B. Lester © Humana Press Inc., Totowa, NJ

2. MAINTENANCE OF PLURIPOTENCY BY DISPARATE BIOCHEMICAL PATHWAYS IN MOUSE AND HUMAN EMBRYONIC STEM CELLS

Mouse embryonic stem (mES) cells have been studied extensively since 1981, when pluripotent cells from mouse blastocysts were first derived using feeder layers *(1,2)*. One of the key characteristics of ES cells is their ability to make the fundamental decision whether to remain pluripotent or differentiate. The biochemical pathways of self-renewal and differentiation for mES have been well described elsewhere *(3)*. ES cell lines derived from nonhuman primates *(4)*, human blastocysts *(5)* and primordial germ cells *(6)* have only recently become available for research, and their intracellular pathways for self-renewal and differentiation are, at this time, largely unknown.

3. BIOCHEMICAL PATHWAYS FOR PLURIPOTENCY IN 129 STRAIN mES CELLS

Maintenance of the undifferentiated state and pluripotency in mES derived from the 129 strain requires the presence of mouse fibroblast feeder layers (mEFs) or leukemia inhibitory factor (LIF). LIF is a member of the interleukin (IL)-6 family of cytokines, which also includes Oncostatin M, ciliary neurotropic factor, IL-11, cardiotrophin-1, and CLC *(7)*. LIF is known to bind to its transmembrane receptor, LIFR, which heterodimerizes with the signal transducing receptor gp130. The pluripotency of mES is dependent on the intracellular signaling events that follow, including phosphorylation by the Janus family of tyrosine kinases (JAK), which activates the signal transducer protein STAT3 *(8)*. The combination of IL-6 and soluble IL-6 receptor also interacts with and activates a homodimer of gp130 to maintain mES cells without involvement of LIFR *(9,10)*.

STAT3 activation is sufficient to maintain mES in the undifferentiated state and inhibition of the gp130-triggered mitogen-activated protein (MAP) kinase (Erk1/2) pathway enhances this effect *(8)*. Activation of Erk1/2, in turn, leads to the loss of pluripotency and onset of differentiation, such that a balance between these opposing signaling pathways determines the fate of the cells *(3,11)*. Recently, it was demonstrated that gp130 signaling has a physiologic role in the process of diapause that occurs naturally in lactating female mice. Mouse embryos arrest at the late blastocyst stage when implantation is prevented. *gp130-/-* embryos are unable to resume development after the end of diapause. The responsiveness of embryonic stem cells to gp130 signaling most likely has its origin in this reaction *(8)*. An interesting observation is that, although 129 strain mES cells respond to LIF, there are LIF-resistant clones from the 129 strain *(3,12)*, other murine ES cells *(3)*, and rat stem cells *(13)* that do not.

4. MAINTENANCE OF HUMAN ES CELLS

As with mES cells, human ES cells (hES) require mEFs to maintain pluripotency. Neither LIF nor IL-6 secreted by the mEFs are responsible for this effect because neither murine LIF nor murine IL-6 act on human receptors *(14,15)*. Additionally, human LIF was not sufficient to maintain hES cell lines in the undifferentiated state *(5,16,17)*. This is also the case with nonhuman primate ES cells *(4)*. One possible explanation of the inability of LIF to maintain pluripotency might relate to deficient cell surface expression of the appropriate cytokine receptors *(18)*. Although gp130 is known to be present on all cells in the body, the LIFR protein is not ubiquitously expressed *(19)*.

Recently, we have shown that STAT3 activation is not sufficient to block differentiation of the recently described hES cell line HSF6 *(20)* when grown on mouse feeder cells or when treated with conditioned media from mEF cells *(21)*. HSF6 cells differentiate in the presence of members of the IL-6 family of cytokines including LIF, IL-6, or in the presence of the designer cytokine hyper IL-6, a complex of soluble IL-6R and IL-6 with greatly enhanced bioactivity *(22)* that has recently been shown to block differentiation in mES cells *(23)* (Fig. 1). Human ES express LIF, IL-6, and gp130 receptors, as well as the downstream signaling molecules (Fig. 2). Undifferentiated mES cells were characterized by activated STAT3, but undifferentiated hES cells in the presence of mEF cells or their conditioned medium were not (Fig. 3). However, stimulation of both human and mES cells with gp130 cytokines resulted in a robust phosphorylation of downstream ERK1, ERK2, and the STAT3 transcription factor (Fig. 3). Loss of the pluripotency markers Nanog, Oct4, and TRA-1-60 was observed in hES cells during gp130-dependent signaling indicating that signaling through this pathway is insufficient to prevent the onset of differentiation (Fig. 4). These data underscore a fundamental difference in requirements of murine versus hES cells for maintenance of the pluripotent state. Furthermore, the data demonstrate the existence of an as-yet unidentified factor in the conditioned media of mouse feeder layer cells that acts in a STAT3-independent manner. Elucidating the molecular mechanisms involved will be necessary to be able to maintain self-renewal and control differentiation into particular cell lineages in human ES.

The inability of hES cells to maintain "stemness" in response to gp130-dependent JAK/STAT signaling is not exclusive to human cells. As described previously, the LIF-responsive clones from the 129 strain of mouse ES cells are themselves unique when compared with LIF-resistant clones from the 129 strain *(3,12)* and other murine ES cells *(3)*, rat stem cells *(13)*, and nonhuman primate ES cells *(4)*. Pluripotent human embryonic germ cells derived from the primordial gonadal ridge are partially dependent on LIF for their propagation; however, differentiated embryoid bodies are also formed and collected in the presence of

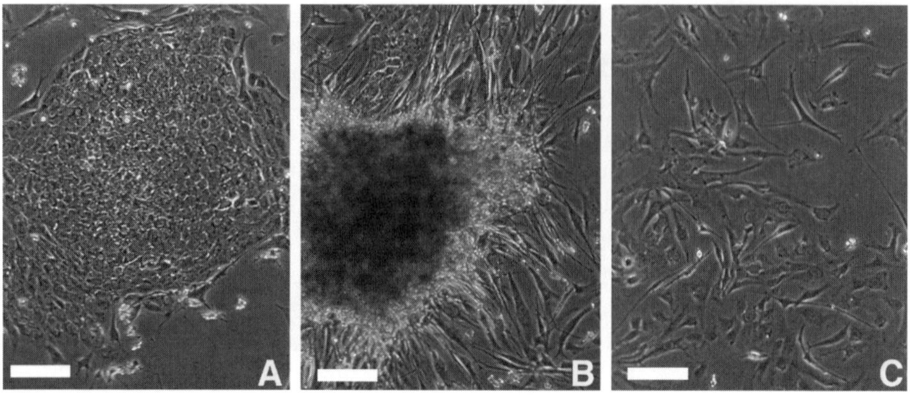

Fig. 1. Comparison of stem cell morphology cultured with conditioned medium from mouse fibroblast feeders (mEF) or in the presence of human leukemia inhibitory factor (hLIF). Phase contrast photomicrographs of HSF6 grown on laminin in the presence of conditioned medium from mEF **(A)**, after 3 days in the presence of hLIF **(B)**, and after 1 week in the presence of hLIF **(C)**. bar = 100 μ*M*. Note the change from a healthy, well defined colony of tightly packed cells in **(A)**, to a colony undergoing differentiation in **(B)**, and a monolayer of differentiated cells in **(C)**.

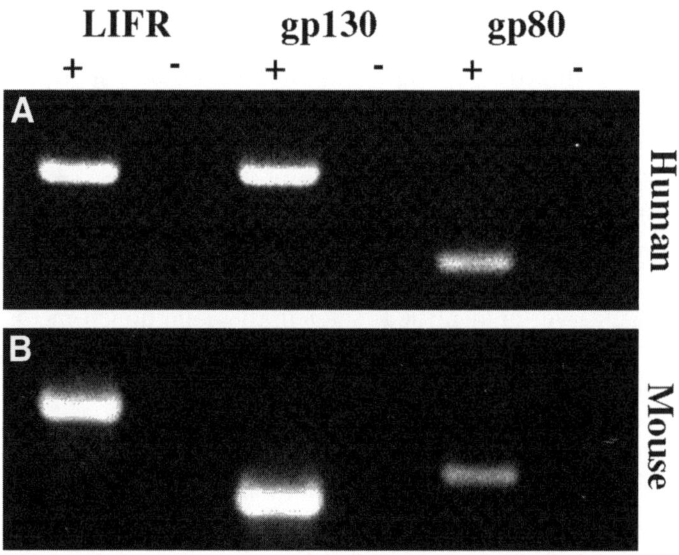

Fig. 2. Expression of leukemia inhibitory factor receptor (LIFR), gp130, and interleukin (IL)-6R (gp80) in human embryonic stem and mouse embryonic stem cells using reverse transcriptase-polymerase chain reaction **(A,B)**. LIFR and gp130 are expressed at high levels in the mouse and human cells **(A,B)**. IL-6 (gp80) is present at lower levels when compared with LIFR and gp130 expression in mouse and human cells **(A,B)**. (Reprinted with permission from AlphaMed Press.)

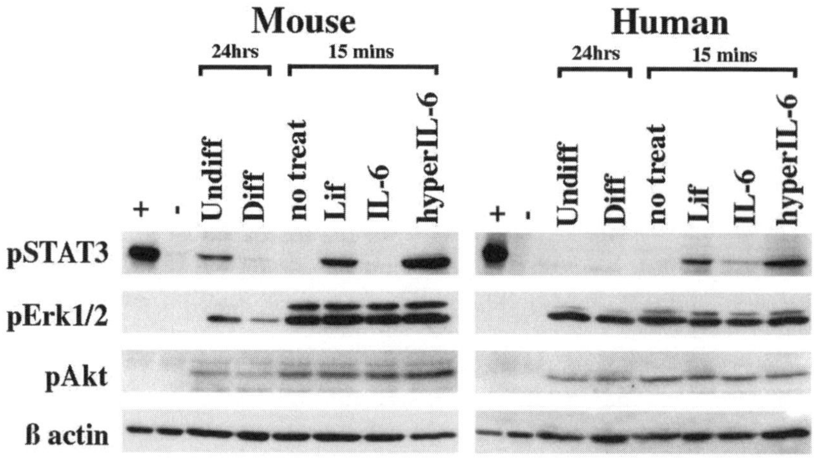

Fig. 3. Chronic and acute stimulation of gp130 signal transduction in mouse embryonic stem (mES) and human embryonic stem (hES) cells. pSTAT3 (Tyr705), pErk1/2 (Thr202/Tyr204), pAkt (Thr308), and β actin were detected on the same blot that contained positive and negative controls for pSTAT3 only. Acute treatment was performed on undifferentiated ES cells for 15 minutes and included no treat: ES cell media (mES: DMEM+FBS; hES: DSR+FGF); or either leukemia inhibitory factor (LIF), IL-6, or hyper IL-6–supplemented ES cell media. Chronic treatment was performed for 24 hours and included: Undiff, undifferentiated mouse and human cells stimulated with ES cell media supplemented with LIF or CM, respectively; or Diff, mouse and human cells stimulated with their respective ES cell media. Western blots are representative of three separate experiments done in duplicate. (Reprinted with permission from AlphaMed Press.)

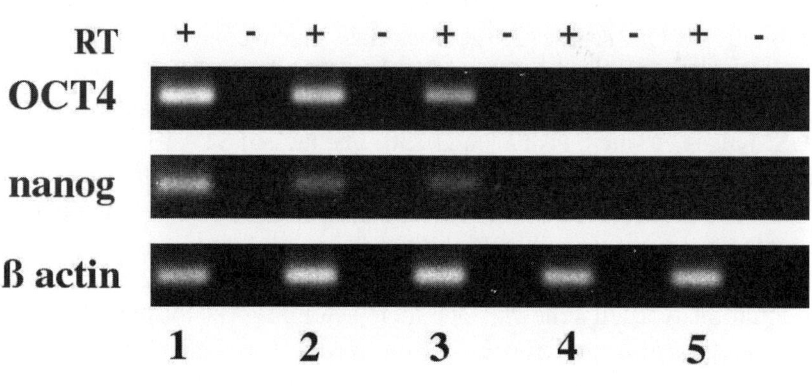

Fig. 4. Semiquantitative reverse transcriptase-polymerase chain reaction of human embryonic stem cells for Oct-4 and Nanog cultured in the presence of conditioned media (lane 1), without culture medium (CM) (lanes 2, 4), or hyper IL-6 (lanes 3, 5). Cells were maintained in CM for 2 weeks in parallel with cells grown without CM or in hyper IL-6. Samples grown without CM or treated with hyper IL-6 cells were collected at 1 week (lanes 2, 3) and at 2 weeks (lanes 4, 5). Both Nanog and Oct-4 expression decreased after 1 week both in the absence of CM and in the presence of hyper IL-6, and was absent at 2 weeks (lanes 4, 5). (Reprinted with permission from AlphaMed Press.)

LIF *(6)*. The inability of LIF to maintain the undifferentiated phenotype has also been observed in the human embryonic carcinoma cell line Ntera/D1, even though all receptor components were expressed *(24)*. In contrast to the hES cells, LIF did not activate STAT3 in the human embryonic carcinoma cells, possibly because of the constitutive expression of the negative feedback protein suppressor of cytokine signaling-1. This suggests that if gp130-dependent signaling could promote hES cell "stemness," the pathway is blocked downstream of STAT3 activation.

This fundamental difference in the maintenance of pluripotency may represent a difference in the developmental stage of each of the stem cell lines. Certainly, gp130 signaling is required for implantation in the mouse because female *Lif* mutants are infertile resulting from implantation failure *(25)*. However, loss of pluripotency is not observed in either *Lif* mutants, which survive into adulthood, or *Lifr* mutants, which die close to parturition because of deficits in the cells derived form the neurectoderm *(26,27)* and *gp130* mutants, which die in mid- to late gestation because of placental, cardiac, hematopoietic, and neuronal malformations *(28,29)*. In the discussion of pluripotency in mES cells, we alluded to the fact that gp130 signaling maintains the preimplantation blastocyst during diapause, a situation in which implantation is delayed because of the physiologic state of the mother, and that the blastocyst remains viable in the uterus for several weeks *(8)*. It is possible that LIF-responsive ES cells resemble the developmental stage at which the late blastocyst enters diapause; ES cells derived from earlier or later stages may not require gp130 signaling for self-renewal.

The factor that is secreted from the mEFs and stimulates hES cell pluripotency remains elusive. One article *(21)* demonstrates that in contrast to mES cells LIF, IL-6, or IL-6 in the presence of soluble IL-6R-induced STAT3 activation via gp130 does not contribute to pluripotency. Other gp130 cytokines such as IL-11 and OSM also activate STAT3 via gp130. The lack of STAT3 activation in the undifferentiated hES cells suggests that, in contrast to mES cells, gp130 activation is not involved in inhibiting differentiation of hES cells. It is likely that not one single ligand is responsible for the maintenance of "stemness," and this may involve the interaction of several signaling events that influence the balance of differentiation over self-renewal. One such factor might be the partially purified, soluble, secreted molecule from a differentiated, LIF-deficient parietal endodermal cell line that supports stem cell pluripotency without STAT3 activation *(3,12)*.

Recent studies show that the newly described gene Nanog, coding for a homeobox protein promoting mES cell renewal, pluripotency, and epiblast formation, may play a leading role in "stemness" *(30,31)*. Nanog is crucial for preimplantation, and although Oct-4 is not required for Nanog expression, Nanog cannot act in its absence. Parallel pathways between Oct-4, Nanog, and STAT3 have been suggested in mES cells; however, Oct-4 and Nanog are obligatory and can maintain pluripotency in the absence and independently of STAT3 activation *(3,30–32)*. Indeed, Nanog expression in the undifferentiated hES cells has been demonstrated *(21)* and progressive loss of nanog on differentiation is also observed in conjunction with the loss of Oct-4. Of particular interest is that Nanog and Oct-4 are expressed in the undifferentiated hES cell in the absence of STAT3 activation. Nanog and Oct-4 expression also occurred in the presence of augmented levels of STAT3 activation. Therefore, the STAT3-independent mechanism for stemness observed in the hES cells may also be a parallel pathway to the well described and possibly redundant STAT3 pathway in mES cells.

One immediate consequence of these findings is to define the STAT3-independent pathway triggered by the contact of hES cells to murine feeder layers or by a soluble factor present in the conditioned media. It can be anticipated that this new pathway will act to activate the transcription factors Oct-4 and Nanog. The molecular definition of stimulators of this new pathway will be extremely helpful in the elucidation of optimal culture conditions for primate and nonprimate ES cells. One such mechanism might be activation of the canonical wnt pathway by as-yet undefined factors secreted by mEFs. It has recently been shown that pluripotency of both murine and hES can be maintained by transient activation of the wnt pathway using a synthetic pharmacologic inactivator of GSK-3, allowing nuclear accumulation of β-catenin and activation of transcription of wnt target genes *(17)*.

5. HUMAN STEM CELLS ARE DIFFERENT FROM EACH OTHER

Although the hES cell lines available through the National Institutes of Health Stem Cell Registry are considered similar, being derived from a 3- to 5-day-old blastocysts, and based on the presence of the stem cell markers, SSEA-4, TRA-1-60, TRA-1-81, Oct-4, and alkaline phosphatase, comparisons have been difficult because, until recently, cell lines from different sources were not studied simultaneously in the same laboratory under the same conditions. It is now becoming apparent that these cell lines exhibit different characteristics from each other. We have studied two such lines, hES3 from ESI International, and HSF6, from the University of California San Francisco. Both cell lines meet the criteria for the use of human embryonic stem cells by federally funded researchers (i.e., they were derived before August 9, 2001 and exhibit all the markers described previously; however, their growth characteristics are very different).

5.1. Growth Conditions

Both cell lines require the presence of mouse feeder layers for proliferation and maintenance of the undifferentiated state. The optimum medium for both is

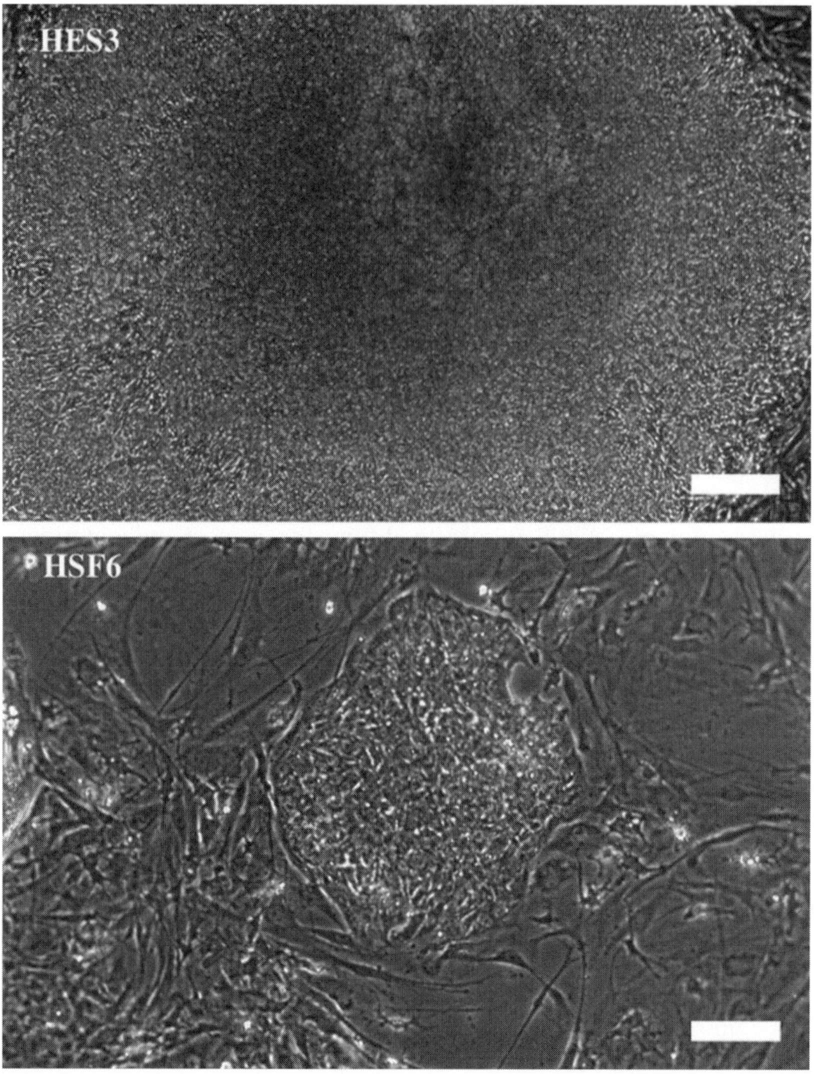

Fig. 5. Comparison of morphology of HES3 and HSF6 stem cell colonies. Phase contrast photomicrographs of HES3 and HSF6 growing on mouse fibroblast feeder layers. Note tightness of colony of HES3 and area of differentiation in the center of the colony. Bar =100 μ*M*.

Dulbecco's modified Eagle's medium, but hES3 requires the addition of fetal bovine serum (FBS) and ITS supplement, whereas HSF6 requires knockout serum replacer and fibroblast growth factor (FGF)2. Morphologically, the cells look very different from each other (Fig. 5). hES3 tends to differentiate spontaneously more easily than HSF6 and grow as three-dimensional colonies on top of the feeder layer that have a central "button" of differentiating cells. HSF6 colonies, on the other hand, are flatter and tend to push out the feeder layers as they proliferate. For undifferentiated self-renewal of HSF6, mouse feeder layers may be replaced by plating the cells on laminin and culturing in conditioned medium from the feeders containing basic FGF2 *(21)*, as has been described for other human stem cell lines *(17,33)*. However the same culture conditions used with hES3 were not successful in our hands or others *(34)*.

5.2. Propagation

Because hES3 is in a continuous state of differentiation, care must be taken when transferring it to a new dish to remove only the undifferentiated areas of the colonies. This is best achieved by cutting the colonies into pieces with a cutting pipette under direct vision using a stereoscope, and removing only the undifferentiated areas. Optimal size of colonies before transfer is 1.5–2 mm diameter. HSF6 are easier to propagate because they do not differentiate as readily and colonies grow in a more uniform condition. Optimal size of colonies at transfer is smaller—less than 500 μ*M* diameter—and collagenase or EGTA-trypsin solution can be used to gently dislodge small clusters of cells from the feeder layers.

5.3. Cryopreservation

Cryopreservation protocols that allow maximal recovery and preservation of stem cell properties of proliferation and pluripotency are an important part of maintenance of stem cells. For hES3 cells, ESI International recommends a procedure that was originally used for cryopreserving embryos *(35)* that uses a combination of dimethyl sulfoxide (DMSO), ethylene glycol, and sucrose in vitrification straws rather than cryovials. This is a tedious process that is very difficult to scale up, because only three or four pieces of a colony can be vitrified at one time. The protocol recommended for HSF6 uses a standard procedure of slow freezing in cryovials in a medium containing 10% DMSO, 90% FBS. We have previously developed a method to cryopreserve islets with excellent survival of endocrine cells. This method involves introducing both DMSO and the disaccharide trehalose into the cells during a controlled cooling process *(36)*. Because trehalose had been used successfully to preserve oocytes *(37)*, we compared all three methods for efficacy of cryopreserving human ES.

Although thawed cells from all three methods showed no difference in level of spontaneous differentiation or ability to form teratomas after transplantation in nude mice, indicating pluripotency was not lost, there were major differences in yields. We found the vitrification method to be unsuitable, both in terms of efficacy and in difficulties in scale-up. For cryopreservation of hES3, the trehalose solution was most efficient, with statistically higher levels of recovery than

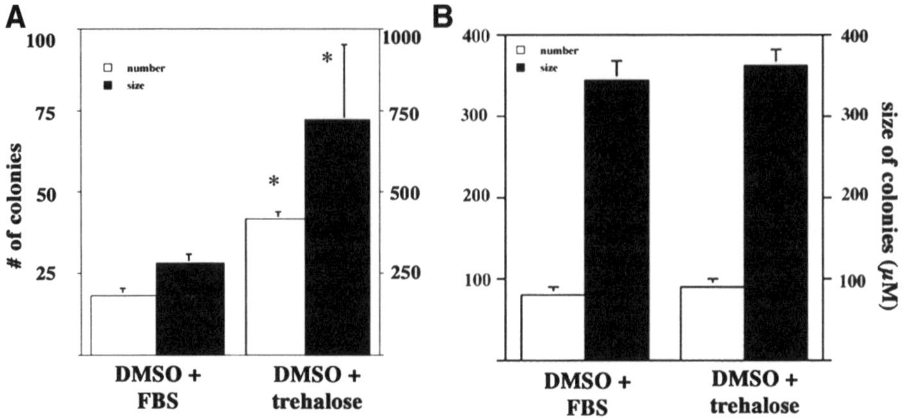

Fig. 6. Representative experiment of comparison of yields from cryopreservation protocols. Analysis of number and size of HES3 (**A**) and HSF6 (**B**) colonies after cryopreservation by two different methods. Embryonic stem cells were thawed and cultured for 1 week, then assayed for number and size of colonies. $*p < 0.05$ compared with treatment with dimethyl sulfoxide fetal bovine serum.

the FBS (Fig. 6A). However, yield of HSF6 cells after thawing was always higher than that for hES3, and the recovery was similar using either trehalose or FBS (Fig. 6B), again demonstrating an underlying difference between the two cell lines.

The reasons for this discrepancy are unknown but may relate to the differences in growth characteristics. hES3 colonies are much more compact, with cells very close together (*see* Fig. 5) and they survive better when transferred in discrete "chunks" rather than in loose cell clusters. Because hES3 remain in larger tighter clusters than HSF6 during the cryoprotection process, it is necessary to get the cryoprotectant medium into the cells inside the clusters. The trehalose strategy used here allows the cells to become transiently porous by exposing them to a thermotropic lipid-phase transition with a high concentration of trehalose outside the cells during the cooling process, enabling the cryoprotectant to enter the cells efficiently, thus stabilizing the cell membranes from the inside. This method facilitates transfer of the cryoprotectant medium into the cells inside the clusters, as well as on the periphery, as we have described for human adult pancreatic islets and fetal islet-like cell clusters *(36)*.

From the discussions here, it is evident that there are no uniform culture conditions for ES cells and that different conditions may lead to different morphologies and phenotypes. It follows that not only the mechanism for self-renewal may be different for each cell type, but also the ability to differentiate into certain cell lineages.

6. ES CELLS AND DIABETES

Islet transplantation as a procedure to induce insulin independence is still a long way from benefiting the population of more than 1 million type 1 diabetic patients in the United States. In addition to the problems involved with immune suppression, a remaining, significant obstacle is the scarcity of human organs for transplantation. For the last 5 years the number of donated pancreases (approximately 6000 per year) has changed little, and of those, only 50% could be expected to produce islet yields suitable for clinical purposes. Also, most transplant recipients require two or more organs to obtain a sufficient islet mass for insulin independence.

Alternative sources of β cells are necessary for endocrine replacement if diabetes is to be a target for cell-based insulin therapies. Potential endocrine replacements from human tissue include adult β cells expanded with growth factors and extracellular matrix components *(38,39)*, putative endocrine precursors from adult pancreases such as ductal cells *(40)*, and fetal pancreatic progenitor cells *(41)*. All of these, however, have limited growth potential. Genetically modified β cells containing transduced oncogenes can be expanded indefinitely, but in addition to their abnormal karyotype, problems with stability and functionality remain a problem *(42)*. An ideal cell replacement for insulin deficient states would be one that has the following properties: unlimited supply, normal karyotype, and functionality of the mature β cell. Embryonic stem cells fulfill the first two criteria, and possibly the third, if they can be induced to differentiate efficiently into mature β cells and release insulin appropriately in response to glucose.

7. ENDOCRINE DIFFERENTIATION OF mES

Induction of endocrine differentiation in rodent ES or progenitor cells has been attempted with varying results. Using mES cells, Lumelsky and colleagues have been able to induce insulin-containing cells using an experimental strategy of stepwise selection through changes in culture conditions *(43)*. The levels of insulin may be increased by using growth inhibitors such as phosphatidylinositol 3-kinase inhibitors *(44)*. However, a recent report questions whether the insulin is actually produced by the stem cells or instead passively transferred from the high insulin content of the medium *(45)*. Soria and his group have obtained an insulin-secreting cell clone from undifferentiated mES cells using a cell trap model to select β-cell precursors, which were subsequently able to secrete insulin in response to glucose in vitro and in vivo *(46)*. After growth and differentiation in nonselective media containing serum, murine ES cells spontaneously differentiated into cells individually expressing each of the four major islet hormones in a study recently reported by Kahan and colleagues.

8. ENDOCRINE DIFFERENTIATION IN HUMAN ES CELLS

Even under the best circumstances of hES culture on mEF, spontaneous differentiation into various cell types occurs, with the default pathway being neurons *(16)*. Only 1–3% of spontaneously differentiated hES cells contain insulin, and, unlike mature β cells, these cells have not been shown to response to glucose *(48)*.

At this time, our laboratory has had little success in replicating the endocrine induction experiments described previously for mES cells. Using the hES cell lines hES3 and HSF6, we have investigated the ability to induce β-cell differentiation using the protocols of selective media with or without growth factor inhibitor used by Lumelsky *(43)* and Hori *(44)* and the nonselective medium used by Kahan *(47)*. Our results show that we were only able to detect immunoreactive C-peptide or PDX-1 in a few (<5%) hES3 cells that had been cultured through the selective media and then exposed to the PI-3 kinase inhibitor. However, the small number of positive cells was no more than hES3 seen differentiating spontaneously into insulin positive cells *(16)*. Analysis by reverse transcriptase-polymerase chain reaction of HSF6 cells treated with selective media showed induction of message for neuroD, and HNF6 (markers of both neuronal and pancreatic endocrine lineage), but no message for PDX-1 or insulin (Fig. 7). Cell clusters stained variously for nestin, neuron-specific β tubulin, vimentin, or pan cytokeratin, indicating mesoderm, endoderm, and ectoderm cell types, were all present. Using the nonselective media, we again saw no evidence of induction of PDX1 or insulin, although transcripts of HNF6 and neuroD were observed. Again, we detected endodermal, ectodermal, and mesodermal cells by immunostaining. Thus, as we have seen for maintenance of stemness, it is apparent that protocols devised for induction of specific differentiation of mouse stem cells may also not be applicable for human cells.

9. FUTURE DIRECTIONS FOR ENDOCRINE INDUCTION

It is not yet known whether any of these methods will eventually be successful with hES cells, but for clinical applications, one of the most significant steps will be the ability to generate pure populations of β cells from hES cells. Separation of β cells from heterogeneous hES cell populations by flow cytometry based on cell surface molecules is one option, but is unlikely to be feasible because hES cells need to be in clusters and do not survive well as single cells *(16)*. Our hypothesis is that generation of pure populations of β cells will require a multistep protocol, involving induction of endoderm followed by selection of endocrine progenitors and culminating in differentiation into mature β cells. This outcome could be achieved by one or more of the following strategies: (1) appropriate use of growth factors and extracellular matrices; (2) selection of endocrine

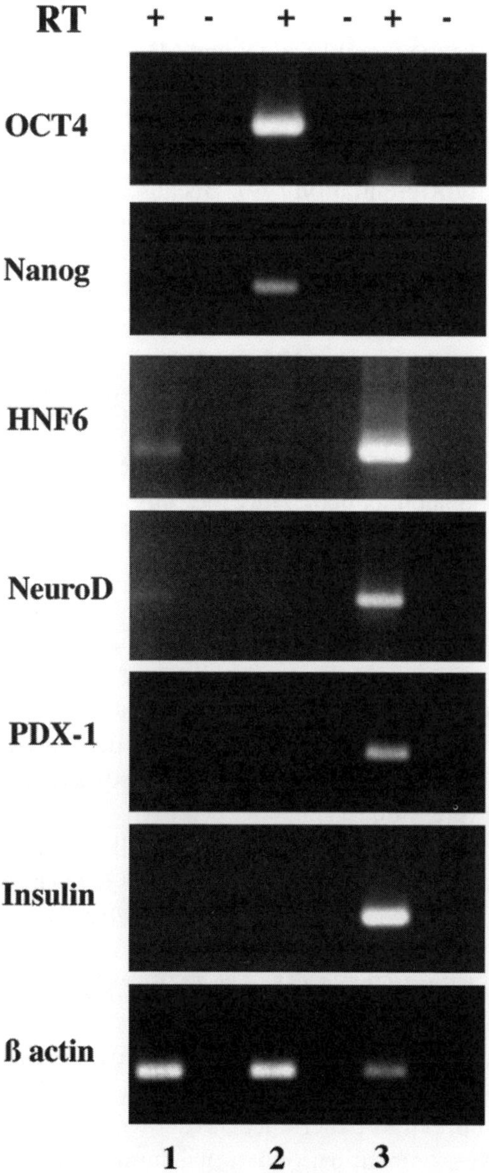

Fig. 7. Semiquantitative reverse transcriptase-polymerase chain reaction of HFS6 cells cultured in the presence of differentiation medium containing phosphatidylinositol 3-kinase inhibitor used by Hori for differentiation of mouse embryonic stem cells (mEF) *(44)* (lane 1), mEF-conditioned media (lane 2), and, for comparison, adult islets (lane 3). Note disappearance of stem cell markers OCT4 and Nanog in human embryonic stem cells in differentiation medium with concomitant appearance of HNF6 and neuroD, but no message for PDX-1 or insulin.

precursors using, for example, cell traps; (3) forced expression of transcription factors necessary for the β cell lineage; and (4) in vivo growth to complete the differentiation process.

Schuldiner and colleagues have examined the effects of several growth factors on in vitro differentiation of hES cells and shown that only two (HGF and NGF) induce endodermal differentiation *(49)*. Because pancreatic tissue arises from the endoderm, treatment with these growth factors could initiate the first step in the differentiation pathway toward β cells. Endodermal lineage could also be induced by transducing transcription factors known to be involved in endodermal differentiation in mammals, such as Gata4 or Gata6 *(50)* .

After endodermal lineage has been induced, endocrine precursors may be further selected on the basis of promoter activity using targeted antibiotic protection and gene traps. This could be achieved by infection of the endodermal cells with viruses containing β-cell, gene-specific promoters driving an antibiotic resistance gene such as neo. Thus the only cells surviving culture in the presence of the antibiotic would be cells expressing the β-cell gene of interest, resulting in a pure population of β-cell precursors. These genes could be promoters for transcription factors present during early stages of β-cell differentiation such as neurogenin 3, PDX-1, or β1/neuroD *(51–53)*. Another alternative would be to force the expression of relevant β-cell transcription factors in endodermal cells by introducing the gene of interest, rather than its promoter, and again use antibiotic selection to obtain a more homogeneous population. This approach has been used successfully by Blyszczuk, who overexpressed PAX4 in mES cells, inducing insulin expression *(54)*.

Extensive genomic and proteomic analysis will be necessary on these transduced lines to ensure that their genetic integrity has not been compromised. After cells containing β cell-specific genes have been selected, further differentiation could be initiated with growth factors or matrices known to induce β-cell maturation, such as exendin-4/GLP-1 *(55–57)*, FGF4 *(58)*, nicotinamide *(59)*, HGF/SF *(19,60)*, or activin A/β-cellulin *(61)*.

Both mES cells and rat fetal pancreatic cells have the ability to become fully mature β cells in vitro *(62,63)*, releasing insulin appropriately in response to glucose. However, previous experience has shown that although it is possible to induce β-cell markers or insulin production in human fetal pancreatic precursors in vitro, these cells are glucose insensitive; the in vivo environment is necessary to achieve glucose responsive insulin release *(57,64)*. The same in vivo signals may be needed for full maturation of hES derived β cells. Clinical application may require some time after transplantation before the cells become responsive to glucose. In vivo treatment with β-cell growth factors such as KGF may also be necessary *(65)*.

10. CONCLUSION

Current culture conditions for ES cells eventually lead to diverse phenotypes with significant intraspecies heterogeneity. Different phenotypes emerge in response to minimal variations in the culture conditions used in different laboratories, reflecting signaling from cell to cell and cell to matrix contacts, as well as from extracellular messages provided by medium or other cells in coculture. Much has been written about the importance of transcriptional profiling to explain the molecular basis of pluripotency in ES cells *(3,66–70)*. These efforts, mainly expended in deriving gene lists to account for "stemness" using microarrays, are a beginning. However, so far the concordance between mouse and human, and even human to human data sets is very low, questioning the validity of such profiling without a uniform initial cell platform on which further developmental steps can be validated biologically. For the field to progress, emphasis should be placed on in vitro and in vivo assay of function of specific gene products and stringent comparison of data from similar cell lines grown in different laboratories under differing conditions. Notwithstanding the inherent difficulties in maintaining stem cells in the laboratory, they are a unique research tool for studying cellular development, and provide a potential cell-based therapy for human diseases such as diabetes.

ACKNOWLEDGMENTS

The authors of this article were supported by a grant from the Larry L. Hillblom Foundation.

REFERENCES

1. Evans MJ, Kaufman MH. Establishment in culture of pluripotential cells from mouse embryos. Nature 1981;292:154–156.
2. Martin GR. Isolation of a pluripotent cell line from early mouse embryos cultured in medium conditioned by teratocarcinoma stem cells. Proc Natl Acad Sci U S A 1981;78:7634–7638.
3. Smith AG. Embryo-derived stem cells: of mice and men. Annu Rev Cell Dev Biol 2001;17:435–462.
4. Thomson JA, Kalishman J, Golos TG, et al. Isolation of a primate embryonic stem cell line. Proc Natl Acad Sci U S A 1995;92:7844–7848.
5. Thomson JA, Itskovitz-Eldor J, Shapiro SS, et al. Embryonic stem cell lines derived from human blastocysts. Science 1998;282:1145–1147.
6. Shamblott MJ, Axelman J, Wang S, et al. Derivation of pluripotent stem cells from cultured human primordial germ cells. Proc Natl Acad Sci U S A 1998;95:13726–13731.
7. Heinrich PC, Behrmann I, Haan S, Hermanns HM, Muller-Newen G, Schaper F. Principles of interleukin (IL)-6-type cytokine signalling and its regulation. Biochem J 2003;374:1–20.
8. Nichols J, Chambers I, Taga T, Smith A. Physiological rationale for responsiveness of mouse embryonic stem cells to gp130 cytokines. Development 2001;128:2333–2339.

9. Herrera P-L, Huarte J, Zufferey R, et al. Ablation of islet endocrine cells by targeted expression of hormone-promoter-driven toxigenes. Proc Natl Acad Sci U S A 1994;91:12999–13003.
10. Yoshida K, Chambers I, Nichols J, et al. Maintenance of the pluripotential phenotype of embryonic stem cells through direct activation of gp130 signalling pathways. Mech Dev 1994;45:163–171.
11. Burdon T, Smith A, Savatier P. Signalling, cell cycle and pluripotency in embryonic stem cells. Trends Cell Biol 2002;12:432–438.
12. Dani C, Chambers I, Johnstone S, et al. Paracrine induction of stem cell renewal by LIF-deficient cells: a new ES cell regulatory pathway. Dev Biol 1998;203:149–162.
13. Vassilieva S, Guan K, Pich U, Wobus AM. Establishment of SSEA-1- and Oct-4-expressing rat embryonic stem-like cell lines and effects of cytokines of the IL-6 family on clonal growth. Exp Cell Res 2000;258:361–373.
14. Van Snick J. Interleukin-6: an overview. Annu Rev Immunol 1990;8:253–278.
15. Owczarek CM, Layton MJ, Metcalf D, et al. Inter-species chimeras of leukaemia inhibitory factor define a major human receptor-binding determinant. EMBO J 1993;12:3487–3495.
16. Reubinoff BE, Pera MF, Fong CY, Trounson A, Bongso A. Embryonic stem cell lines from human blastocysts: somatic differentiation in vitro. Nat Biotechnol 2000;18:399–404.
17. Sato N, Meijer L, Skaltsounis L, Greengard P, Brivanlou AH. Maintenance of pluripotency in human and mouse embryonic stem cells through activation of Wnt signaling by a pharmacological GSK-3-specific inhibitor. Nat Med 2004;10:55–63.
18. Rose-John S. GP130 stimulation and the maintenance of stem cells. Trends Biotechnol 2002;20:417.
19. Taga T, Kishimoto T. Gp130 and the interleukin-6 family of cytokines. Annu Rev Immunol 1997;15:797–819.
20. Abeyta MJ, Clark AT, Rodriguez RT, Bodnar MS, Pera RA, Firpo MT. Unique gene expression signatures of independently-derived human embryonic stem cell lines. Hum Mol Genet 2004;13:601–608.
21. Humphrey R, Beattie GM, Lopez AD, King CC, Bucay N, Hayek A. Maintenance of pluripotency in human embryonic stem cells is STAT3 independent. Stem Cells 2004;22:522–530.
22. Fischer M, Goldschmitt J, Peschel C, et al. I. A bioactive designer cytokine for human hematopoietic progenitor cell expansion. Nat Biotechnol 1997;15:142–145.
23. Viswanathan S, Benatar T, Rose-John S, Lauffenburger DA, Zandstra PW. Ligand/receptor signaling threshold (LIST) model accounts for gp130-mediated embryonic stem cell self-renewal responses to LIF and HIL-6. Stem Cells 2002;20:119–138.
24. Schuringa JJ, van der Schaaf S, Vellenga E, Eggen BJ, Kruijer W. LIF-induced STAT3 signaling in murine versus human embryonal carcinoma (EC) cells. Exp Cell Res 2002;274: 119–129.
25. Stewart CL, Kaspar P, Brunet LJ, et al. Blastocyst implantation depends on maternal expression of leukaemia inhibitory factor. Nature 1992;359:76–79.
26. Li M, Sendtner M, Smith A. Essential function of LIF receptor in motor neurons. Nature 1995;378:724–727.
27. Ware CB, Horowitz MC, Renshaw BR, et al. Targeted disruption of the low-affinity leukemia inhibitory factor receptor gene causes placental, skeletal, neural and metabolic defects and results in perinatal death. Development 1995;121:1283–1299.
28. Yoshida K, Taga T, Saito M, et al. Targeted disruption of gp130, a common signal transducer for the interleukin 6 family of cytokines, leads to myocardial and hematological disorders. Proc Natl Acad Sci U S A 1996;93:407–411.

29. Nakashima K, Wiese S, Yanagisawa M, et al. Developmental requirement of gp130 signaling in neuronal survival and astrocyte differentiation. J Neurosci 1999;19:5429–5434.
30. Chambers I, Colby D, Robertson M, et al. Functional expression cloning of Nanog, a pluripotency sustaining factor in embryonic stem cells. Cell 2003;113:643–655.
31. Mitsui K, Tokuzawa Y, Itoh H, et al. The homeoprotein Nanog is required for maintenance of pluripotency in mouse epiblast and ES cells. Cell 2003;113:631–642.
32. Constantinescu S. Stemness, fusion and renewal of hematopoietic and embryonic stem cells. J Cell Mol Med 2003;7:103–112.
33. Xu C, Inokuma MS, Denham J, et al. Feeder-free growth of undifferentiated human embryonic stem cells. Nat Biotechnol 2001;19:971–4.
34. Richards M, Fong CY, Chan WK, Wong PC, Bongso A. Human feeders support prolonged undifferentiated growth of human inner cell masses and embryonic stem cells. Nat Biotechnol 2002;20:933–936.
35. Vajta G, Holm P, Kuwayama M, et al. Open Pulled Straw (OPS) vitrification: a new way to reduce cryoinjuries of bovine ova and embryos. Mol Reprod Dev 1998;51:53–58.
36. Beattie GM, Crowe JH, Lopez AD, Cirulli V, Ricordi C, Hayek A. Trehalose: a cryoprotectant that enhances recovery and preserves function of human pancreatic islets after long-term storage. Diabetes 1997;46:519–523.
37. Al-aghbari AM, Menino AR. Survival of oocytes recovered from vitrified sheep ovarian tissues. Anim Reprod Sci 2002;71:101–110.
38. Hayek A, Beattie GM, Cirulli V, Lopez AD, Ricordi C, Rubin JS. Growth factor/matrix-induced proliferation of human adult beta-cells. Diabetes 1995;44:1458–1460.
39. Beattie GM, Montgomery AM, Lopez AD, et al. A novel approach to increase human islet cell mass while preserving beta-cell function. Diabetes 2002;51:3435–3439.
40. Bonner-Weir S, Taneja M, Weir GC, et al. In vitro cultivation of human islets from expanded ductal tissue. Proc Natl Acad Sci U S A 2000;97:7999–8004.
41. Hayek A, Beattie GM. Processing, storage and experimental transplantation of human fetal pancreatic cells. Ann Transplant 1997;2:46–54.
42. Dufayet De La Tour D, Halvorsen T, Demeterco C, et al. beta-Cell differentiation from a human pancreatic cell line in vitro and in vivo. Mol Endocrinol 2001;15:476–483.
43. Lumelsky N, Blondel O, Laeng P, Velasco I, Ravin R, McKay R. Differentiation of embryonic stem cells to insulin-secreting structures similar to pancreatic islets. Science 2001;292: 1389–1394.
44. Hori Y, Rulifson IC, Tsai BC, Heit JJ, Cahoy JD, Kim SK. Growth inhibitors promote differentiation of insulin-producing tissue from embryonic stem cells. Proc Natl Acad Sci U S A 2002;99:16105–16110.
45. Rajagopal J, Anderson WJ, Kume S, Martinez OI, Melton DA. Insulin staining of ES cell progeny from insulin uptake. Science 2003;299:363.
46. Soria B, Roche E, Berna G, Leon-Quinto T, Reig JA, Martin F. Insulin-secreting cells derived from embryonic stem cells normalize glycemia in streptozotocin-induced diabetic mice. Diabetes 2000;49:157–162.
47. Kahan BW, Jacobson LM, Hullett DA, et al. Pancreatic precursors and differentiated islet cell types from murine embryonic stem cells: an in vitro model to study islet differentiation. Diabetes 2003;52:2016–2024.
48. Assady S, Maor G, Amit M, Itskovitz-Eldor J, Skorecki KL, Tzukerman M. Insulin production by human embryonic stem cells. Diabetes 2001;50:1691–1697.

49. Schuldiner M, Yanuka O, Itskovitz-Eldor J, Melton DA, Benvenisty N. From the cover: effects of eight growth factors on the differentiation of cells derived from human embryonic stem cells. Proc Natl Acad Sci U S A 2000;97:11307–11312.
50. Fujikura J, Yamato E, Yonemura S, et al. Differentiation of embryonic stem cells is induced by GATA factors Genes Dev 2002;16:784–789.
51. Gu G, Dubauskaite J, Melton DA. Direct evidence for the pancreatic lineage: NGN3+ cells are islet progenitors and are distinct from duct progenitors. Development 2002;129:2447–2457.
52. Edlund H. Developmental biology of the pancreas. Diabetes 2001;50(Suppl. 1):S5–S9.
53. German M, Aschroft S, Docherty K, et al. The insulin gene promoter. A simplified nomenclature. Diabetes 1995;44:1002–1004.
54. Blyszczuk P, Czyz J, Kania G, et al. Expression of Pax4 in embryonic stem cells promotes differentiation of nestin-positive progenitor and insulin-producing cells. Proc Natl Acad Sci U S A 2003;100:998–1003.
55. Hui H, Wright C, Perfetti R. Glucagon-like peptide 1 induces differentiation of islet duodenal homeobox-1-positive pancreatic ductal cells into insulin-secreting cells. Diabetes 2001;50: 785–796.
56. Stoffers DA, Kieffer TJ, Hussain MA, et al. Insulinotropic glucagon-like peptide 1 agonists stimulate expression of homeodomain protein IDX-1 and increase islet size in mouse pancreas. Diabetes 2000;49:741–748.
57. Movassat J, Beattie GM, Lopez AD, Hayek A. Exendin 4 up-regulates expression of PDX 1 and hastens differentiation and maturation of human fetal pancreatic cells. J Clin Endocrinol Metab 2002;87:4775–4781.
58. Wells JM, Melton DA. Early mouse endoderm is patterned by soluble factors from adjacent germ layers. Development 2000;127:1563–1572.
59. Otonkoski T, Beattie GM, Mally MI, Ricordi C, Hayek A. Nicotinamide is a potent inducer of endocrine differentiation in cultured human fetal pancreatic cells. J Clin Invest 1993;92:1459–1466.
60. Otonkoski T, Beattie GM, Rubin JS, Lopez AD, Baird A, Hayek A. Hepatocyte growth factor/scatter factor has insulinotropic activity in human fetal pancreatic cells. Diabetes 1994;43:947–953.
61. Demeterco C, Beattie GM, Dib SA, Lopez AD, Hayek A. A role for activin A and betacellulin in human fetal pancreatic cell differentiation and growth. J Clin Endocrinol Metab 2000;85:3892–3897.
62. Soria B. In-vitro differentiation of pancreatic beta-cells. Differentiation 2001;68:205–219.
63. Hellerstrom C, Swenne I. Functional maturation and proliferation of fetal pancreatic b-cells. Diabetes 1991;40:89–93.
64. Hayek A, Beattie GM. Experimental transplantation of human fetal and adult pancreatic islets. J Clin Endocrinol Metab 1997;82:2471–2475.
65. Movassat J, Beattie GM, Lopez AD, Portha B, Hayek A. Keratinocyte growth factor and beta-cell differentiation in human fetal pancreatic endocrine precursor cells. Diabetologia 2003;46:822–829.
66. Ivanova NB, Dimos JT, Schaniel C, Hackney JA, Moore KA, Lemischka IR. A stem cell molecular signature. Science 2002;298:601–604.
67. Ramalho-Santos M, Yoon S, Matsuzaki Y, Mulligan RC, Melton DA. "Stemness": transcriptional profiling of embryonic and adult stem cells. Science 2002;298:597–600.
68. Fortunel NO, Otu HH, Ng HH, et al. Comment on " 'Stemness': transcriptional profiling of embryonic and adult stem cells" and "a stem cell molecular signature". Science 2003;302:393; author reply 393.

69. Sato N, Sanjuan IM, Heke M, Uchida M, Naef F, Brivanlou AH. Molecular signature of human embryonic stem cells and its comparison with the mouse. Dev Biol 2003;260:404–413.
70. Sperger JM, Chen X, Draper JS, et al. Gene expression patterns in human embryonic stem cells and human pluripotent germ cell tumors. Proc Natl Acad Sci U S A 12003;00:13350–13355.

II Translational Research

6 Islet Precursor Cells in Adult Pancreatic Islets

Gladys Teitelman and Irem Nasir

CONTENTS

1. INTRODUCTION

The search for new sources of β cells is driven by the shortage of islets of Langerhans suitable for replacement therapy for type I diabetes. Recent advances in stem cell research, described in other sections of this book, have led to promising sources of insulin-producing cells *(1–5)*. In addition, significant progress in the elucidation of the molecular program that guides the differentiation of islet cells during development *(6–22)* will certainly provide tools to expand the population of embryonic β-precursor cells and promote their differentiation into mature, insulin-producing cells. The adult pancreas is another potential source of β-precursor cells. The existence of islet progenitor cells in mature pancreas can be inferred from the fact that new islets are normally formed during postnatal life *(23,24)* and that a dramatic increase in islet number occurs in response to various stimuli *(25–27)*. The presence of "endocrine stem/progenitor cells" could not only provide a source of cells suitable for transplantation, but also could replenish the β-cell population that has been depleted by injury or disease.

From: *Contemporary Endocrinology: Stem Cells in Endocrinology*
Edited by: L. B. Lester © Humana Press Inc., Totowa, NJ

However, there is scant information regarding the identity and location of precursor cells in adult pancreas. The fact that, during development, islets derive from precursors present in the pancreatic duct *(7,28)* raised the possibility that cells within the duct, or the ductal cells themselves, retain the potency to form β cells in adults. In agreement with this possibility, there is evidence suggesting that precursors present in the pancreatic duct play a role in the restitution of islet number after the experimental reduction in the size of the pancreas *(29–31)*. Cells producing insulin were also derived from pancreatic ducts of nonobese diabetic (NOD) mice and from human ductal tissue in vitro *(32,33)*. Another source of putative β-progenitor cells are cells expressing nestin, an intermediate filament characteristic of neuronal precursors, that were located in pancreatic islet of adults *(34)*. In vitro, nestin+ cells proliferate and generate insulin-producing cells *(34)*. Whether the nestin+ cells of islets display a regenerative potential in vivo remains to be determined. Finally, cells expressing the proendocrine gene neurogenin-3 were detected in adult islets *(7)*, supporting the view that islets contain β-precursor cells that could participate in islet cell renewal or growth. Our laboratory is interested in testing the potential of non-β cells of the islet to transdifferentiate into β cells in response to injury or exogenous growth factors. To address this question, we first characterized the phenotype of islet cells in embryos at different stages of development and then examined whether cells expressing embryonic traits appeared in islets during islet growth and regeneration.

2. DIFFERENTIATION OF ISLET CELLS DURING EMBRYONIC DEVELOPMENT

The mammalian pancreas is a mixed exocrine and endocrine gland that produces digestive enzymes and hormones. The enzymes are produced by cells of the exocrine portion, whereas the hormones are synthesized by cells that are clustered in the islets of Langerhans. The pancreas develops from fusion of dorsal and ventral primordia, which appear as buds from the embryonic gut. Each primordium is formed by an endodermally derived pancreatic duct containing undifferentiated precursor cells that migrate away from the duct to generate both islet and acinar cells. In mice, islets achieve a typical mature configuration after birth. Insulin (IN) containing β cells form the core of the islets and the other three classical endocrine cell types, the α, δ, and pancreatic polypeptide (PP) cells, which synthesize glucagon (GLU), somatostatin (SOM), and PP, respectively, are located in the periphery of the islet.

The first indication of morphogenesis of the pancreas occurs around day 9.5 in mice (22–25 somites) when the dorsal endoderm evaginates and is surrounded by condensed mesoderm. One day later, the ventral anlagen differentiates. Endocrine cell differentiation, which begins while the pancreatic cell precursors are still within the pancreatic duct *(35–37)*, depends on interactions between the endodermal epithelium and the surrounding mesenchyme *(6,14,38,39)*. The epithelial cells proliferate and branch, forming the primitive pancreatic duct. The two primitive glands grow independently, forming both endocrine and exocrine tissues, and finally merge at embryonic (e)-10.5 in mouse and e-11.5 in rat *(28)*. The different endocrine cell types appear sequentially during development. GLU^+ and IN^+ cells were first seen at days 9.5 and 10, respectively; SOM at day 15; and PP at postnatal day 1 *(35–37,40,41)*, whereas acinar cell differentiation starts at e-15 *(28,42)*.

The process that guides the differentiation of the endocrine cells is believed to involve the sequential activation and inactivation of transcription factors *(14,22)*. The homeodomain proteins pancreas transcription factor-1 (*ptf-1*) and pancreas-duodenum (*pdx-1*) are the earliest markers of pancreatic development *(15,41,42)*. Although *ptf-1* confers pancreatic fate to the foregut endoderm *(15)*, expression of *pdx-1* marks the endocrine, exocrine, and duct cells of the pancreas *(9,41)*. Accordingly, *pdx-1* null mice are apancreatic *(6,43)*. A subset of Pdx-1 precursors initiate the expression of neurogenin 3 (ngn3), a member of the basic helix–loop–helix family of proneural genes, and become endocrine progenitor cells *(8,9,17)*. Ngn3 is expressed by islet precursors during development but not in mature islet cells *(17)*. This observation and the fact that ablation of ngn3 expression results in the absence of endocrine cells *(8)*, whereas its ectopic expression in the embryonic epithelium induces the appearance of a large number of hormone-producing cells *(10)*, led to the hypothesis that ngn3 functions as a proendocrine gene driving islet cell differentiation *(14,16,22)*. Endocrine precursors expressing Pdx-1/Ngn3 activate neuroD, another member of the family of proneural basic helix–loop–helix *(44,45)*. This step is presumably followed by the inhibition of ngn3 and the transformation of the precursor population into mitotically quiescent, hormone-containing cells *(13)*. Several transcription factors are presumed to play a role in determining the different islet cell types. Among these genes are Nkx2.2, Nkx 6.1, Pax 4, and Pax 6 (reviewed in ref. *14*). The identity of the extrinsic signals regulating islet cell differentiation is poorly understood *(14,16)*. It also remains to be determined whether the early islet precursor cells are depleted during development or if they can be reactivated in adults and induced to generate endocrine cells.

Although analysis of transcription factor expression reveals the identity of factors required for the differentiation of the islet cell types, it does not address the cell lineage relationship of pancreatic islet cells (reviewed in refs. *14,22,41*). Recent studies in which transcripts produced by individual precursor cells present in the pancreatic duct were examined indicated that these cells were pluripotent *(20)*. Our proposed model, illustrated in Fig. 1, incorporates findings by us and others *(35–37,42,46–49)*. This model postulates that during embryonic develop-

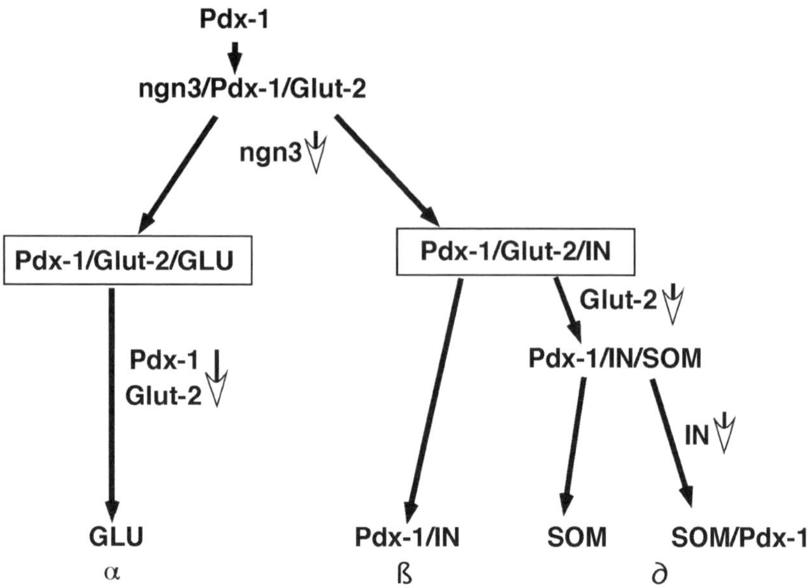

Fig. 1. The proposed cell lineage relationship of pancreatic islet cells is indicated. Cells coexpressing hormones are considered intermediate cell types in the cell lineage pathway, whereas adult cells are monospecific. The downregulation of markers in each pathway of differentiation are indicated by arrows. Cells indicated with asterisks also appear in islets of adults following islet injury. We hypothesize that these cells are putative precursor cells that transdifferentiate into IN+ cells. Not included in this graph is the proposed cell lineage of exocrine cells, pancreatic polypeptide cells of islets, and the timetable of expression of other transcription factors involved in islet differentiation

ment islet cells undergo a gradual process of differentiation during which they coexpress more than one hormone, Pdx-1, and the low-affinity glucose transporter 2 (Glut-2). These cells are considered intermediate cell types in the cell lineage pathway. Eventually, islet cells become restricted in their potential and become mono-specific *(41,42)*. Expression of Pdx-1 becomes restricted to the β cells and to a fraction of the δ cells (16%) and PP cells (9%) *(40–42)*, whereas Glut-2 is only expressed by β cells *(47,51)*.

3. ISLET CELL NEOGENESIS IN ADULT MICE

The observation that embryonic islet cells coexpressing several markers generate mature islet cells that contain only one hormone prompted us to ascertain whether β cells that differentiate during neogenesis undergo a similar process of stepwise differentiation. We hypothesized that depletion of all IN+ cells of the islets was required for the activation and differentiation of the putative progenitor cells. The ablation of the existing β cell population was achieved with the injection of high-dose streptozotocin (SZ), a specific β-cell toxin *(52,53)*, which induced massive β-cell death *(51)*. Mice were severely diabetic 24 hours after SZ injection *(51)*. Pancreatic islets from these mice contained a new subset of cells that immunostained with antibodies to insulin (Fig. 2C,D). Importantly, the number of β cells that reappeared in islets of SZ treated mice increased significantly when normoglycemia was restored by exogenous insulin treatment *(51)*.

A series of experiments were performed to demonstrate that the new β cells visualized after SZ treatment were newly differentiated IN^+ cells rather than "old" β cells that evaded the effect of the toxin. Because chronic hyperglycemia results in β-cell degranulation and decreased levels of insulin, it could be argued that acute hyperglycemia, such as that found in mice 1 day after the injection of the drug (at 1 day post-SZ), had similar effect. If "old" β cells survived the effect of the toxin, these cells would become degranulated at 1 day post-SZ, thus evading detection by immunohistochemical staining. After the reestablishment of normoglycemia by exogenous insulin injection, these cells would have restored the intracellular insulin concentration to normal levels and would stain again for insulin. To address this issue, we stained islets from 1 day post-SZ mice with aromatic L-amino acid decarboxylase (AADC), a neuronal enzyme localized in the cytoplasm of all the endocrine cells of the islet *(51)*. AADC stained all the islet cells of normoglycemic control mice and the degranulated β cells of diabetic obese mice (Fig. 3A), indicating that AADC levels did not decrease with hyperglycemia. In hyperglycemic 1 day post-SZ mice, $AADC^+$ cells were found in the periphery but not in the center of the islets, where β cells are normally found (Fig. 3B), confirming that in most, if not all β cells, the endocrine cells present in this location were deleted by the toxin.

To ascertain the effect of blood glucose levels on β-cell neogenesis, we compared pancreata from mice that remained hyperglycemic (H) throughout the duration of the study (H-X days post-SZ) with pancreata from mice that received SZ at day 0, exogenous insulin starting at day 1 of the experiment and achieved normoglycemia by day 2. At 2 days post-SZ, some of these mice were sacrificed, whereas the remainder received insulin implants. Mice that became normoglycemic (N) after receiving the implants were sacrificed at day 4 or 6 after SZ (N – X days post-SZ).

Pancreata of H – 2 days post-SZ mice had islets that were almost completely devoid of β cells and contained peroxidase staining cellular debris (Fig. 2B). In contrast to the hyperglycemic mice, more than half of the N – 2 days post-SZ mice (25 of 40) had islets that contained 5–60 insulin cells per islet section (Fig. 2C,D). Some of those islets contained IN^+ cells only in the periphery whereas, in other islets, IN^+ cells were also located in the core. The cores of these islets lacked cellular debris seen in the hyperglycemic mice. The debris were replaced by a bed

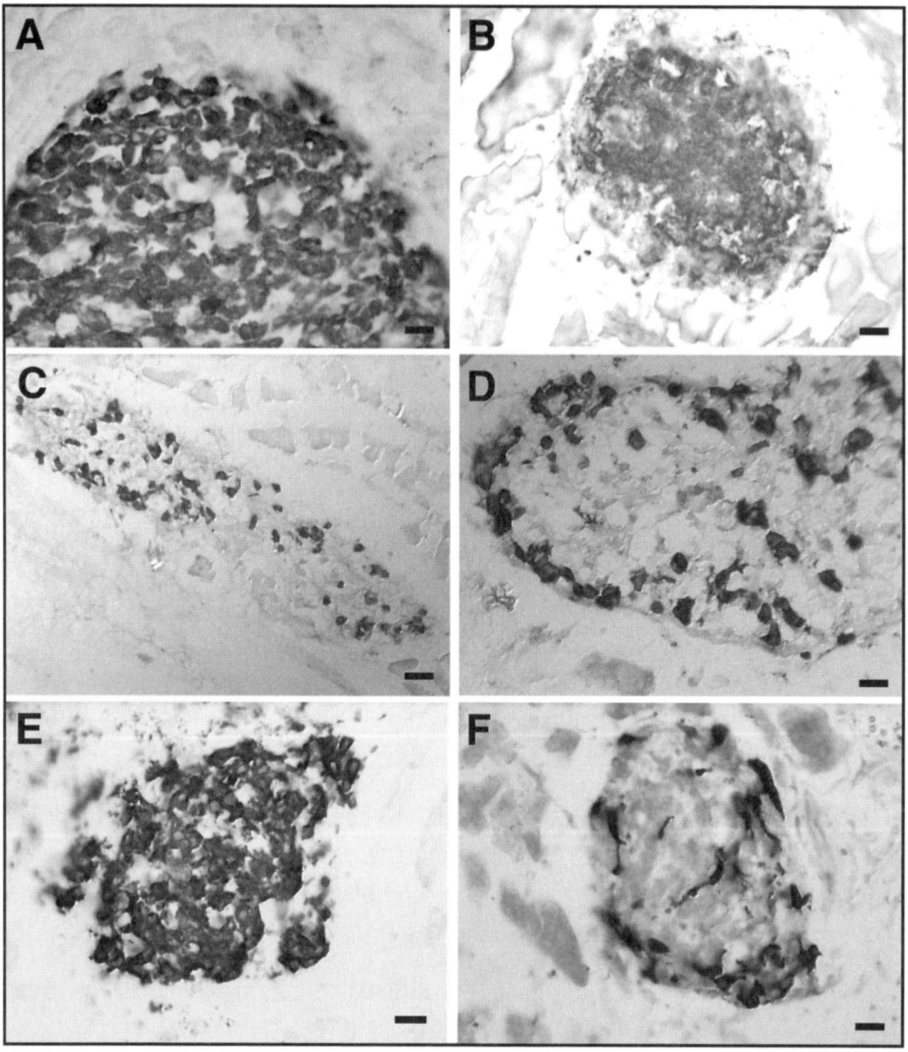

Fig. 2. β-cell neogenesis photomicrograph. **(A–E)** Islets stained for insulin. **(A)** Islet of control mouse. **(B)** Islet of a hyperglycemic 2 days post-streptozotocin (SZ) mouse. Most, if not all, of the stained material in the islet is cell debris. Bar: 60 μm. **(C,D)** Photomicrograph of islets of a normoglycemic 2 days post-SZ mouse. Note the presence of many stained β cells. Bar in **(C)**: 100 μm. Bar in **(D)**: 60 μm. **(E)** Islet of 6 days post-SZ normoglycemic mice. The pancreas contained other islets of larger size, similar to that shown in **(C)**, but that were completely filled by β cells. Bar: 60 μm. **(F)** Islet of normoglycemic 6 days post-SZ mouse shown in **(E)**, stained for somatostatin. Note that some δ cells are located in the core of the islet and that the stained cells do not form a uniformly shaped rim, suggesting an islet in the process of reformation. Bar: 60 μm.

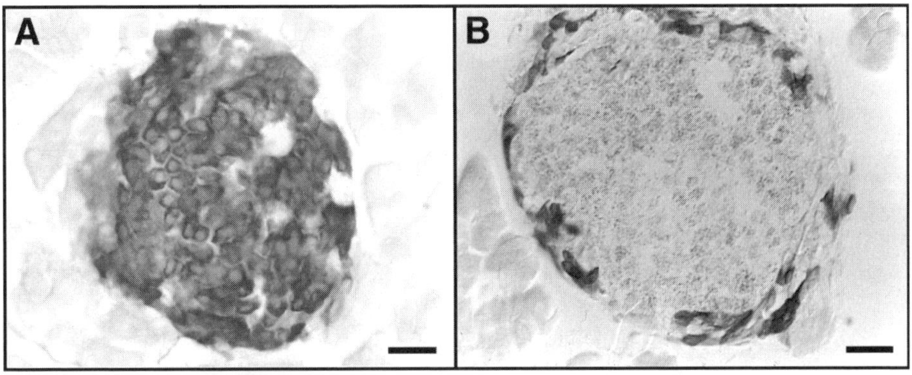

Fig. 3. Absence of endocrine cells in the core of islets of 1 day post-streptozotocin (SZ) mice. **(A,B)** Islets of obese mice and 1 day post-SZ/200 mice stained with aromatic L-amino acid decarboxylase (AADC). Note the presence of darkly stained cells in **(A)** and that the core of the islet shown in **(B)** lacks AADC⁺ cells, a characteristic of all pancreatic islets of 1 day post-SZ/200 mice. Bar: 30 μm.

of fibroblast-like unstained cells (*see* Fig. 2), suggesting that the restoration of normoglycemia facilitated the removal of dead cells by invading macrophages.

The relative β-cell volume per tissue increased from 2% of untreated, normoglycemic control values at 2 days post-SZ to 40% of control values at 6 days post-SZ (Fig. 4). These findings indicate that insulin-induced normoglycemia may have promoted an early burst in β-cell regeneration; however, the number of newly formed β cells per islet did not reached control levels during the study. In addition, the success of recovery was not uniform among normoglycemic mice. Because SZ damages many tissues in addition to the pancreas *(53)*, it is probable that in most SZ-treated mice, its deleterious effect was only partially reversed by the exogenous insulin treatment.

We then sought to determine whether cells expressing embryonal traits reappeared in pancreatic islets after SZ treatment, possibly marking a precursor cell generating the new IN+ cells. The percentage of PDX-1/SOM⁺ cells, one of the cell types expressing immature traits found in pancreas during development, was higher in islets of N – 2 days post-SZ (60%) than in islets of H – 2 days post-SZ (30%) (Fig. 5) *(50, 51)*. In contrast, no difference was found in the percentage of PDX-1/GLU⁺ and PDX-1/PP⁺ cells between experimental animals and untreated controls *(50,51)*. Triple label immunofluorescence from pancreatic islets of N – 2 days SZ mice revealed PDX-1⁺ cells coexpressing SOM and IN *(51)*. Although some islets contained several PDX-1/SOM/IN⁺ cells in addition to the cells containing only SOM, other islets in the same pancreas were populated mainly by monospecific β and δ cells *(51)*. PDX/SOM/IN⁺ cells were not

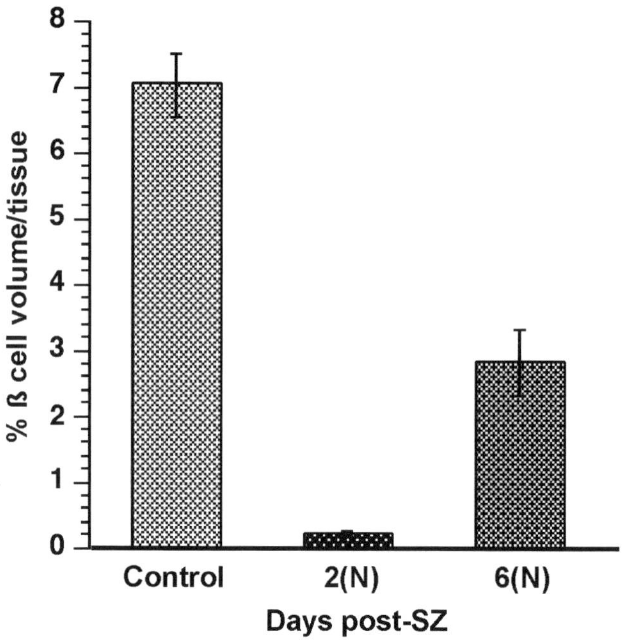

Fig. 4. Relative β-cell volume per tissue increased during insulin treatment. The relative β-cell volume was measured in randomly selected sections from three mice per experimental group. Bar graphs indicate results for controls and 2 and 6 days post-streptozotocin (SZ). Relative β-cell volume of hyperglycemic 2 days post-SZ (2×10^{-4}) was not included in the graph. Absolute islet mass in controls is obtained by multiplying the relative β-cell volume by the weight of the pancreas (0.15 ± 0.01, $n = 5$). Weight of pancreas from experimental animals was not determined. More than 5000 points were scored for each experimental group. Values are expressed as mean ± standard error of the mean. $p < 0.001$ vs controls.

detected in islets of controls *(51)*. No cells expressing GLU/IN or PP/IN were seen after SZ treatments or in controls *(51)*. These results suggest that new β cells could be generated by transdifferentiation of SOM^+ cells. We postulate that the process of transformation of SOM^+ cells into insulin-containing β cells in normoglycemic SZ-treated mice occurs in at least three separate stages. The first stage is the activation of PDX-1 expression in SOM^+ cells. The second stage is the initiation of insulin expression by PDX-1/SOM^+ cells; and, in the third stage of the conversion, SOM^+/IN cells downregulate SOM^+ expression and differentiate into fully mature Glut-2+ β cells.

In addition to the PDX-1/SOM^+ cells, a second set of immature islet cell was detected in islets of SZ-treated mice. These were GLU-positive cells expressing Glut-2, a cell type found in embryonic pancreas *(51)*. Glut-2/GLU^+ cells reappeared in islets of N – 2 days post-SZ mice *(51)*. At this time point, most of the

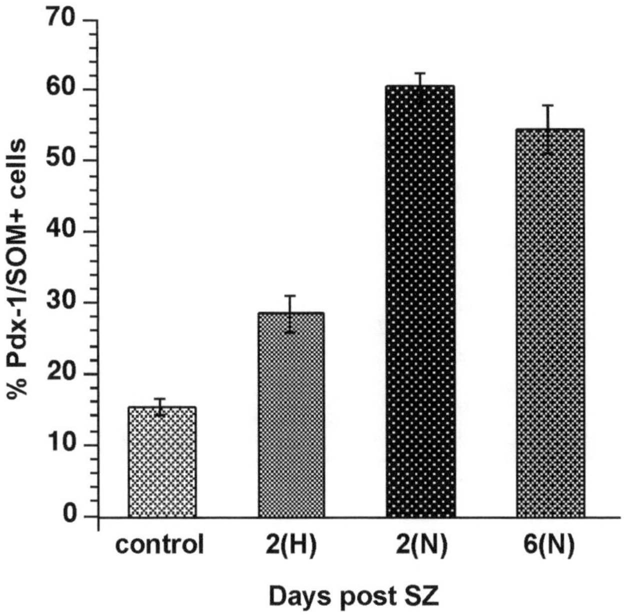

Fig. 5. The percentage of PDX-1/SOM$^+$ cells increased in normoglycemic streptozotocin (SZ) +and insulin (IN)-treated islets The percentage of PDX-1/SOM$^+$ cells at different times after injection of SZ and IN is compared between controls, 2 and 6 days post-SZ mice. At least three pancreata per stage were examined in controls and in normoglycemic 2 and in 6 days post-SZ mice. These tissues did not show hemorrhage or necrosis. Total number of cells scored for the PDX-1/SOM$^+$ combination in islets of control and hyperglycemic 2 days post-SZ mice was 1234 from 15 islets and 2353 from 42 islets, respectively. Total number of cells scored for the PDX-1/SOM$^+$ combination for normoglycemic mice at 2 and 6 post-SZ were 1924 from 30 islets and 1419 from 19 islets. The number of cells expressing PDX-1 and SOM is expressed as the mean ± standard error of the mean of the cells immunoreactive for SOM. In this figure, the number of days after SZ injection = x days post-SZ. Insulin was injected 24 hours after the injection of SZ. $*p < 0.001$ vs controls. H, hyperglycemic; N, normoglycemic.

Glut-2$^+$ cells coexpressed glucagon *(51)*. Glut-2 expression by GLU cells persisted in islets of pancreata with suboptimal regeneration even at 6 days post-SZ, but was transient in pancreata with fully reformed islets *(51)*. This observation suggested that the inhibition of Glut-2 expression by GLU correlated with the success of the regeneration process. In contrast to N-mice, Glut-2/GLU cells were not seen in islets of H – 2 days post-SZ mice raising the possibility that the appearance of this cell type is inhibited by high circulating blood glucose levels. No Glut-2 cells expressed SOM. As expected, β, but not α cells of controls expressed Glut-2 *(51)*.

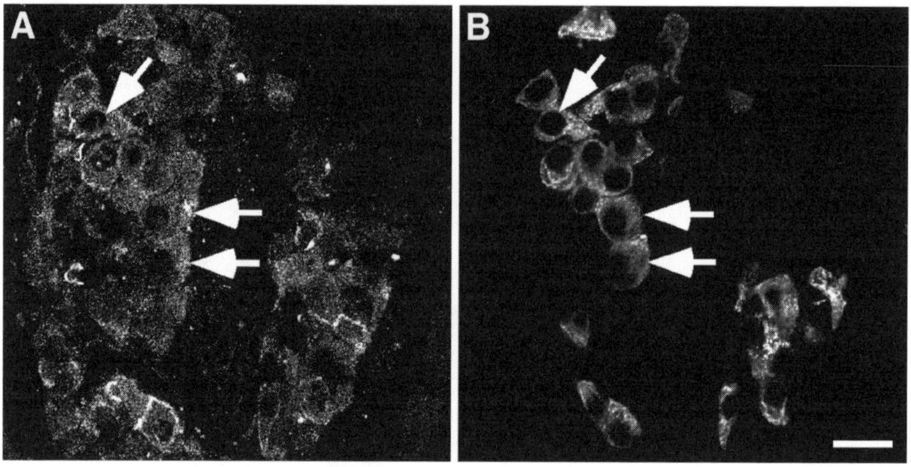

Fig. 6. Reappearance of Glut-2/IN⁺ cells during regeneration. **(A-C)** Photomicrographs of an islet of a normoglycemic 4 days post-streptozotocin mouse costained with Glut-2 **(A)** and insulin **(B)**. Many cells are doubly labeled, some of these cells indicated with arrows. Bar: 20 μm.

In islets of N – 2 days post-SZ mice, some of the Glut-2^+ cells coexpressed IN *(51)* and the number of IN/Glut-2 cells increased over time (Fig. 6) *(51)*. We postulate that GLU/Glut-2^+ cells present in islets of SZ-treated normoglycemic mice are a second set of intra-islet β-cell precursors and that these cells turn off GLU expression before the initiation of IN synthesis. This timing of GLU expression inhibition would account for the absence of double-labeled GLU/IN^+ cells in regenerating islets. In contrast to islets of normoglycemic mice, islets of hyperglycemic 6 days post-SZ mice contained IN^+ cells but only a few of these cells had diffuse and poorly localized Glut-2 staining (not shown). It is likely that acinar cells did not generate new β cells (NBCs) because sections of pancreas of N mice processed for visualization of IN and amylase failed to reveal the presence of doubly labeled cells.

4. PROTRACTED HYPERGLYCEMIA HAD A DETRIMENTAL EFFECT ON β-CELL NEOGENESIS

The observation that IN injected at day 1 post-SZ promoted β-cell neogenesis raised the question as to whether the hormone would have a similar effect after a protracted hyperglycemic period. This possibility is of obvious importance because it could determine the outcome in patients with a long history of diabetes. We found that an extended period of hyperglycemia did not inhibit the appearance of NBCs *(54)*. However, the presence of these cells was transient and they quickly disappeared from the islets (Fig. 7). These observations suggest that

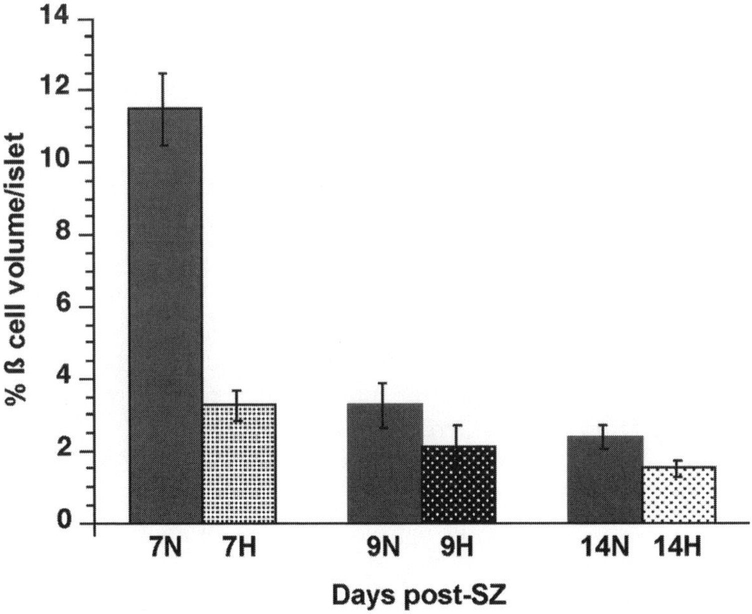

Fig. 7. Insulin injection promoted a transient increase in β-cell volume per islet. Six days post-streptozotocin (SZ) mice were injected with SZ at day 1, with insulin at day 6, and their blood glucose levels was tested at day 7. A group of normoglycemic (N) 7 days post-SZ mice ($n = 7$) were killed and their pancreas examined. Other normoglycemic 7 days post-SZ mice received insulin pellets and were examined 2 and 7 days later (9N and 14N, respectively). Mice that did not receive insulin therapy remained hyperglycemic (H) and were examined at 7, 9, and 14 days post-SZ (7H, 9H, and 14H, respectively). Randomly selected islets were analyzed, three mice per group. At least 5000 points were scored for each group. The number of β cells per islet area is expressed as mean ± standard error of the mean. Note that there is a threefold difference in the β-cell volume per islets from 7N and 7H mice ($p < 0.001$) and that the β-cell volume in normoglycemic mice decreased with time (i.e., 9N and 14N). p of 9N vs 9H and of 14N vs 14 H < 0.05.

the demise of the NBCs was due to alterations in the microenvironment of the islet affected by the long exposure to high glucose levels. These results also suggest that the survival of the newly formed β cells is dependent on the early detection of diabetes followed by prompt reestablishment of euglycemia by insulin therapy.

5. β-CELL NEOGENESIS IS CURTAILED IN ISLETS OF NOD MICE

The finding of putative β-precursor cells in islets of our CD-1 outbred mice prompted us to ascertain whether similar cells populate islets of NOD mice, a strain in which islets are eliminated by an autoimmune process similar to that occurring in type I diabetes in humans (reviewed in ref. *55*). In NOD mice, the inflammatory insulinitis leads to diabetes between 13 and 30 weeks of age *(55)*. We examined islets of mutant 1- to 4-month-old NOD mice for the presence of two putative β-precursor cells, the PDX-1/SOM$^+$ and the Glut2/GLU$^+$ cells. All 1-month-old NOD mice examined were normoglycemic and contained islets that had an apparent normal morphology, whereas 2-month-old NOD mice, which were still normoglycemic, had islets with mild to severe insulinitis. At 4 months, one of the NOD mice analyzed had mild hyperglycemia (blood glucose 156 mg/dL), whereas the other three mice were severely hyperglycemic (blood glucose >400 mg/dL). Pancreata of both normoglycemic and hyperglycemic 4-month-old NOD mice contained islets with different degrees of lymphocyte infiltration and β-cell number. As expected, the number of affected islets was greater in hyperglycemic animals. The percentage of SOM$^+$PDX-1$^+$ cells was always higher in islets of NOD mutants than in islets of littermate controls (Fig. 8).

Islets of NOD mice also contained the second putative precursor cell, the Glut-2/GLU$^+$ cells. Glut-2/GLU$^+$ cells appeared in islets of prediabetic mice and in mice with mild hyperglycemia (Fig. 9A,B). Islets of diabetic (blood glucose >500 mg/dL) NOD mice lacked Glut-2 and Glut-2/GLU$^+$ cells and had GLU$^+$ cells with abnormal morphology *(51)*. These results confirmed previous reports by others indicating a decrease in Glut-2 levels in mice with autoimmune diabetes *(56)*.

However, the progenitors found in islets of NOD mice failed to generate PDX-1/SOM/IN$^+$ or Glut-2/IN$^+$ cells and eventually vanished during progression of the autoimmune disease. We speculate that intra-islet precursors of NOD mice, like those of their nondiabetic counterparts, are capable of regenerating the β-cell population and will do so if the immunologic insult to the islets is circumvented.

6. β-CELL PRECURSORS CONTRIBUTE TO β-CELL HYPERPLASIA DURING PREGNANCY

To ascertain whether putative β-precursor cells contribute to the formation of new β cells during normal islet growth, we examined islets of pregnant mice to study development of islet hyperplasia that is characteristic of gestation *(57,58)*. The percentage of non-β-cell populations coexpressing PDX-1/SOM$^+$ at day (D) 10 of gestation, D15, and postpartum day 7 was examined. The percentage of PDX-1/SOM$^+$ cells increased twofold at D10 and then gradually returned to control levels by the end of gestation. In contrast, the percentages of PDX-1/GLU cells did not change (Nasir and Teitelman, unpublished).

If PDX-1/SOM$^+$ cells are precursors, it is predicted that they will proliferate to replenish the population of δ cells as well as new cells expressing insulin. Examination of islets processed for immunostaining and autoradiography indi-

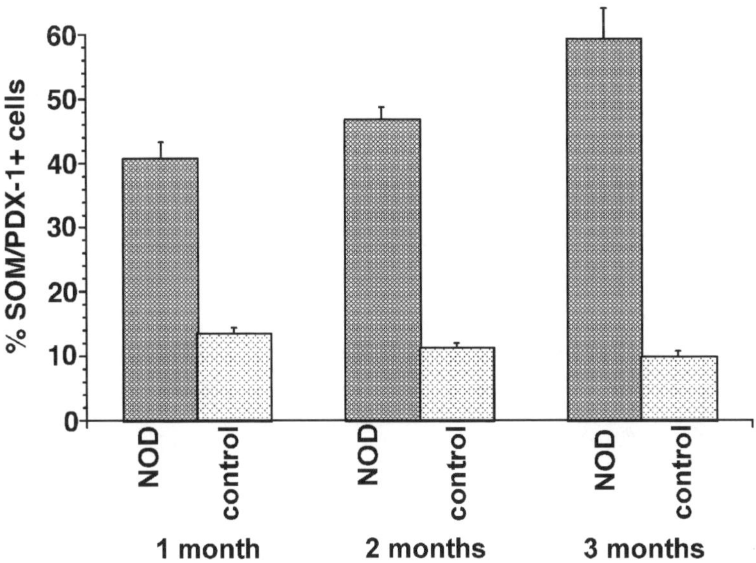

Fig. 8. Sections of nonobese diabetic pancreas were processed for double immunostaining and the percentage of $SOM^+PDX\text{-}1^+$ cells over the total number of SOM^+ cells scored.

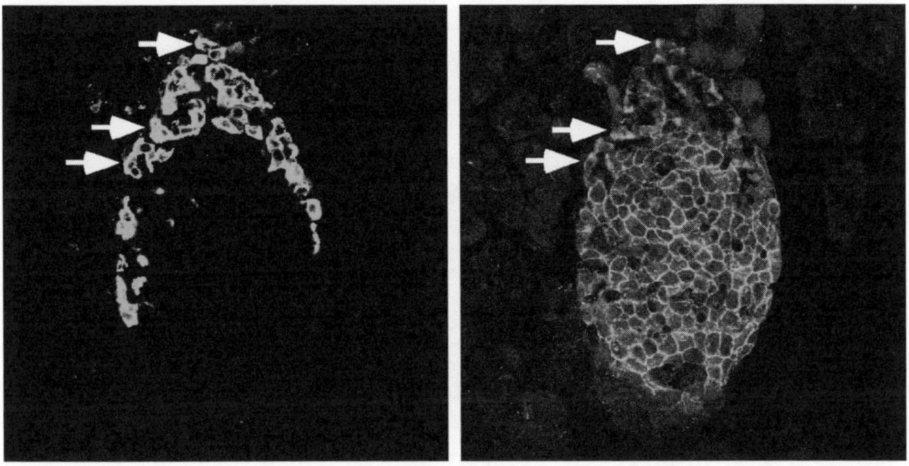

Fig. 9. Confocal microscopic analysis of an islet of female nonobese diabetic (NOD) mice. **(A,B)** Islet of prediabetic 2-month-old NOD mice illustrates the presence cells expressing both glucagon **(A)** and Glut-2 **(B)**. Some of the Glut-2/Glu^+ cells are indicated with arrows.

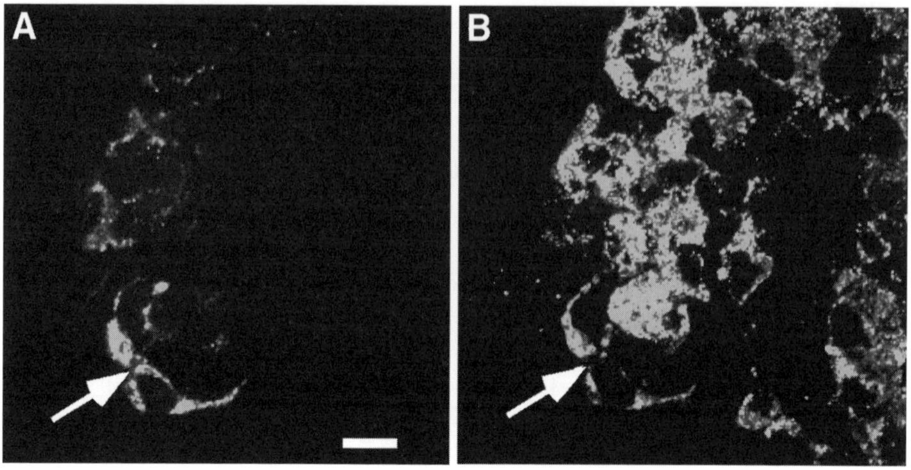

Fig. 10. Cells coexpressing PDX-1/SOM/IN differentiated in pancreatic islets during gestation. Photomicrograph illustrates a section of pancreas of a mouse at day 15 of pregnancy processed for visualization of PDX-1/SOM (**A**) and IN (**B**) and examined by confocal microscopy. Cells coexpressing PDX-1/SOM/IN are indicated by arrows. Bar: 20 μm.

cated that there was a twofold increase in the ^{3}H-thymidine labeling index of SOM cells during early gestation, returning to control levels during the perinatal period. The rate of GLU$^+$ cells proliferation also increases 1.4-fold during pregnancy. However, in contrast to SOM cells, the augmentation in the number of replicating α cells occurred during late gestation (Nasir and Teitelman, unpublished).

We then compared pancreata of control, D10, D15, and D17 mice with pregnant mice pancreata to determine whether SOM cells coexpressed IN and PDX-1. Cells coexpressing PDX-1/SOM/IN were found in islets of pregnant mice at all stages of gestation (Fig. 10), comprising 1–2% of all SOM$^+$ cells. These islets, however, lacked cells coexpressing GLU and IN. In controls, PDX-1/IN$^+$ cells did not contain SOM or GLU.

We then asked whether prolactin, a gestational hormone known to play a key role in the regulation of islet function during pregnancy *(56)* induced the expression of PDX-1/SOM/IN+ cells in islets during gestation. We compared islets of virgin females infused for 1 week with saline or with prolactin at levels found in pregnant mice. The percentage of PDX-1/SOM$^+$ and PDX-1/SOM/IN$^+$ cell types was similar in both groups of mice, suggesting that prolactin is not involved in the differentiation of the putative β-cell precursors.

7. SUMMARY

Taken together, the findings in the three mouse models examined—the SZ-treated, NOD, and pregnant mice—support the view that precursor cells populating the islets have the ability to generate new β cells. Identification of cues inducing the differentiation of the putative β-precursor cells still remain to be elucidated. Conceivably, the signal molecules could be hormones reported to affect islet size and function during pregnancy *(58)* or cytokines activated by islet injury.

The source of precursor cells responsible for generating the new β cells is unresolved. One possible source is non-β cells of the islet that transdifferentiate into insulin-producing cells. Another source could be undifferentiated precursors or nestin$^+$ cells reported to populate murine islets that produce the new β cells, presumably going through the intermediate stages of differentiation found in embryonic and regenerating pancreas. It is also possible that the original β-cell precursors are the α cells of the islet. Glucagon cells, known to express "stem" cell properties *(59)*, could generate all the intermediate and mature cell types of the β-cell lineage. Studies in progress in our laboratory are designed to ascertain the lineage of the new β cells using cell-independent genetic markers. In addition, we are actively investigating the identity of the signals responsible for the initiation of β-cell neogenesis in islets of adults. An understanding of these issues may lead to the exciting possibility of promoting β-cell regeneration in patients with type I diabetes.

ACKNOWLEDGMENTS

Supported by grants from the National Institute of Health (NIDDK), the Juvenile Diabetes Foundation, and the American Diabetes Association.

REFERENCES

1. Assady S, Maor G, Amit M, Itskovitz-Eldor J, Skorecki KL, Tzukerman M. Insulin production by human embryonic stem cells. Diabetes 2001;50:1691–1697.
2. Cornelius JG, Tchernev V, Kao K-J, Pech AB. In vitro-generation of islets in long term cultures of pluripotent stem cells from adult mouse pancreas. Horm Metab Res 1997; 29:271–277.
3. Lumelsky N, Blondel O, Laeng P, Velasco I, Ravin R, McKay R. Differentiation of embryonic stem cells to insulin secreting structures similar to pancreatic islets. Science 2001;292:1389–1394.
4. Ramiya VK, Maraist M, Arfors KE, Schatz DA, Peck AB, Cornelius JG. Reversal of insulin-dependent diabetes using islets generated in vitro from pancreatic stem cells. Nat Med 2000;6:278–282.
5. Soria B, Roche E, Berna G, Leon-Quinto T, Reig JA, Martin F. Insulin secreting cells derived from embryonic stem cells normalize glycemia in streptozotocin-induced diabetic mice. Diabetes 2000;49:1–6.

6. Edlund H. Pancreatic organogenesis—developmental mechanisms and implications for therapy. Nat Rev Genet 2002;3:524–532.
7. Gu G, Brown JR, Melton DA. Direct lineage tracing reveals the ontogeny of pancreatic cell fates during mouse embryogenesis. Mech Dev 2003;120:35–43.
8. Gradwohl G, Dierich A, LeMeur M, Guillemot F. Neurogenin 3 is required for the development of the four endocrine cell lineages of the pancreas. Proc Natl Acad Sci USA 2000;97:1607–1611.
9. Gu G, Dubauskaite J, Melton DA. Direct evidence for the pancreatic lineage: Ngn3+ cells are islet progenitors and are distinct from duct progenitors. Development 2002;129:2447–2457.
10. Grappin-Botton A, Majithia AR, Melton DA. Key events of pancreas formation are triggered in gut endoderm by ectopic expression of pancreatic regulatory genes. Genes Dev 2001;15:444–454.
11. Hart A, Papadopoulou S, Edlund H. Fgf10 maintains notch activation, stimulates proliferation and blocks differentiation of pancreatic epithelial cells. Dev Dyn 2003;228:185–193.
12. Cleaver O, Melton DA. Endothelial signaling during development. Nat Med 2003;9:661–668.
13. Jenssen J, Heller RS, Funder-Nielsen T, et al. Independent development of pancreatic α and β cells from neurogenin-3 expressing precursors. Diabetes 2000;49:163–176.
14. Jensen J. Gene regulatory factors in pancreatic development. Dev Dyn 2004;229:176–200.
15. Kawaguchi Y, Cooper B, Gannon M et al. The role of transcriptional regulator Ptf1a in converting intestinal to pancreatic progenitors. Nat Genet 2002;32:128–134.
16. Murtaugh LC, Melton DA. Genes, signals, and lineages in pancreas development. Annu Rev Cell Dev Biol 2003;19:71–89.
17. Schwittzgebel VM, Scheel DW, Conners JR, et al. Expression of neurogenin 3 reveals an islet cell precursor population in the pancreas. Development 2000;127:3533–3542.
18. St-Onge L, Sosa-Pineda B, Chowdhury K, Mansouri A, Gruss P. Pax 6 is required for differentiation of glucagon-producing a cells in the mouse pancreas. Nature 1997;387:406–409.
19. Sosa-Pineda B, Chowdhury K, Torres M, Oliver G, Gruss P. The Pax4 gene is essential for differentiation of insulin-producing β cells in the mammalian pancreas. Nature 1997;386: 99–402.
20. Chiang MK, Melton DA. Single cell transcript analysis of pancreas development. Dev Cell 2003;4:383–393.
21. Sussel L, Kalamaras J, Hartigan-O'Connor DJ, et al. Mice lacking the homeodomain transcription factor Nkx2.2 have diabetes due to arrested differentiation of pancreatic beta cells. Development 1998;125:2213–2221.
22. Wilson ME, Scheel D, German MS. Gene expression cascades in pancreatic development. Mech Dev 2003;120:5–80.
23. Hellestrom C, Swenne I. Growth pattern of pancreatic islet cells in animals. In: Volk BV, Arquilla ER, eds. The Diabetic, 2nd ed. New York, Plenum Medical Book Co., 1985, pp. 53–80.
24. Bonner-Weir S. Perspective—postnatal pancreatic β cell growth. Endocrinology. 2000;141: 1926–1929.
25. Lipsett M, Finegood DT. β cell neogenesis during prolonged hyperglycemia in rats. Diabetes 2002;51:1834–1841.
26. Song SY, Gannon M, Washington MK, et al. Expansion of Pdx-1 expressing pancreatic epithelium and islet neogenesis in transgenic mice over-expressing transforming growth factor alpha. Gastroenterology 1999;117:1416–1426.
27. Garcia-Ocana A, Takane KK, Syed MA, Philbrick WM, Vasavada RC, Stewart AF. Hepatocyte growth factor overexpression in the islet of transgenic mice increases beta cell proliferation, enhances islet mass and induces mild hyperglycemia. J Biol Chem 2000;275:1226–1232.

28. Pictet R, Rutter WJ. Development of the embryonic pancreas. In: Steiner DF, Frenkel N, eds. Handbook of Physiology, Section 7. Washington, DC, American Physiological Society, 1972, pp 25–66.
29. Bonner-Weir S, Baxter LA, Schuppin GT, Smith FE. A second pathway for regeneration of adult exocrine and endocrine pancreas: a possible recapitulation of embryonic development. Diabetes 1993;42:1715–1720.
30. Rooman I, Lardon J, Bowens L. Gastrin stimulates β cell neogenesis and increases islet mass from transdifferentiated but not from normal exocrine pancreas tissue. Diabetes 2002;51:686–690.
31. Rooman I, Hereman Y, Heimberg H, Bowens L. Modulation of rat pancreatic acinoductal transdifferentiation and expression of Pdx-1 in vitro. Diabetologia 2000;43:907–914.
32. Bonner-Weir S, Taneja M, Weir G, et al. In vitro cultivation of human islets from expanded ductal tissue. Proc Natl Acad Sci USA 2000;97:7999–8005.
33. Gao R, Ustinov J, Pulkkinen MA, Lundin K, Korsgren O, Otonkoski T. Characterization of endocrine progenitor cells and critical factors for their differentiation in human adult pancreatic cell culture. Diabetes 2003;52:2007–2015.
34. Zulewski H,Abraham EJ, Gerlach MJ, et al. Multipotential nestin-positive stem cells isolated from adult pancreatic islets differentiate ex-vivo into pancreatic endocrine, exocrine and hepatic phenotypes. Diabetes 2001;50:521–533.
35. Alpert S, Hanahan D, Teitelman G. Hybrid insulin genes reveal a developmental lineage for pancreatic endocrine cells and imply a relationship with neurons. Cell 1988;53:295–308.
36. Gittes GK, Rutter WJ. Onset of cell-specific gene expression in the developing mouse pancreas. Proc Natl Acad Sci USA 1992;89:1128–1132.
37. Herrera PL, Huarte J, Sanvito F, Meda P, Orci L, Vassalli JD. Embryogenesis of the murine endocrine pancreas; early expression of the pancreatic polypeptide gene. Development 1991;113:1257–1265.
38. Golosow N, Grobstein C. Epitheliomesenchymal interaction in pancreatic morphogenesis. Dev Biol 1962;4:242–255.
39. Wessels NK, Cohen JH. Early pancreas organogenesis: morphogenesis, tissue interactions, and mass effects. Dev Biol 1967;15:237–270.
40. Upchurch B, Aponte GW, Leiter AB. Expression of peptide YY in all four islet cell types in the developing mouse pancreas suggests a common peptide YY producing progenitor. Development 1994;120:245–252.
41. Gannon M, Wright CVE. Endodermal patterning and organogenesis. In: Mood S, ed. Cell Lineage and Fate Determination. New York, Academic Press, 1999, pp. 583–615.
42. Guz Y, Montminy MR, Stein R, et al. Expression of murine stf-1, a putative insulin gene transcription factor, in β cells of pancreas, duodenal epithelium and pancreatic exocrine and endocrine progenitors during ontogeny. Development 1995;121:11–18.
43. Offield MF, Jetton TL, Labosky PA, et al. PDX-1 is required for pancreatic outgrowth and differentiation of the rostral duodenum. Development 1996;122:983–995.
44. Naya FJ, Stellrecht CM, Tsai MJ. Tissue-specific regulation of the insulin gene by a novel basic helix-loop-helix transcription factor. Genes Dev 1995;9:1009–1019.
45. Naya FJ, Huang HP, Qui Y, et al. Diabetes, defective pancreatic morphogenesis, and abnormal enteroendocrine differentiation in BETA2-NeuroD-deficient mice. Genes Dev 1997;11: 2323–2334.
46. Herrera PL. Adult insulin and glucagon-producing cells differentiate from two independent lineages. Development 2000;127:317–2322.

47. Pang K, Mukonoweshuro C, Wong GC. Beta cells arise from glucose transporter type 2(Glut-2)-expressing epithelial cells of the developing rat pancreas. Proc Natl Acad Sci USA 1994;91:9559–9563.
48. Teitelman G, Alpert S, Polak JM, Martinez A, Hanahan D. Precursor cells of mouse endocrine pancreas coexpress insulin,glucagon,and the neuronal proteins tyrosine hydroxylase and neuropeptide Y, but not pancreatic polypeptide. Development 1993;118:1031–1039.
49. Vincent M, Guz Y, Rozenberg M, et al. Abrogation of protein convertase 2 (PC-2) activity results in delayed islet cell differentiation and maturation, increase in alpha cell proliferation and islet neogenesis. Endocrinology 2003;144:4061–4069.
50. Fernandes A, King LC, Guz Y, Stein R, Wright CVE, Teitelman G. Differentiation of new insulin producing cells is induced by injury in adult pancreatic islets. Endocrinology 1997;138:1750–1762.
51. Guz Y, Nasir I, Teitelman G. Regeneration of pancreatic β cells from intra-islet precursor cells in an experimental model of diabetes. Endocrinology 2001;142:4956–4969.
52. Like AA, Rossini AA. Streptozotocin-induced pancreatic insulinitis: new model of diabetes mellitus. Science 1976;193:415–418.
53. Rodrigues B, Poucheret P, Batell ML, McNeill JH. In: McNeill JH, ed. Streptozotocin-induced diabetes: induction, mechanisms(s), and dose dependency. Experimental Models of Diabetes. Boca Raton, FL, CRC Press, 1999, pp. 3–14.
54. Guz Y, Torres A, Teitelman G. Detrimental effect of protracted hyperglycaemia on beta-cell neogenesis in a mouse murine model of diabetes. Diabetologia 2002;45:1689–1696.
55. Leiter EH, Gerling IC, Flynn JC. Spontaneous insulin-dependent diabetes mellitus (IDDM) in nonobese diabetic(NOD) mice: comparison with experimentally induced IDDM. In: McNeill JH, ed. Experimental Models of Diabetes. Boca Raton, FL, CRC Press, 1999, pp. 257–294.
56. Reddy S, Young M, Poole CA, JM Ross. Loss of glucose transporter-2 precedes insulin loss in the non-obese diabetic and the low-dose streptozotocin mouse models: a comparative immunohistochemical study by light and confocal microscopy. Gen Comp Endocrinol 1998;111:9–19.
57. Sorenson RL, Brejle TC. Adaptation of islets of Langerhans to pregnancy: β cell growth, enhanced insulin secretion and the role of lactogenic hormones. Horm Metab Res 1996;29:301–307.
58. Nielsen JH, Galsgaard ED, Moldrup A, et al. Regulation of β cell mass by hormones and growth factors. Diabetes 2001;50(Suppl. 1):S25–S29.
59. Wang J, Webb G, Cao Y, Steiner DF. Contrasting patterns of expression of transcription factors in pancreatic alpha and beta cells. Proc Natl Acad Sci USA 2003;100:12660–12665.

7 Transcription Factor-Directed Differentiation of Stem Cells Along an Endocrine Lineage

William L. Lowe, Jr.

CONTENTS

1. INTRODUCTION

Loss of endocrine gland function from a variety of causes (e.g., autoimmune destruction, infection, injury) is commonly encountered in clinical endocrinology. Although hormone replacement is generally adequate to replace the basic function of the gland and maintain viability, it typically cannot reproduce the intricate regulation of hormone secretion. Thus, despite the availability of hormone replacement, those who require it are often at risk for the development of long-term problems (e.g., microvascular complications or severe hypoglycemia in diabetes, complications of long-term overreplacement of hydrocortisone or inadequate hydrocortisone replacement during times of stress). Thus cell replacement therapy capable of restoring endocrine function similar to that of the native gland would represent a major therapeutic advance. To that end, the differentiation of stem cells to generate new endocrine cells offers great potential.

As described in other chapters, a number of different approaches can be employed to differentiate embryonic or other stem cells along a specific lineage. One approach that has been employed is forced differentiation. This can

From: *Contemporary Endocrinology: Stem Cells in Endocrinology*
Edited by: L. B. Lester © Humana Press Inc., Totowa, NJ

be accomplished by expressing a gene important for cell lineage determination to direct stem cell differentiation along a specific pathway. Typically, these genes initiate a hierarchical cascade of gene expression that ultimately results in cell differentiation. Beyond providing a means to develop cells capable of being used for cell replacement therapy, this approach of using transcription factor expression to direct stem cell differentiation also provides important insight into the genetic programs directed by different transcription factors and the developmental program of different cell types. This chapter will describe how this approach has been used to develop partially or fully differentiated cells capable of replacing cell function.

2. TRANSCRIPTION FACTOR-DIRECTED DIFFERENTIATION OF NONENDOCRINE CELL TYPES

Multiple approaches have been used to successfully transfer DNA into stem cells and permit expression of specific genes (e.g., stable transfection of DNA after electroporation, use of adenoviral or lentiviral vectors). To date, the approach of directed differentiation via transcription factor expression in stem cells has been used to greatest effect to generate nonendocrine cells. Thus, a few examples of directed differentiation of stem cells into nonendocrine cells are described.

2.1. Hematopoietic Cells

Removing embryonic stem (ES) cells from feeder cells or leukemia inhibitory factor, both of which inhibit ES cell differentiation, and placing them on a nonadherent surface results in the formation of clusters of cells referred to as embryoid bodies. Within embryoid bodies, ES cells spontaneously differentiate and generate cells from all three germ layers (i.e., mesoderm, ectoderm, and endoderm). Among the cell types formed in embryoid bodies are blood elements. However, the differentiation of blood elements in embryoid bodies appears to recapitulate primitive hematopoiesis, which occurs in the yolk sac, and not definitive hematopoiesis, which is mediated by definitive hematopoietic stem cells and persists throughout life (reviewed in ref. *1*). Given the inability to generate definitive hematopoietic stem cells from ES cells, long-term stable engraftment of ES-derived hematopoietic cells in bone marrow after transplantation into irradiated recipients has not been accomplished. To address the problem of generating definitive hematopoietic stem cells, screens to define factors important for hematopoietic stem cell development have been undertaken. From these screens, strategies have been developed to generate transplantable ES cell-derived hematopoietic stem cells capable of engrafting in the bone marrow of irradiated mice.

Among the factors identified in these screens was the transcription factor HoxB4 *(1)*. HoxB4 is a homeobox transcription factor and a member of a family of genes that are transcribed from four clusters referred to as *HoxA*, *HoxB*, *HoxC*, and *HoxD (2)*. Several members of this large family of genes, including *HoxB4*, are important for hematopoietic lineage commitment. A second factor identified in the screens was the transcription factor Stat5 *(3)*. Stat5 is a member of a family of transcription factors that are present in the cytoplasm and form homo- or heterodimers following tyrosine phosphorylation *(4)*. The phosphorylated dimers translocate to the nucleus where they mediate a program of gene expression. The Stats are activated by a variety of cytokines and other peptides, including those that are important for hematopoiesis. Stat5 is downstream of the Bcr/Abl oncogene, which is important in the pathogenesis of chronic myelogenous leukemia and regulates definitive hematopoietic stem cells *(3,5)*.

To determine the impact of either HoxB4 or Stat5 expression on the differentiation of ES cells, ES cells capable of doxycycline-inducible expression of one of the two transcription factors were developed *(3,6)*. In the case of Stat5, a mutant form of the protein which is constitutively active was expressed. In both cases, the transcription factors were expressed from day 4 to day 6 of cell differentiation in embryoid bodies. Expression of both transcription factors enhanced the formation of hematopoietic colony-forming cells. Importantly, subsequent culturing of the cells on stromal cells in the presence of cytokines and doxycycline generated hematopoietic blast cells. Transplantation of the HoxB4- and Stat5-induced ES-derived hematopoietic cells into irradiated syngeneic mice had different outcomes. HoxB4-induced cells were able to home to the bone marrow, contribute to myeloid and lymphoid lineages, and be represented in the hematopoietic stem cell pool *(6)*. Stat5-expressing cells were able to engraft only in the presence of the continued induced expression of Stat5, and, even under these conditions, their contribution to hematopoietic lineages was lost after 8 weeks *(1)*. Despite the more limited potential of these cells, Stat5 expression clearly augmented commitment of ES cells to a hematopoietic pathway. These studies demonstrate the potential utility of manipulating gene expression as a means to direct cell differentiation, and, in the case of cells expressing Stat5, demonstrate that activation of an effector of specific signaling pathways was able to direct ES cell differentiation.

2.2. Neural Cells

Several different approaches have been employed to direct or augment the differentiation of ES cells into neural cells. Among the earliest genes to be expressed in neuroepithelium during differentiation of neural cells are basic helix–loop–helix transcription factors that are members of the NeuroD/neurogenin family *(7)*. NeuroD3 is expressed early, followed by expression of NeuroD1 and NeuroD2. Stable transfection of ES cells with vectors that express a member of the NeuroD family followed by growth under conditions that promote ES cell differentiation resulted in differentiation along a neural lineage *(8)*.

Depending on the transcription factor that was expressed, the phenotype of the cells varied. Expression of NeuroD3 resulted in primitive-appearing neural cells that were bipolar with short, branched processes. In contrast, cells expressing NeuroD2 were unipolar with longer processes.

The SOX proteins are a family of transcription factors that contain an HMG-box DNA binding domain *(9)*. Members of this family, including SOX1, SOX2, and SOX3, appear to contribute to cell fate decisions in the developing nervous system *(9)*. SOX1 expression occurs at the time of neural induction, suggesting that it may direct cells toward a neural fate *(10)*. Indeed, in embryonal carcinoma cells, which, as with ES cells, are capable of differentiating into all three germ layers, treatment with retinoic acid induces neural differentiation and stimulates SOX1 expression *(10)*. Similarly, expression of a *Sox1* cDNA in embryonal carcinoma cells results in neural differentiation, as reflected by the expression of neuroepithelial and neuronal markers *(10)*. Importantly, SOX1 was expressed in an inducible fashion in the embryonal carcinoma cells, and only transient expression of SOX1 was required to induce neural differentiation. In this example of using a transcription factor to direct differentiation, SOX1 expression was able to substitute for a known inductive factor, retinoic acid. In other tissues, the genetic programs responsible for tissue development and cell differentiation are being elucidated, but the inductive factors that stimulate them remain more obscure. This example suggests that expressing genes that initiate and direct genetic programs stimulated by inductive factors is one approach to direct differentiation along a specific pathway.

In addition to using transcription factor expression to initiate a genetic program that directs stem cell differentiation, transcription factor expression can also be used to augment the differentiation of ES cells along a specific pathway. Cells of potential clinical importance are midbrain neurons that secrete dopamine, because they offer a potential therapy for Parkinson's disease. The generation of these cells has been accomplished by modifying a previously devised method for the differentiation of ES cells into neurons. Specifically, the proportion of neurons capable of producing dopamine was increased by treating cells late in the differentiation process with fibroblast growth factor 8 and sonic hedgehog *(11)*. Among the transcription factors induced by treatment with sonic hedgehog and fibroblast growth factor 8 is nuclear receptor related-1 (Nurr1) *(11)*. To augment the differentiation of cells into dopamine-secreting neurons, a cDNA-encoding Nurr1 was stably and constitutively expressed in ES cells, and the cells were then subjected to the same differentiation protocol. This increased the proportion of neurons expressing tyrosine hydroxylase, the enzyme responsible for conversion of tyrosine to dopamine, from approximately 20% to 78% *(12)*. Consistent with this, these cultures produced greater amounts of dopamine and expressed higher levels of mRNA encoding proteins important for the development and function of dopamine neurons. Most important, the differentiated Nurr1-expressing cells were more effective in correcting abnormal behaviors when transplanted into rodents in which a Parkinson's disease-like syndrome had been induced *(12)*.

2.3 Endoderm Development

Endocrine glands such as the pancreas and thyroid are derived from endoderm. To date, differentiation of ES cells into cells of endodermal origin has proven more challenging than differentiation into cells of mesodermal or ectodermal origin. Among the transcription factors expressed in early endoderm layers from which the pancreas arises are Foxa1 and Foxa2 (previously referred to as hepatocyte nuclear factor 3α [HNF3α] and 3b [HNF3β], respectively) *(13–15)*. Mice with a null mutation of *Foxa2* fail to develop foregut and mid-gut endoderm *(16,17)*. When ES cells overexpressing HNF3β were differentiated in embryoid bodies, increased expression of genes present in endoderm-derived tissues, including albumin and the cystic fibrosis transmembrane conductance regulator, was observed, although genes expressed late in endoderm differentiation (e.g., α1-antitrypsin and phosphoenolpyruvate carboxykinase) were expressed either at low levels or not all *(15)*. Overexpression of HNF3α markedly increased cystic fibrosis transmembrane conductance regulator expression, but had only a small effect on albumin expression *(15)*. These studies demonstrate that expression of specific transcription factors is able to initiate a series of regulatory events that directs differentiation along an endoderm lineage. Such an approach may hold promise for facilitating the differentiation of ES cells into endocrine glands.

3. USE OF TRANSCRIPTION FACTORS TO DIRECT DIFFERENTIATION ALONG AN ENDOCRINE CELL LINEAGE

Examples of using transcription factors to direct the differentiation of stem cells along an endocrine lineage are more limited. To date, most effort has been directed toward the development of insulin-secreting cells, although this approach has also been used to generate cells capable of steroid hormone synthesis. These efforts are described in the following sections.

3.1. Insulin-Secreting Cells

Type 1 diabetes occurs secondary to the autoimmune-mediated destruction of insulin-producing β-cells in pancreatic islets. In contrast, insulin resistance is important in the development of type 2 diabetes, although β-cell dysfunction characterized by an inability to secrete adequate amounts of insulin to overcome insulin resistance also contributes to the pathogenesis of type 2 diabetes. Thus the development of insulin-secreting cells would provide an effective therapy for type 1 and, possibly, type 2 diabetes.

3.1.1. Pancreas Development

The molecular mechanisms of pancreatic development provide insight into the transcription factors needed to initiate the hierarchical cascade of gene expression that results in differentiation along an islet cell lineage. This knowledge will facilitate developing strategies to generate insulin-secreting cells from stem cells. The molecular and cellular mechanisms important for pancreatic development have been the subject of several recent reviews *(14,18–20)*. A brief overview is presented here.

Pancreatic islet development is a complex process dependent on multiple factors, including expression of a series of transcription factors important for cell differentiation and transmission of signals generated from surrounding mesenchyme and blood vessels. Differentiation of endoderm precursor cells into islets is controlled by a cascade of transcriptional events directed by a series of transcription factors that are expressed in a temporal and cell-specific pattern (Fig. 1). Expression of Pdx-1, a homeodomain protein, is important for early pancreatic development, because mice and humans homozygous for mutations in the *Pdx1* gene are apancreatic. Subsequently, neurogenin3 (ngn3) expression is important for the differentiation of pancreatic endocrine cell types. Null mutations of the *ngn3* gene abrogate islet development in mice *(21,22)*. Additional transcription factors, including NeuroD1/β 2 and Pax 6, also affect islet cell development, whereas Pax 4, Nkx2.2, and Nkx6.1 are important for β-cell development, although some of these factors also contribute to the differentiation of α, δ, or pancreatic polypeptide cells in islets. As indicated in Fig. 1, many of these transcription factors are expressed not only during development but also in differentiated adult islet cells.

3.1.2. Insulin-Secreting Cells From ES Cells

As described elsewhere (Chapter 8), protocols to induce the differentiation of ES cells into insulin-secreting cells have been developed *(23–25)*. To date, the efficiency of generating insulin-secreting cells using these protocols has been low, and the cells have, in general, been relatively hypofunctional compared with native islets. One approach to enhance the differentiation process has been to express transcription factors important in islet development.

The impact of constitutively expressing either Pdx-1 or Pax4 in ES cells was recently described *(26)*. Pdx-1 functions at multiple levels of pancreatic development. It is important not only for development of the exocrine and endocrine pancreas, but it is also important for maintaining the differentiated β-cell phenotype, as it regulates the expression of several genes important for β-cell function, including the genes that encode insulin, the glucose transporter GLUT2, and glucokinase *(14,18–20)*. Pax4 is a paired domain homeobox transcription factor that is important for committing endocrine precursor cells along the β- and δ-cell

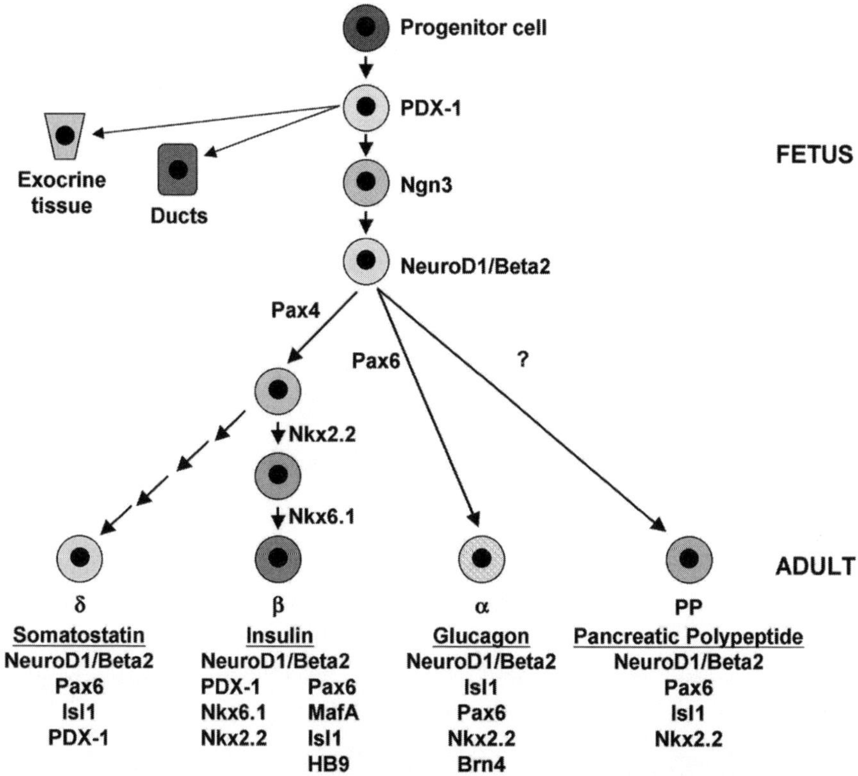

Fig. 1. Model for the role of transcription factors during islet differentiation. The proposed role for different transcription factors in islet differentiation is shown. For simplicity, the association of a single transcription factor with different developmental events is based on the timing of their expression or the timing of their predominant role in differentiation. Any given factor likely functions at multiple steps during differentiation, and expression of multiple factors is probably required at each step of differentiation. Also shown are differentiated adult islet cells. Below each cell is the hormonal product of that cell type and the transcription factors that are expressed in the differentiated adult δ, β, α, and pancreatic polypeptide cells.

lineage, because islets from mice with a null mutation of the Pax4 gene lack β and δ cells *(14,18–20)*. Three different approaches have been used to differentiate native ES cells and ES cells expressing either Pdx-1 or Pax4: (1) spontaneous differentiation in embryoid bodies followed by adherent culture in standard medium, (2) selection of nestin-positive cells and differentiation using a protocol similar to that described by Lumelsky et al. *(24)*, and (3) use of nestin-positive cells in histotypic culture that promotes the generation of spheroids *(26)*. In cells undergoing spontaneous differentiation, Pax4- and Pdx-1-expressing cells generally showed increased expression of genes encoding transcription factors and other proteins important for or characteristic of differentiated islet cell function. Moreover, the amount of insulin mRNA and percentage of cells expressing insulin was increased in the Pdx-1- and Pax4-expressing cells, although the impact of Pax4 was greater than that of Pdx-1. After the selection and differentiation of nestin-positive cells, approximately 80% of Pax4-expressing cells produced insulin. Growth of cells in histotypic culture resulted in spheroids containing cells with insulin-positive granules, albeit at a density lower than that present in adult β cells. When transplanted into diabetic mice, differentiated nestin-positive Pax4-expressing and wild-type ES cells were equally efficacious in restoring euglycemia. Thus expression of transcription factors important for β-cell development and differentiation augments the in vitro differentiation of ES cells into insulin-secreting cells, although the functional consequences in vivo remain unclear. One problem with the approach described previously is that transcription factor expression during development is dynamic. Indeed, Pax4 is important for β-cell differentiation during development, but it is essentially absent in adult murine β cells *(27)*. Pdx-1 expression is relatively uniform early in development, but is later heterogeneous with high levels in β cells and lower levels in undifferentiated precursor cells (19). Thus constitutive expression fails to reproduce the dynamic regulation of transcription factor expression characteristic of cellular differentiation.

3.1.3. Insulin-Secreting Cells From Tissue Stem Cells

An alternative approach to using ES cells is to redirect the differentiation of adult stem cells along an islet lineage. One means of accomplishing this has been to use cells of endodermal origin. This has been attempted using IEC-6 cells, which are immature rat intestinal stem cells that exhibit an undifferentiated morphology and limited expression of intestinal-specific genes *(28)*. Various approaches have been used to direct the differentiation of these cells into insulin-secreting cells. Stable and constitutive expression of Pdx-1 in IEC-6 cells caused them to assume an enteroendocrine cell phenotype capable of expressing serotonin, cholecystokinin, gastrin, and somatostatin *(29)*. To direct these cells along an islet cell lineage, the Pdx-1-expressing cells were subsequently treated with betacellulin *(30,31)*. Betacellulin is a member of the epidermal growth factor family of peptides that is expressed in adult and fetal pancreas, signals through the ErbB family of tyrosine kinase receptors, and stimulates the proliferation of multiple cell types, including β cells *(32,33)*. Several lines of evidence suggest that betacellulin plays a key role in islet cell proliferation or differentiation. Betacellulin enhances pancreatic regeneration after a 90% pancreatectomy by increasing β-cell proliferation and mass *(34)*. It also increases DNA synthesis in human fetal pancreatic epithelial cells and enhances β-cell development in fetal murine pancreatic explant cultures *(33,35)*. Treatment of PDX-1-expressing IEC-6 cells with betacellulin resulted in insulin expression and the formation of secretory granules. However, insulin secretion was neither glucose-dependent nor stimulated by arginine *(30,31)*. Among the transcription factors induced by betacellulin treatment was Isl-1. Isl-1 is an LIM homeodomain factor that is important early in pancreatic development and is expressed in pancreatic epithelium and mesenchyme surrounding the pancreas *(36)*. It is also expressed later in development in postmitotic endocrine cells and is present in mature islet cells *(36)*. Its role in islet function is unclear. Overexpression of Isl-1 in Pdx-1-expressing cells also resulted in insulin expression *(30,31)*. Transplantation of IEC-6 cells expressing both Pdx-1 and Isl-1 into diabetic rats transiently decreased the blood glucose level, although euglycemia was not restored *(30)*. These studies suggest that expressing specific transcription factors in tissue stem cells can redirect their differentiation along an islet lineage, but that additional factors will be needed to fully differentiate the cells.

Liver is a second endoderm-derived tissue that has been used as a source of cells that can be directed to differentiate into islets. Like pancreas, liver is derived from ventral endoderm, and both tissues express members of the hepatocyte nuclear family and exhibit glucose responsiveness *(37)*. Indeed, it has been suggested that there is an endodermal progenitor cell common to liver and pancreas *(38)*. In vivo expression of transcription factors has been used to differentiate liver cells into insulin-secreting cells *(37)*. Adenoviral-mediated expression of Pdx-1 has successfully generated insulin-producing cells in liver *(39,40)*. After expression of Pdx-1, liver produced not only insulin, but also other islet genes, including those encoding glucagon, somatostatin, and islet amyloid polypeptide. Expression of these genes, as well as the *Pdx1* gene, was prolonged as Pdx-1, insulin, and somatostatin expression was present 6–8 months after the initial infection. Glucagon expression was extinguished after about 4 months. Prolonged expression of Pdx-1, and presumably other islet proteins, appeared to be due to auto-induction of the native *Pdx1* gene by Pdx-1 expressed from the adenoviral vector *(40)*. After Pdx-1 expression, the insulin content of the liver was increased 10- to 30-fold, but this was still only 1.3–3% of the insulin content of pancreas *(40)*. Insulin produced by the liver was functional in that it was able to treat and prevent diabetes induced by streptozotocin, a β-cell toxin *(39,40)*. The cells producing insulin were distinct from those that produced glucagon and were localized in proximity to the central vein. Mature hepatocytes reside in this region of the liver, although, because only a small percentage of infected cells expressed insulin, only a small subpopulation of cells appears to be capable of transdifferentiation. The nature of these cells that undergo transdifferentiation is not clear.

A similar approach has been used to develop insulin-producing cells from epithelial progenitor cells derived from fetal liver *(41)*. These cells express markers of hepatocytes, bile ducts, and oval cells and are capable of differentiating into mature hepatocytes in vivo *(42)*. Oval cells are thought to represent hepatic stem cells *(43)*. Transduction of these progenitor cells with a lentivirus that constitutively expresses mRNA encoding Pdx-1 results in partial differentiation along an islet lineage *(41)*. Despite expression of Pdx-1, these cells continued to express hepatocyte markers, including glycogen, dipeptidyl peptidase IV, and γ-glutamyl transpeptidase. Autoinduction of the endogenous *Pdx1* gene was again evident, and some transcription factors present in adult β cells (e.g., NeuroD1, Nkx6.1) were also expressed, whereas others such as Nkx2.2 and Pax6 were absent *(41)*. Interestingly, neurogenin3, which is present in developing but not mature islets, was also present. Finally, insulin and the prohormone convertases PC1/3 and PC2 as well as islet amyloid polypeptide, glucagon, pancreatic polypeptide, and elastase were expressed. Thus proteins present in both the endocrine and exocrine pancreas were produced. It has not been established whether these different hormones and enzymes are coexpressed by the same or different cells. Importantly, these cells exhibit glucose-stimulated insulin secretion, albeit with a curve that is shifted to the right compared with native islets. This may reflect a lack of expression of GLUT2 and glucokinase and expression of only the Kir6.2 subunit of the ATP-sensitive potassium channel that is important for insulin secretion. Importantly, these cells appeared to secrete mature processed insulin and were able to reverse streptozotocin-induced diabetes.

In studies using an adenoviral vector capable of higher and more prolonged expression, in vivo Pdx-1 expression in the liver had a different effect. In this circumstance, insulin-producing cells were present, but cells exhibiting characteristics of exocrine cells, including expression of trypsin, were also present *(44,45)*. Interestingly, insulin and trypsin were coexpressed by the same cells, and the latter induced a severe hepatitis *(44,45)*. In contrast, use of this same adenoviral vector to express the transcription factor NeuroD1/Beta2 and betacellulin resulted in the formation of islet clusters capable of reversing streptozotocin-induced diabetes *(44,45)*. The islet-like clusters were, in general, localized immediately underneath the liver capsule. Thus the cells from which islet-like structures were generated appeared to be distinct from those in the proximity of the central vein that differentiated into insulin-secreting cells following Pdx-1 expression. After expression of NeuroD1 and betacellulin, glucagon, somatostatin, and pancreatic polypeptide were also present in the islet-like structures. Unlike native islets, individual cells in the islet-like structures produced multiple hormones. Other genes characteristic of mature islets were also expressed, including those encoding the prohormone convertases PC1/3 and

PC2 and the Kir6.2 and SUR1 subunits of the ATP-sensitive potassium channel *(44,45)*. Insulin granules were also present in the cells.

3.2. Steroidogenic Cells

Another endocrine gland susceptible to destruction by autoimmunity, infection, and bleeding is the adrenal gland. Because oral replacement of cortisol does not accurately reproduce the pattern of cortisol secretion by the native adrenal gland, the generation of adrenal cells from stem cells would be of therapeutic benefit.

The only transcription factor that has been expressed in ES cells to help direct differentiation along a steroidogenic cell lineage is steroidogenic factor 1 (SF-1) *(46)*. SF-1 is an orphan member of the steroid receptor superfamily (reviewed in *(47)*. It is expressed in a variety of tissues, including the adrenal cortex, testis (Sertoli cells), ovary (granulosa and theca cells), the placenta, and the pituitary and hypothalamus. During development, SF-1 is expressed in the urogenital ridge as early as embryonic day 9 in mice, and its role in the differentiation of steroidogenic tissues is demonstrated by the absence of adrenal glands and gonads in mice with a null mutation of the SF-1 gene *(48,49)*. In humans, mutations in SF-1 are associated with hypogonadism and hypoadrenalism *(47)*. Among the targets of SF-1 are the genes that encode the steroidogenic cytochrome P450 enzymes *(47)*.

Given the role of SF-1, it is not surprising that its expression in ES cells directs their differentiation toward a steroidogenic phenotype *(46)*. The morphology of ES cells stably transfected with a vector expressing SF-1 changes from birefringent spheres into flat, phase-dull sheets despite the continued presence of mouse embryo fibroblast feeder cells and leukemia inhibitory factor, both of which prevent ES cell differentiation. Among the factors known to induce steroidogenesis in steroidogenic cell lines are retinoic acid and cyclic adenosine 5′-monophosphate, which is the downstream effector of hormones such as adrenocorticotropic and luteinizing hormones. Treatment of the SF-1–expressing ES cells with a cyclic adenosine 5′-monophosphate analogue with or without retinoic acid markedly increased expression of the rate-limiting steroidogenic enzyme P450 side-chain cleavage ($P450_{scc}$), an effect not observed in native ES cells *(46)*. Moreover, in cells provided with 20α-hydroxycholesterol, a substrate for $P450_{scc}$, progesterone was synthesized in amounts proportional to the expression of $P450_{scc}$ mRNA. It is important to note that this change in cell phenotype occurred despite the continued presence of mouse embryo fibroblasts and leukemia inhibitory factor. Thus SF-1 expression is capable of initiating a program that converts ES cells into steroidogenic cells and may serve to augment the development of steroidogenic tissues from stem cells.

4. CONCLUSION

The studies described here indicate that transcription factor expression has the potential to direct or augment stem cell differentiation. As demonstrated, expression of a specific transcription factor can initiate a genetic program typically activated by inductive factors elaborated in vivo by surrounding tissues and cells, thus allowing differentiation to proceed in vitro. One of the problems with this approach, however, is that the constitutive expression of transcription factors is not able to reproduce the dynamic expression of transcription factors that is characteristic of the differentiation process. This may interfere with the final maturation of cells or alter cell function. Approaches that have been used to address this concern are using vectors (e.g., adenoviral vectors) in which expression is time-limited or vectors that allow inducible expression of the gene of interest. Clearly, expressing transcription factors in differentiating stem or progenitor cells will provide important insight into the genetic programs responsible for differentiation along specific cell lineages and has the potential to facilitate ongoing efforts to develop means to differentiate stem cells into specific hormone-secreting cells that will be available for cell replacement therapy.

REFERENCES

1. Kyba M, Daley GQ. Hematopoiesis from embryonic stem cells: lessons from and for ontogeny. Exp Hematol 2003;31:994–1006.
2. Payne KJ, Crooks GM. Human hematopoietic lineage commitment. Immunol Rev 2002;187: 48–64.
3. Kyba M, Perlingeiro RC, Hoover RR, Lu CW, Pierce J, Daley GQ. Enhanced hematopoietic differentiation of embryonic stem cells conditionally expressing Stat5. Proc Natl Acad Sci USA 2003;100(Suppl. 1):11904–11910.
4. Ihle JN. The Stat family in cytokine signaling. Curr Opin Cell Biol 2001;13:211–117.
5. Shuai K, Halpern J, ten Hoeve J, Rao X, Sawyers CL. Constitutive activation of STAT5 by the BCR-ABL oncogene in chronic myelogenous leukemia. Oncogene 1996;13:247–254.
6. Kyba M, Perlingeiro RC, Daley GQ. HoxB4 confers definitive lymphoid-myeloid engraftment potential on embryonic stem cell and yolk sac hematopoietic progenitors. Cell 2002;109:29–37.
7. Lee JE. Basic helix-loop-helix genes in neural development. Curr Opin Neurobiol 1997;7:13–20.
8. O'Shea KS. Neuronal differentiation of mouse embryonic stem cells: lineage selection and forced differentiation paradigms. Blood Cells Mol Dis 2001;27:705–712.
9. Wilson M, Koopman P. Matching SOX: partner proteins and co-factors of the SOX family of transcriptional regulators. Curr Opin Genet Dev 2002;12:441–446.
10. Pevny LH, Sockanathan S, Placzek M, Lovell-Badge R. A role for SOX1 in neural determination. Development 1998;125:1967–1978.
11. Lee SH, Lumelsky N, Studer L, Auerbach JM, McKay RD. Efficient generation of midbrain and hindbrain neurons from mouse embryonic stem cells. Nat Biotechnol 2000;18:675–679.
12. Kim JH, Auerbach JM, Rodriguez-Gomez JA, et al. Dopamine neurons derived from embryonic stem cells function in an animal model of Parkinson's disease. Nature 2002;418:50–56.

13. Ang SL, Wierda A, Wong D, et al. The formation and maintenance of the definitive endoderm lineage in the mouse: involvement of HNF3/forkhead proteins. Development 1993;119:1301–1315.
14. Chakrabarti SK, Mirmira RG. Transcription factors direct the development and function of pancreatic beta cells. Trends Endocrinol Metab 2003;14:78–84.
15. Levinson-Dushnik M, Benvenisty N. Involvement of hepatocyte nuclear factor 3 in endoderm differentiation of embryonic stem cells. Mol Cell Biol 1997;17:3817–3822.
16. Ang SL, Rossant J. HNF-3 beta is essential for node and notochord formation in mouse development. Cell 1994;78:561–574.
17. Weinstein DC, Ruiz i Altaba A, Chen WS, et al. The winged-helix transcription factor HNF-3 beta is required for notochord development in the mouse embryo. 1994;Cell 78:575–588.
18. Kemp DM, Thomas MK, Habener JF. Developmental aspects of the endocrine pancreas. Rev Endocr Metab Disord 2003;4:5–17.
19. Murtaugh LC, Melton DA. Genes, signals, and lineages in pancreas development. Annu Rev Cell Dev Biol 2003;19:71–89.
20. Jensen J. Gene regulatory factors in pancreatic development. Dev Dyn 2004;229:176–200.
21. Gradwohl G, Dierich A, LeMeur M, Guillemot F. neurogenin3 is required for the development of the four endocrine cell lineages of the pancreas. Proc Natl Acad Sci USA 2000;97:1607–1611.
22. Schwitzgebel VM, Scheel DW, Conners JR, et al. Expression of neurogenin3 reveals an islet cell precursor population in the pancreas. Development 2000;127:3533–3542.
23. Soria B, Roche E, Berna G, Leon-Quinto T, Reig JA, Martin F. Insulin-secreting cells derived from embryonic stem cells normalize glycemia in streptozotocin-induced diabetic mice. Diabetes 2000;49:157–162.
24. Lumelsky N, Blondel O, Laeng P, Velasco I, Ravin R, McKay R. Differentiation of embryonic stem cells to insulin-secreting structures similar to pancreatic islets. Science 2001;292:1389–1394.
25. Hori Y, Rulifson IC, Tsai BC, Heit JJ, Cahoy JD, Kim SK. Growth inhibitors promote differentiation of insulin-producing tissue from embryonic stem cells. Proc Natl Acad Sci USA 2002;99:16105–16110.
26. Blyszczuk P, Czyz J, Kania G, et al. Expression of Pax4 in embryonic stem cells promotes differentiation of nestin-positive progenitor and insulin-producing cells. Proc Natl Acad Sci USA 2003;100:998–1003.
27. Smith SB, Ee HC, Conners JR, German MS. Paired-homeodomain transcription factor PAX4 acts as a transcriptional repressor in early pancreatic development. Mol Cell Biol 1999;19: 8272–8280.
28. Quaroni A, May RJ. Establishment and characterization of intestinal epithelial cell cultures. Meth Cell Biol 1980;21B:403–427.
29. Yamada S, Kojima H, Fujimiya M, Nakamura T, Kashiwagi A, Kikkawa R. Differentiation of immature enterocytes into enteroendocrine cells by Pdx1 overexpression. Am J Physiol Gastrointest Liver Physiol 2001;281:G229–G236.
30. Kojima H, Nakamura T, Fujita Y, et al. Combined expression of pancreatic duodenal homeobox 1 and islet factor 1 induces immature enterocytes to produce insulin. Diabetes 2002;51:1398–1408.
31. Yoshida S, Kajimoto Y, Yasuda T, et al. PDX-1 induces differentiation of intestinal epithelioid IEC-6 into insulin-producing cells. Diabetes 2002;51:2505–2513.
32. Dunbar AJ, Goddard C. Structure-function and biological role of betacellulin. Int J Biochem Cell Biol 2000;32:805–815.
33. Huotari MA, Miettinen PJ, Palgi J, et al. ErbB signaling regulates lineage determination of developing pancreatic islet cells in embryonic organ culture. Endocrinology 2002;143:4437–4446.

34. Li L, Seno M, Yamada H, Kojima I. Promotion of beta-cell regeneration by betacellulin in ninety percent-pancreatectomized rats. Endocrinology 2001;142:5379–5385.
35. Demeterco C, Beattie GM, Dib SA, Lopez AD, Hayek A. A role for activin A and betacellulin in human fetal pancreatic cell differentiation and growth. J Clin Endocrinol Metab 2000;85:3892–3897.
36. Ahlgren U, Pfaff SL, Jessell TM, Edlund T, Edlund H. Independent requirement for ISL1 in formation of pancreatic mesenchyme and islet cells. Nature 1997;385:257–260.
37. Meivar-Levy I, Ferber S. New organs from our own tissues: liver-to-pancreas transdifferentiation. Trends Endocrinol Metab 2003;14:460–466.
38. Grompe M. Pancreatic-hepatic switches in vivo. Mech Dev 2003;120:99–106.
39. Ferber S, Halkin A, Cohen H, et al. Pancreatic and duodenal homeobox gene 1 induces expression of insulin genes in liver and ameliorates streptozotocin-induced hyperglycemia. Nat Med 2000;6:568–572.
40. Ber I, Shternhall K, Perl S, et al. Functional, persistent, and extended liver to pancreas transdifferentiation. J Biol Chem 2003;278:31950–1957.
41. Zalzman M, Gupta S, Giri RK, et al. Reversal of hyperglycemia in mice by using human expandable insulin-producing cells differentiated from fetal liver progenitor cells. Proc Natl Acad Sci USA 2003;100:7253–7258.
42. Malhi H, Irani AN, Gagandeep S, Gupta S. Isolation of human progenitor liver epithelial cells with extensive replication capacity and differentiation into mature hepatocytes. J Cell Sci 2002;115:2679–2688.
43. Petersen BE. Hepatic "stem" cells: coming full circle. Blood Cells Mol Dis 2001;27:590–600.
44. Chan L, Fujimiya M, Kojima H. In vivo gene therapy for diabetes mellitus. Trends Mol Med 2003;9:430–435.
45. Kojima H, Fujimiya M, Matsumura K, et al. NeuroD-betacellulin gene therapy induces islet neogenesis in the liver and reverses diabetes in mice. Nat Med 2003;9:596–603.
46. Crawford PA, Sadovsky Y, Milbrandt J. Nuclear receptor steroidogenic factor 1 directs embryonic stem cells toward the steroidogenic lineage. Mol Cell Biol 1997;17:3997–4006.
47. Parker KL, Rice DA, Lala DS, et al. Steroidogenic factor 1: an essential mediator of endocrine development. Recent Prog Horm Res 2002;57:19–36.
48. Sadovsky Y, Crawford PA, Woodson KG, et al. Mice deficient in the orphan receptor steroidogenic factor 1 lack adrenal glands and gonads but express P450 side-chain-cleavage enzyme in the placenta and have normal embryonic serum levels of corticosteroids. Proc Natl Acad Sci USA 1995;92:10939–10943.
49. Luo X, Ikeda Y, Parker KL. A cell-specific nuclear receptor is essential for adrenal and gonadal development and sexual differentiation. Cell 1994;77:481–490.

8 Generation of Islet-Like Structures From ES Cells

Nadya Lumelsky

Contents

1. INTRODUCTION

Type 1 and type 2 diabetes, though different diseases, both involve inadequate cell mass of insulin-producing β cells, the most abundant cell type of pancreatic islets of Langerhans. Insulin injections alleviate hyperglycemia in the majority of diabetic patients. However, insulin therapy cannot provide the finely tuned control of glucose homeostasis afforded by native pancreatic islets. As a result, diabetic patients commonly develop multiple life-threatening complications, such as cardiovascular and kidney disease, neuropathy, and blindness. Recent successes in pancreatic islet transplantation *(1)* fueled new hope that this procedure could significantly improve the quality of life for diabetic patients. Unfortunately, because the islets needed for transplantation are obtained from cadaveric donors only, few patients can receive this therapy. The shortage of islets could potentially be overcome by deriving them from alternative sources such as embryonic stem (ES) cells. This chapter will provide a review of the recent progress in generating islet-like hormone-producing cell clusters from ES cells.

From: *Contemporary Endocrinology: Stem Cells in Endocrinology*
Edited by: L. B. Lester © Humana Press Inc., Totowa, NJ

2. PANCREATIC ISLET: A MINIORGAN

The mammalian pancreas is composed of the exocrine acini, endocrine islets, and pancreatic ducts. The exocrine pancreas makes digestive enzymes, which are released into the digestive system through pancreatic ductal system. The islets, which constitute about 1–2% of the total pancreatic cell mass, are distributed in the exocrine tissue. They produce endocrine hormones required for utilization of glucose. An islet is not merely an aggregate of cells, but rather a miniorgan containing different hormone producing and other types of cells that participate in functionally important cell–cell interactions *(2)*. The hormone-producing cells of the islets are α, β, δ, and pancreatic polypeptide cells. They secrete glucagon, insulin, somatostatin, and pancreatic polypeptide, respectively. Insulin-producing β cells are the most abundant hormone-producing cell type of the islet. Among nonhormonal cell types, islets contain peripheral neurons, mesenchymal, and peri-islet Schwann cells as well as endothelial and smooth muscle cells that compose islet vasculature *(3,4)*. Also residing in the islets may be a population of pancreatic stem and progenitor cells *(5–7)*. It has been suggested that these stem and progenitor cells may have the capacity to generate new islet cells to compensate for cell loss during normal cell turnover and after islet damage. In view of the functional importance of islet complexity, it is likely that islet-like structures approximating this complexity would provide a better alternative to purified β cells for therapeutic applications.

3. ES CELLS, UNLIMITED EXPANSION CAPACITY, AND PLURIPOTENCY

Mouse ES cells were derived more than 20 years ago by Evans and Kaufman from the inner cells mass of the blastocyst stage embryo *(8)*. This pioneering work and that which followed identified several important properties of ES cells. It was found, in particular, that when cultured in vitro, these cells could be propagated indefinitely in the undifferentiated state. Also, they could shift from proliferation to differentiation mode by simple change of culture medium. The differentiated progeny of ES cells composes cells of all three germ layers: endoderm, mesoderm, and ectoderm. Moreover, it is thought that during in vitro differentiation, the ES cells may be recapitulating normal embryonic development *(9)*. When ES cells are injected into mouse blastocysts in vivo, they colonize all tissues of the developing embryo derived from this blastocyst, including the germ line *(10,11)*. This property, called pluripotency, has been used extensively for introducing specific mutations into the mouse genome. In line with their pluripotency, when injected into the immunodeficient nude mice, ES cells generate heterogeneous tumors called teratomas, which are composed of different cell types derived from all three germ layers *(12)*.

The capacity of ES cells for multilineage differentiation in vitro has attracted considerable interest after recent derivation of ES cells from human blastocysts *(13)*. It turns out that, similarly to mouse cells, human ES cells can be continually propagated in vitro in the undifferentiated state, and also induced to differentiate into multiple cell lineages. It was thus realized that human ES cells could potentially provide an unlimited source of transplantable material for treatment of a variety of diseases resulting from the loss of differentiated cell mass, including diabetes. However, before ES cell-based therapies will become practical reality, several important obstacles will need to be overcome. These are discussed in the following sections.

4. ES CELL DIFFERENTIATION: THE ISSUE OF CONTROL

One of the main difficulties in introducing ES cell technology into clinical practice stems from our insufficient knowledge of mechanisms that control the cell fate determination in ES cell cultures. Although several protocols have been proposed describing directed differentiation of ES cells into specific lineages, such as neural *(14,15)*, hematopoietic *(16)*, endothelial, smooth muscle *(17)*, and cardiac muscle *(18)*, in addition to the cell type of interest, a variety of other cell types are always generated in a typical ES cell culture. None of the existing differentiation protocols result in a fully controlled and uniform pattern of differentiation. Another complicating issue is a potential tumorigenicity of ES cell-derived cell populations. Because the undifferentiated ES cells are tumorigenic, even a small fraction of cells that escape differentiation would create a potential source of tumors after transplantation in vivo.

Several approaches to improve control over ES cell differentiation have been proposed. For example, because in vitro differentiation the ES cells is thought to approximate normal embryonic development, the exposure of ES cell cultures to growth factors, extracellular matrix components, and cell–cell interactions controlling normal development might promote and streamline the differentiation process *(19,20)*. Additionally, the enrichment of ES cell cultures with the desired cell type can be achieved using positive selection to purify the cells of interest, or using negative selection to remove the heterologous cells *(21,22)*. Such selection approaches can also aid in purging ES cell cultures from undifferentiated tumorigenic cells. Still another way to eliminate tumorigenic cells is to genetically modify the ES cells to express suicide genes: this would render them sensitive to specific pharmacological toxins *(23,24)*. It is likely that a combination of several approaches will be used in the future ES cell-based clinical protocols.

5. PANCREATIC SPECIFICATION AND DEVELOPMENT

The existing protocols of pancreatic differentiation of ES cells suffer from low efficiency, high rate of cell death accompanying differentiation, and experiment-to-experiment variability. It is widely recognized that improvement of these protocols will be critically dependent on the progress in our understanding of the mechanisms of pancreatic development. These mechanisms will be discussed briefly. Several recent reviews are available for in-depth discussion on this topic *(25–27)*.

The pancreas develops from endoderm, which in the mouse is specified to pancreatic fate around embryonic day 8.5 (E8.5). Although the exact mechanisms of pancreatic specification are still poorly understood, recent results obtained in the chicken system suggest that the signals responsible for patterning of the endoderm to become pancreas are generated by the mesoderm adjacent to the prospective pancreatic endoderm *(28)*. Moreover, the results of the same work indicate that several members of the transforming growth factor-β (TGF-β) superfamily may be responsible for this inducing activity. After specification, the pancreas develops in dorsal and ventral portions, which are in close proximity with two mesodermal tissues: notochord (dorsal pancreas) and cardiac mesoderm (ventral pancreas) (Fig. 1). The notochord and the cardiac mesoderm govern survival and differentiation of the pancreas by generating permissive signals produced by fibroblast growth factor (FGF), TGF-β, and the hedgehog families of growth factors *(29–31)*. In addition to pancreas, the neural tube contacts notochord during early embryogenesis. Consequently, the dorsal pancreas and the neural tube are exposed to the same signaling molecules. It is therefore not surprising that pancreatic and neural development are controlled by similar mechanisms *(25,32)*. Recently, it was established that, in addition to notochord, the dorsal aorta, which is another mesodermal derivative (and is juxtaposed with dorsal pancreas after its separation from the notochord), generates signals essential for pancreatic development *(33–35)*. Later in embryogenesis, the dorsal and ventral pancreatic buds fuse and the pancreas becomes embedded in the surrounding pancreatic mesenchyme. During the late stages of development, the mesenchyme serves as a source of signals for pancreatic growth, differentiation, and morphogenesis *(32)*.

Pancreatic transcription factors are outlined in Fig. 2A,B. It is noteworthy that the majority of pancreatic transcription factors are also involved in nervous system development *(25,27)*. Homeodomain transcription factors, Hb9 (encoded by Hlxb9 gene), PDX-1 (also called Ipf1), and a helix–loop–helix transcription factor, neurogenin3 (ngn3), are among the earliest markers of pancreatic development. Recently another transcription factor, Ptf1a/P48, was added to the list of essential transcriptional regulators of early pancreatic development *(34,36)*.

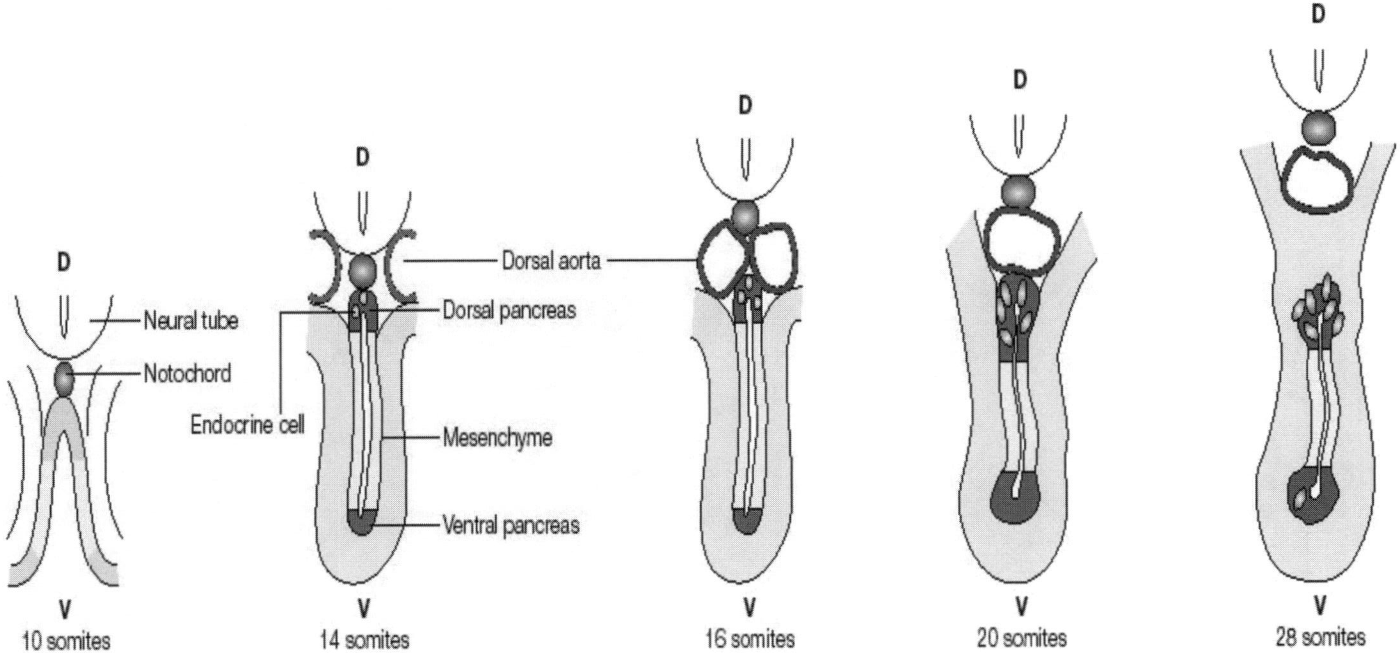

Fig. 1. Scheme of early steps of pancreatic organogenesis. Shown are cross sections through a mouse embryo at the level of developing pancreas. The 10-somite stage roughly corresponds to E8; the 28-somite stage, to E10 in mouse. D, dorsal; V, ventral. (From ref. *31*.)

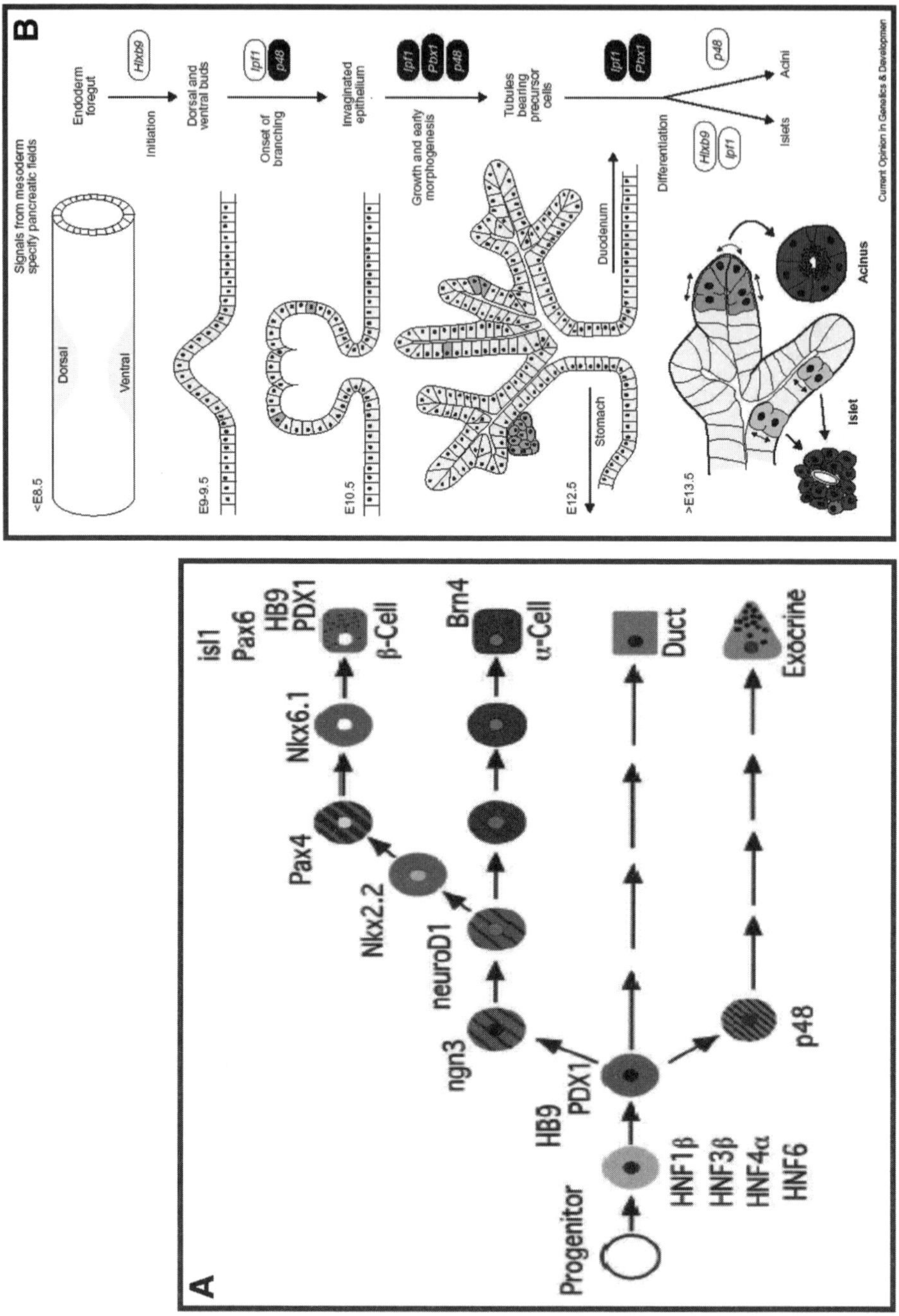
A
Progenitor
HNF1β
HNF3β
HNF4α
HNF6
HB9
PDX1
ngn3
neuroD1
Nkx2.2
Pax4
Nkx6.1
isl1
Pax6
HB9
PDX1
β-Cell
Brn4
α-Cell
Duct
p48
Exocrine
B
Signals from mesoderm specify pancreatic fields
<E8.5
Dorsal
Ventral
Endoderm foregut
Hlxb9
Initiation
Dorsal and ventral buds
E9-9.5
Ipf1
p48
Onset of branching
Invaginated epithelium
E10.5
Ipf1
Pbx1
p48
Growth and early morphogenesis
Tubules bearing precursor cells
E12.5
Stomach
Duodenum
Ipf1
Pbx1
Differentiation
Hlxb9
Ipf1
p48
Islets
Acini
>E13.5
Islet
Acinus
Current Opinion in Genetics & Development

Advances in microarray technology have allowed generation of global pancreatic transcriptional profiles *(37,38)*. Because this analysis allows simultaneous screening of many genes, it is expected that it will facilitate discovery of new elements regulating pancreatic development. This information will be essential for designing novel strategies for pancreatic differentiation of ES cells.

The existing protocols for generating endocrine hormone-producing cells from ES cells can be divided into two groups (Fig. 3). The first group of protocols takes advantage of the capacity of ES cells to undergo spontaneous pancreatic differentiation in fetal bovine serum-containing medium. These protocols may or may not include a genetic selection step to enrich the cultures for hormone-producing cells. Protocols of the second type attempt to induce pancreatic differentiation with specific growth factors and extracellular matrix molecules in defined culture medium.

6. SPONTANEOUS PANCREATIC DIFFERENTIATION OF ES CELLS

6.1. Differentiation Without Selection

Assady and coworkers *(39)* have studied a pattern of pancreatic gene expression during spontaneous differentiation of human ES cells. They carried out these experiments with two culture techniques: in suspension, where ES cells form simple cell aggregates called embryoid bodies (EBs), and in adherent cultures grown at high cell density. Insulin expression was examined by immunohistochemistry in the 19-day-old EBs. The authors have found insulin-expressing cells scattered throughout EBs and in small clusters within EBs. They also found that as the EBs matured, the number of insulin-expressing cells gradually increased. To characterize the insulin-producing cells further, they measured insulin secretion from 20- to 22-day-old EBs and 22- and 31-day-old, high-density adherent cultures in the presence of 5.5 m*M* and 25 m*M* glucose. Insulin secretion into the medium was detected in both types of cultures but this insulin secretion was not sensitive to increasing glucose concentration. The reverse transcriptase-polymerase chain reaction (RT-PCR) analysis of a panel of pancre-

Fig. 2. (*opposite page*) **(A)** A model depicting the role of islet transcription factors in endocrine differentiation during development. The proposed position for each transcription factor is based on its time of expression, functional role, or both. Although some transcription factors function at several steps, only single steps are shown for simplicity. (From ref. *27*.) **(B)** A model depicting the role of the key pancreatic transcription factors during different steps of pancreatic organogenesis. (From ref. *25*.) Ipf1 in **(B)** and Pdx1 in **(A)** designate the same transcription factor.

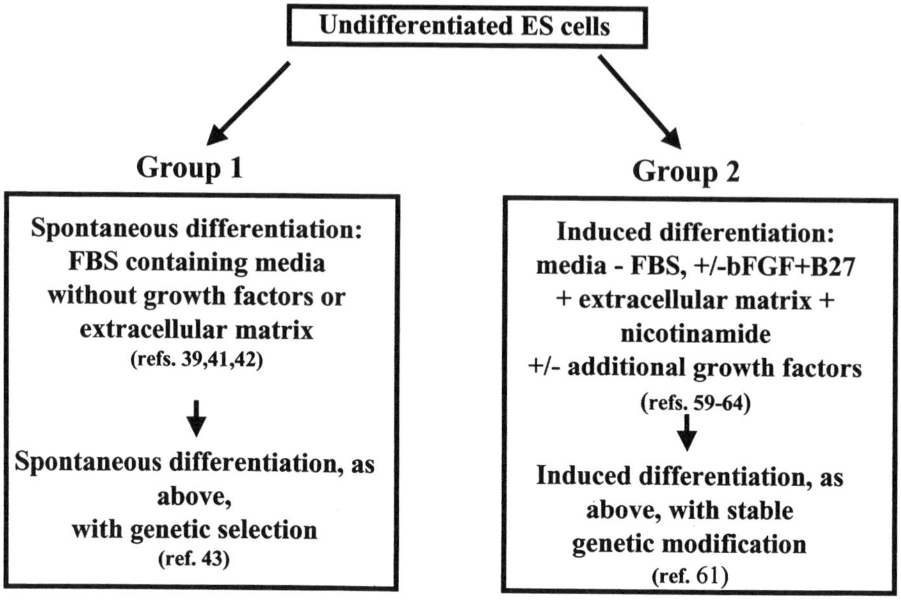

Fig. 3. Summary of current pancreatic endocrine differentiation protocols.

atic endocrine genes was also carried out. Their results showed that insulin, PDX-1, ngn3, glucokinase, and the β-cell-specific glucose transporter, Glut2, are all induced in EB and in adherent cultures. During the course of the culture, the expression of PDX-1 and ngn3 preceded expression of insulin, Glut2, and glucokinase. These results suggest that, similarly to normal pancreatic development, PDX-1 and ngn3 may control expression of insulin, Glut2, and glucokinase in human ES cell cultures *(40)*.

Shiroi et al. have investigated spontaneous pancreatic differentiation of mouse ES cells *(41)*. After EB formation, they platted the EBs on tissue culture plates to allow cell outgrowth. The authors used the zinc-chelating agent dithizone, which selectively stains β cells, to observe emergence of insulin-positive cell clusters. After 21 days, the first cells faintly stained with dithizone became visible; the intensity of staining became more apparent by day 28. Dithizone-positive cell clusters were isolated from the culture dishes and subjected to RT-PCR analysis for expression of several pancreatic markers; insulin, glucagon, pancreatic polypeptide, but not somatostatin expression was observed. Also, expression of Glut2, PDX-1, and a marker of endoderm, hepatocyte nuclear factor-3β, was detected.

Kahan at al. used a similar nonselective differentiation protocol to analyze the pattern of gene expression during pancreatic differentiation of mouse ES cells *(42)*. In agreement with the results of other investigators, they found progressive accumulation of hormone expressing cells in their cultures. The RT-PCR analysis showed that gene expression of several pancreatic transcription factors was induced in their cultures. They also found that early in the culture the majority of hormone positive cells coexpressed different islet hormones. At the end of the experiment, however, the majority of cells expressed only a single hormone. The authors argued that this dynamic pattern of gene expression might be a reflection of normal islet differentiation.

Although the results of these experiments shows that spontaneous pancreatic differentiation can occur in mouse and human ES cell cultures, the efficiency of this process is undoubtedly too low to be of practical value for generating significant numbers of hormone-producing cells.

6.2. Selection of Insulin-Producing Cells From Spontaneously Differentiating ES Cell Cultures

It has been shown previously that genetic selection against heterologous cell types generated during the course of spontaneous ES cell differentiation can result in enrichment for the cell types of interest. For example, this approach has been used to obtain purified cardiomyocyte- and neural-like cells from mouse ES cell cultures *(21,22)*. Soria and coworkers used a similar strategy to select insulin-producing cells from spontaneously differentiating mouse ES cells *(43)*. They introduced into the ES cells a plasmid conferring resistance to two antibiotics. The first antibiotic-resistance gene was under control of a constitutive promoter, and the second gene was under control of an insulin promoter. During the first stage of the culture the undifferentiated ES cells were selected for resistance to the first antibiotic. This allowed generation of a stable cell line in which every cell carried the plasmid. After this step, the ES cells were transferred into differentiation medium containing the second antibiotic. Because the second antibiotic resistance gene was under control of insulin promoter, only cells producing insulin survived this round of selection. The authors report that the insulin content of the ES cell-derived progeny obtained with this protocol was approximately 90% of the insulin content of normal mouse islets. When the insulin release in response to glucose and other agonists was measured in vitro, the cells showed stimulated release. Moreover, when implanted into diabetic mice, the insulin-producing cells normalized hyperglycemia. This normalization disappeared, however, after 12 weeks in about 40% of transplanted animals. The comparison of glucose tolerance of the transplanted animals with that of the nondiabetic controls showed that in the transplanted animals the plasma glucose levels were significantly elevated, and the recovery to normal glucose levels was delayed.

The results of this work suggest that spontaneous differentiation protocols combined with genetic selection can enrich ES cell cultures for insulin-producing cells. One can envision these protocols being further improved by placing the second antibiotic resistance gene under control of promoters active in pancreatic progenitor cells such as PDX-1 or ngn3 promoters. A potential advantage of such a strategy is that it would allow selection of a pancreatic cell type that, unlike terminally differentiated insulin producing cells, would have high proliferative potential *(44)*. These pancreatic progenitor cells could then be selectively expanded and induced to differentiate into insulin producing cells.

7. INDUCED PANCREATIC DIFFERENTIATION OF ES CELLS

7.1. Differentiation of ES Cells Into Endoderm

Although it has been shown that all three embryonic germ layers, including endoderm, are generated during spontaneous differentiation of human ES cells *(45)*, the efficiency of endodermal differentiation is known to be low. In the mouse ES cell system, the enhancement of endodermal differentiation has been accomplished using gene transfer of hepatocyte nuclear factor 3-α and 3-β genes, which are normally expressed early in the endoderm development *(46)*. This genetic modification resulted in the induction of several additional endodermal genes, such as albumin, α1-antitrypsin, transthyretin, and phosphoenolpyruvate carboxykinase.

7.2. Effect of Growth Factors on Pancreatic Differentiation of ES Cells

To investigate the potential of human ES cells for directed differentiation, Benvenisty and coworkers studied the effect of eight growth factors on expression of a wide panel of genes characteristic of ectoderm, mesoderm and endoderm *(47)*. In particular, they tested the effect of nerve growth factor, basic FGF (bFGF), activin-A, TGF-β1, hepatocyte growth factor, epidermal growth factor, bone morphogenetic protein 4, and retinoic acid. Among the endodermal genes, expression of albumin, α1-antitrypsin, amylase, PDX-1, and insulin were examined. When the gene expression of cells cultured without addition of growth factor were analyzed, only amylase mRNA was detected. In the nerve growth factor-treated cells, PDX-1 and amylase, but not insulin, were expressed. None of the other growth factors induced pancreatic gene expression in human ES cells. The authors argued that their work represented the first step toward directed differentiation of human ES cells. Achieving this goal will likely require a combination of growth factor treatment and specific cell-selection approaches.

7.3. Application of Neural Differentiation Protocols to Pancreatic Differentiation of ES Cells

Considering their different embryologic origins, the common developmental control mechanisms and overlap in gene expression between neural and pancreatic cells *(25,32)* are quite intriguing. In addition to common developmental mechanisms, there also exists a functional overlap between neural and pancreatic cells. For example, the release of insulin by β cells and release of neurotransmitters by neurons is accomplished through similar mechanisms *(48)*. These similarities suggest a common ancestral origin of insulin producing cells and neurons. In fact, in Drosophila, the ablation of insulin-producing cell clusters located in the brain leads to a phenotype reminiscent of diabetes *(49)*. Moreover, it has been reported that a patient with a brain tumor of a neuroectodermal origin has developed severe hypoglycemia resulting from insulin production by the tumor *(50)*.

Another common feature of pancreatic and neural cells is expression of a marker of neural progenitor cells, nestin *(51)*. It has been suggested that nestin might also be a marker of pancreatic progenitor cells *(7,52,53)*. Conclusive evidence for nestin as a marker of pancreatic progenitor cells is lacking *(54,55)*. In fact, this hypothesis has been challenged in several works, which claim mesenchymal rather than epithelial origin of nestin-expressing cells found in the pancreas *(31,56,57)*.

Because of the similarities between pancreatic and neural development, we hypothesized that the culture conditions, which are known to promote neural differentiation of ES cells *(14,15,19,58)*, might also promote their pancreatic differentiation. Therefore, we tested pancreatic phenotype of ES cell-derived progeny cultured under a modified ES cell neural differentiation protocol *(59)*. As outlined in Fig. 4, our basic protocol consisted of five stages: expansion of undifferentiated ES cells (stage 1), generation of EBs (stage 2), selective enrichment of cultures for nestin-expressing cells in fetal bovine serum-free medium (stage 3), expansion of a nestin-enriched cell population in the presence of bFGF (stage 4), and differentiation by bFGF withdrawal (stage 5). We have found that, in addition to neurons, cells expressing insulin, glucagon, and somatostatin are generated using this protocol. It is noteworthy that in these cultures the hormone-producing cells aggregate to form cell clusters with the insulin-positive cells in the interior and the glucagon- and somatostatin-positive cells at the periphery of the clusters. This cell arrangement is characteristic of normal rodent islets. As expected, neurons were also abundantly generated under these culture conditions. These neurons were primarily localized to the periphery of the islet-like clusters and were found in a close association with hormone-expressing cells. When tested in vitro for response to glucose and other insulin-release agonists and antagonists, the cell clusters secreted insulin in the medium in a

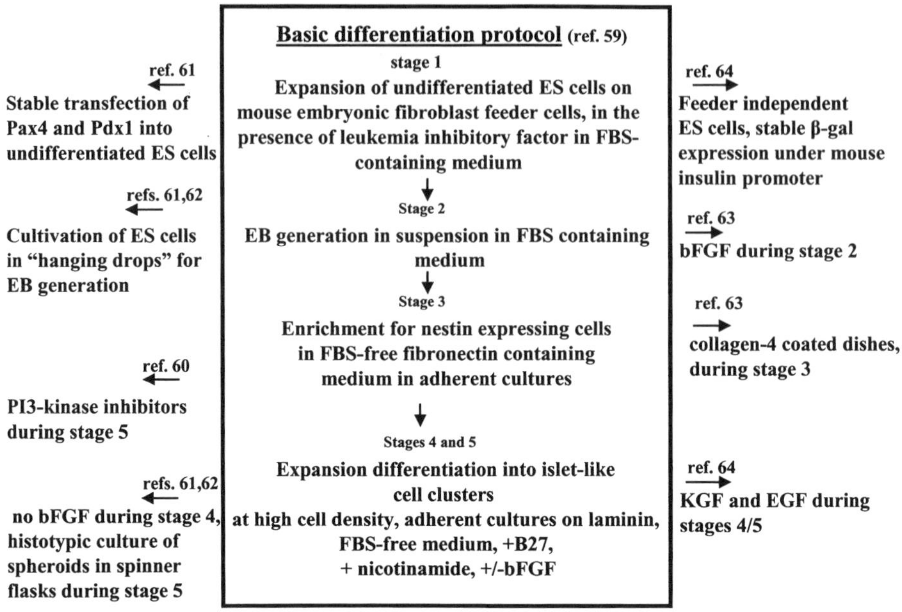

Fig. 4. Induced differentiation of mouse embryonic stem cells into islet-like cell clusters.

regulated fashion suggesting that they use physiologic mechanisms of insulin release.

These results indicate that neural differentiating protocols may be useful for enhancing pancreatic differentiation of ES cells. However, we have also found that the ES cell-derived cell clusters are lacking important features of normal islets. For example, expression of PDX-1 diminished rather than increased with culture maturation. These results may suggest that the ES cell-derived insulin-producing cells are unstable and could be undergoing apoptosis. Also, the insulin content of the clusters was significantly below that of the normal islets. Consequently, when injected into diabetic mice, the cell clusters, although surviving and continuing to express insulin, were unable to correct hyperglycemia.

As shown in Fig. 4, the basic ES cell differentiation protocol has been recently extended by several groups of investigators *(60–64)*. Hori et al. found that when an inhibitor of phosphoinositide 3-kinase (PI-3K) was added to stage 5 cultures, the endocrine cell number and the insulin content of mouse ES cell-derived islet-like clusters was increased. The insulin content of β-like cells obtained in the presence of the inhibitor was 30-fold greater than those in its absence. It was also found that the PI-3K inhibitor arrested proliferation of the ES cell-derived cell progeny. It was thus concluded that this treatment may help to eliminate potentially tumorigenic cells from the culture. When transplanted into diabetic mice, the PI-3K inhibitor-treated cells significantly reduced hyperglycemia. Importantly, the hyperglycemia reemerged after removal of the graft implying that the grafted cells were directly responsible for the observed effect.

To increase efficiency of the basic differentiation system, Blyszczuk et al. *(61,62)* constitutively overexpressed β-cell-specific transcription factors Pax4 and Pdx1 in the ES cells. Additionally, they cultured islet-like clusters (spheroids) in suspension in spinner bottles, referred to in this work as histotypic maturation. These modifications allowed generation of spheroids containing insulin-like secretory granules, as determined by electron microscopy. The spheroids were able to normalize glucose levels when transplanted under the kidney capsule of diabetic mice. However, the glucose normalization was monitored only for 2 weeks after transplantation. No nephrectomy was performed to test the direct contribution of the grafted cells to glucose normalization.

Moritoh et al. *(64)* have investigated pancreatic differentiation of mouse ES cells adapted to feeder-free growth in the undifferentiated state. To trace the insulin promoter activity during the course of the ES cell culture, the ES cells were stably transfected with the β galactosidase (LacZ) gene driven by a mouse insulin 2 promoter. The results of this work show that a proportion of cells have expressed insulin at the end of the culture. It was also found that insulin and LacZ immunoreactivity overlapped, and that Pdx1 is expressed in the nucleus of insulin producing cells. Unlike normal β-cells, however, insulin-producing cells coexpressed glucagon, suggesting that they might be developmentally immature. Nevertheless, the islet-like cell clusters had released insulin into the medium in response to glucose. On the basis of their results the authors argue that the ES cell-derived insulin producing cells are similar to normal β cells.

In still another modification of the basic protocol, Kim et al. *(63)* added bFGF into the culture medium during EB formation. The islet like clusters that were generated released insulin in response to glucose and, when implanted into diabetic nude mice, were able to reduce hyperglycemia for 20 days after cell implantation. As in the work of Moritoh et al. *(64)*, no graft removal was carried out. The electron microscopic analysis of the differentiated cells suggested the presence of insulin granules.

The recent report by Rajagopal et al. *(65)* has brought a considerable amount of controversy to the field of pancreatic differentiation of ES cells. The authors report that their attempt to reproduce the basic differentiation protocol *(59)* with human and mouse ES cells resulted in a significant insulin signal as detected by immunocytochemistry, but only in a minimal insulin gene expression signal as determined by RT-PCR. They argued that the absorption of insulin from the growth medium significantly contributed to the overall level of insulin, which they detected by immunocytochemistry. The authors caution that to avoid possible artifacts of insulin detection, several different methods should be combined for analysis of in vitro pancreatic differentiation of ES cell cultures.

Although it cannot be ruled out that a portion of insulin signal detected by several laboratories in the ES cell cultures could have resulted from insulin absorbed from the culture medium, this artifactual phenomenon is unlikely to be solely responsible for the observed pancreatic endocrine phenotype of these cultures. The finding by different independent groups of glucose-stimulated insulin secretion, expression of multiple islet genes by RT-PCR, alleviation of hyperglycemia in diabetic mice, and the insulin promoter-mediated LacZ expression strongly suggest that pancreatic differentiation indeed takes place in these ES cell cultures. The current debate is evidently a reflection of the rapid growth of this still young field. It is also a reflection of the relative inefficiency and the experiment-to-experiment variability of the existing protocols. These issues will certainly be resolved by further technical refinement driven by progress in our understanding of pancreatic development.

8. CONCLUSION

Human ES cells have the potential to provide a virtually unlimited supply of functional cells for treatment of different degenerative diseases, including type 1 and type 2 diabetes. Recent results suggest that ES cells can be directed to differentiate into pancreatic endocrine hormone producing cells. Furthermore, the differentiated cells can self-organize into cell clusters with structure and cellular composition approximating that of pancreatic islets. However, before application of ES cell-based technologies to treat diabetes can become a reality, a number of serious obstacles such as poor control and inefficiency of pancreatic differentiation, apoptosis of the differentiated cell populations, and potential tumorigenicity of the cells need to be overcome. Progress in this field will be highly dependent on advances in understanding normal pancreatic development and, especially, of the instructive signals responsible for commitment to endodermal and pancreatic fate. Additional improvements of pancreatic ES cell-based protocols will come from advances in cell-selection techniques. Discovery of new pancreatic markers, particularly, cell surface markers characteristic of different stages of pancreatic development, will facilitate these advances. Further, development of the new tissue-engineering strategies to improve generation and to extend survival of the organ-like islet structures will move the field forward.

REFERENCES

1. Shapiro AM, Lakey JR, Ryan EA, et al. Islet transplantation in seven patients with type 1 diabetes mellitus using a glucocorticoid-free immunosuppressive regimen. N Engl J Med 2000;343:230–238.

2. Kanno T, Gopel SO, Rorsman P, Wakui M. Cellular function in multicellular system for hormone-secretion: electrophysiological aspect of studies on alpha-, beta- and delta-cells of the pancreatic islet. Neurosci Res 2002;42:79–90.
3. Sunami E, Kanazawa H, Hashizume H, Takeda M, Hatakeyama K, Ushiki T. Morphological characteristics of Schwann cells in the islets of Langerhans of the murine pancreas. Arch Histol Cytol 2001;64:191–201.
4. Teitelman G, Guz Y, Ivkovic S, Ehrlich M. Islet injury induces neurotrophin expression in pancreatic cells and reactive gliosis of peri-islet Schwann cells. J Neurobiol 1998;34:304–318.
5. Bonner-Weir S, Sharma A. Pancreatic stem cells. J Pathol 2002;197:519–526.
6. Lechner A, Habener JF. Stem/progenitor cells derived from adult tissues: potential for the treatment of diabetes mellitus. Am J Physiol Endocrinol Metab 2003;284:E259–E266.
7. Lechner A, Leech CA, Abraham EJ, Nolan AL, Habener JF. Nestin-positive progenitor cells derived from adult human pancreatic islets of Langerhans contain side population (SP) cells defined by expression of the ABCG2 (BCRP1) ATP-binding cassette transporter. Biochem Biophys Res Commun 2002;293:670–674.
8. Evans MJ, Kaufman MH. Establishment in culture of pluripotential cells from mouse embryos. Nature 1981;292:154–156.
9. Keller GM. In vitro differentiation of embryonic stem cells. Curr Opin Cell Biol 1995;7:862–869.
10. Rosenthal N. Prometheus's vulture and the stem-cell promise. N Engl J Med 2003;349:267–274.
11. Loebel DA, Watson CM, De Young RA, Tam PP. Lineage choice and differentiation in mouse embryos and embryonic stem cells. Dev Biol 2003;264:1–14.
12. Rossant J, Papaioannou VE. The relationship between embryonic, embryonal carcinoma and embryo-derived stem cells. Cell Differ 1984;15:155–161.
13. Thomson JA, Itskovitz-Eldor J, Shapiro SS, et al. Embryonic stem cell lines derived from human blastocysts. Science 1998;282:1145–1147.
14. Okabe S, Forsberg-Nilsson K, Spiro AC, Segal M, McKay RD. Development of neuronal precursor cells and functional postmitotic neurons from embryonic stem cells in vitro. Mech Dev 1996;59:89–102.
15. Lee SH, Lumelsky N, Studer L, Auerbach JM, McKay RD. Efficient generation of midbrain and hindbrain neurons from mouse embryonic stem cells. Nat Biotechnol 2000;18:675–679.
16. Wiles MV, Keller G. Multiple hematopoietic lineages develop from embryonic stem (ES) cells in culture. Development 1991;111:259–267.
17. Yamashita J, Itoh H, Hirashima M, et al. Flk1-positive cells derived from embryonic stem cells serve as vascular progenitors. Nature 2000;408:92–96.
18. Boheler KR, Czyz J, Tweedie D, Yang HT, Anisimov SV, Wobus AM. Differentiation of pluripotent embryonic stem cells into cardiomyocytes. Circ Res 2002;91:189–201.
19. Kim JH, Auerbach JM, Rodriguez-Gomez JA, et al. Dopamine neurons derived from embryonic stem cells function in an animal model of Parkinson's disease. Nature 2002;418:50–56
20. Czyz J, Wobus A. Embryonic stem cell differentiation: the role of extracellular factors. Differentiation 2001;68:167–174.
21. Klug MG, Soonpaa MH, Koh GY, Field LJ. Genetically selected cardiomyocytes from differentiating embryonic stem cells form stable intracardiac grafts. J Clin Invest 1996;98:216–224.
22. Li M, Pevny L, Lovell-Badge R, Smith A. Generation of purified neural precursors from embryonic stem cells by lineage selection. Curr Biol 1998;8:971–974.
23. Fareed MU, Moolten FL. Suicide gene transduction sensitizes murine embryonic and human mesenchymal stem cells to ablation on demand—a fail-safe protection against cellular misbehavior. Gene Ther 2002;9:955–962.

24. Schuldiner M, Itskovitz-Eldor J, Benvenisty N. Selective ablation of human embryonic stem cells expressing a "suicide" gene. Stem Cells 2003;21:257–265.
25. Kim SK, MacDonald RJ. Signaling and transcriptional control of pancreatic organogenesis. Curr Opin Genet Dev 2002;12:540–547.
26. Kumar M, Melton D. Pancreas specification: a budding question. Curr Opin Genet Dev 2003;13:401–407.
27. Wilson ME, Scheel D, German MS. Gene expression cascades in pancreatic development. Mech Dev 2003;120:65–80.
28. Kumar M, Jordan N, Melton D, Grapin-Botton A. Signals from lateral plate mesoderm instruct endoderm toward a pancreatic fate. Dev Biol 2003;259:109–122.
29. Kim SK, Hebrok M, Melton DA. Notochord to endoderm signaling is required for pancreas development. Development 1997;124:4243–4252.
30. Zaret KS. Hepatocyte differentiation: from the endoderm and beyond. Curr Opin Genet Dev 2001;11:568–574.
31. Edlund H. Pancreatic organogenesis—developmental mechanisms and implications for therapy. Nat Rev Genet 2002;3:524–532.
32. Slack JM. Developmental biology of the pancreas. Development 1995;121:1569–1580.
33. Lammert E, Cleaver O, Melton D. Induction of pancreatic differentiation by signals from blood vessels. Science 2001;294:564–567.
34. Yoshitomi H, Zaret KS. Endothelial cell interactions initiate dorsal pancreas development by selectively inducing the transcription factor Ptf1a. Development 2004;131:807–817.
35. Lammert E, Cleaver O, Melton D. Role of endothelial cells in early pancreas and liver development. Mech Dev 2003;120:59–64.
36. Kawaguchi Y, Cooper B, Gannon M, Ray M, MacDonald RJ, Wright CV. The role of the transcriptional regulator Ptf1a in converting intestinal to pancreatic progenitors. Nat Genet 2002;32:128–134.
37. Chiang MK, Melton DA. Single-cell transcript analysis of pancreas development. Dev Cell 2003;4:383–393.
38. Gu G, Wells JM, Dombkowski D, Preffer F, Aronow B, Melton DA. Global expression analysis of gene regulatory pathways during endocrine pancreatic development. Development 2004;131:165–179.
39. Assady S, Maor G, Amit M, Itskovitz-Eldor J, Skorecki KL, Tzukerman M. Insulin production by human embryonic stem cells. Diabetes 2001;50:1691–1697.
40. Schwitzgebel VM, Scheel DW, Conners JR, et al. Expression of neurogenin3 reveals an islet cell precursor population in the pancreas. Development 2000;127:3533–3542.
41. Shiroi A, Yoshikawa M, Yokota H, et al. Identification of insulin-producing cells derived from embryonic stem cells by zinc-chelating dithizone. Stem Cells 2002;20:284–292.
42. Kahan BW, Jacobson LM, Hullett DA, et al. Pancreatic precursors and differentiated islet cell types from murine embryonic stem cells: an in vitro model to study islet differentiation. Diabetes 2003;52:2016–2024.
43. Soria B, Roche E, Berna G, Leon-Quinto T, Reig JA, Martin F. Insulin-secreting cells derived from embryonic stem cells normalize glycemia in streptozotocin-induced diabetic mice. Diabetes 2000;49:157–162.
44. Soria B. In-vitro differentiation of pancreatic beta-cells. Differentiation 2001;68:205–219.
45. Drukker M, Katz G, Urbach A, et al. Characterization of the expression of MHC proteins in human embryonic stem cells. Proc Natl Acad Sci USA2002; 99:9864–9569.

46. Levinson-Dushnik M, Benvenisty N. Involvement of hepatocyte nuclear factor 3 in endoderm differentiation of embryonic stem cells. Mol Cell Biol 1997;17:3817–3822.
47. Schuldiner M, Yanuka O, Itskovitz-Eldor J, Melton DA, Benvenisty N. From the cover: effects of eight growth factors on the differentiation of cells derived from human embryonic stem cells. Proc Natl Acad Sci USA 2000;97:11307–11312.
48. Komatsu M, Yokokawa N, Takeda T, Nagasawa Y, Aizawa T, Yamada T. Pharmacological characterization of the voltage-dependent calcium channel of pancreatic B-cell. Endocrinology 1989125:2008–2014.
49. Rulifson EJ, Kim SK, Nusse R. Ablation of insulin-producing neurons in flies: growth and diabetic phenotypes. Science 2002;296:1118–1120.
50. Nakamura T, Kishi A, Nishio Y, et al. Insulin production in a neuroectodermal tumor that expresses islet factor-1, but not pancreatic-duodenal homeobox 1. J Clin Endocrinol Metab 2001;86:1795–1800.
51. Lendahl U, Zimmerman LB, McKay RD. CNS stem cells express a new class of intermediate filament protein. Cell 1990;60:585–595.
52. Zulewski H, Abraham EJ, Gerlach MJ, et al. Multipotential nestin-positive stem cells isolated from adult pancreatic islets differentiate ex vivo into pancreatic endocrine, exocrine, and hepatic phenotypes. Diabetes 2001;50:521–533.
53. Abraham EJ, Leech CA, Lin JC, Zulewski H, Habener JF. Insulinotropic hormone glucagon-like peptide-1 differentiation of human pancreatic islet-derived progenitor cells into insulin-producing cells. Endocrinology 2002;143:3152–3161.
54. Delacour A, Nepote V, Trumpp A, Herrera PL. Nestin expression in pancreatic exocrine cell lineages. Mech Dev 2004;121:3–14.
55. Esni F, Stoffers DA, Takeuchi T, Leach SD. Origin of exocrine pancreatic cells from nestin-positive precursors in developing mouse pancreas. Mech Dev 2004;121:15–25.
56. Selander L, Edlund H. Nestin is expressed in mesenchymal and not epithelial cells of the developing mouse pancreas. Mech Dev 2002;113:189–192.
57. Lardon J, Rooman I, Bouwens L. Nestin expression in pancreatic stellate cells and angiogenic endothelial cells. Histochem Cell Biol 2002;117:535–540.
58. Bain G, Kitchens D, Yao M, Huettner JE, Gottlieb DI. Embryonic stem cells express neuronal properties in vitro. Dev Biol 168:1995;342–357.
59. Lumelsky N, Blondel O, Laeng P, Velasco I, Ravin R, McKay R. Differentiation of embryonic stem cells to insulin-secreting structures similar to pancreatic islets. Science 2001;292:1389–1394.
60. Hori Y, Rulifson IC, Tsai BC, Heit JJ, Cahoy JD, Kim SK. Growth inhibitors promote differentiation of insulin-producing tissue from embryonic stem cells. Proc Natl Acad Sci USA 2002;99:16105–16110.
61. Blyszczuk P, Czyz J, Kania G, et al. Expression of Pax4 in embryonic stem cells promotes differentiation of nestin-positive progenitor and insulin-producing cells. Proc Natl Acad Sci USA 2003;100:998–1003.
62. Kania G, Blyszczuk P, Czyz J, Navarrete-Santos A, Wobus AM. Differentiation of mouse embryonic stem cells into pancreatic and hepatic cells. Methods Enzymol 2003;365:287–303.
63. Kim D, Gu Y, Ishii M, et al. In vivo functioning and transplantable mature pancreatic islet-like cell clusters differentiated from embryonic stem cell. Pancreas 2003;27:e34–e41.
64. Moritoh Y, Yamato E, Yasui Y, Miyazaki S, Miyazaki J. Analysis of insulin-producing cells during in vitro differentiation from feeder-free embryonic stem cells. Diabetes 2003;52:1163–1168.
65. Rajagopal J, Anderson WJ, Kume S, Martinez OI, Melton DA. Insulin staining of ES cell progeny from insulin uptake. Science 2003;299:363.

9 The Therapeutic Potential of Liver Repopulation for Metabolic or Endocrine Disorders

Sanjeev Gupta

CONTENTS

1. INTRODUCTION

Liver repopulation with transplanted cells should be of significant interest for multiple genetic and acquired disorders. The regenerative potential of liver cells offers many opportunities for genetic manipulations and cell transplantation research. The general consideration is that use of mature hepatocytes or stem/progenitor cells for this purpose will provide effective ways to ameliorate specific diseases. Recent progress in various aspects of liver-directed cell therapy has been highly promising. For instance, it has become clear that transplanted cells can engraft efficiently and proliferate under suitable conditions to repopulate significant portions of the liver. Moreover, specific disorders can be corrected by hepatocyte transplantation. Also, genetic manipulation of cells before transplantation offers further opportunities for treating diseases. However, a variety of relevant issues still need to be resolved, including the types of cells that will be most efficacious for clinical applications, effective ways to cryopreserve cells for use at short notice, and abrogation of allograft rejection by nontoxic means. Contemplating liver-directed cell therapy for major endocrine disorders

From: *Contemporary Endocrinology: Stem Cells in Endocrinology*
Edited by: L. B. Lester © Humana Press Inc., Totowa, NJ

such as type 1 diabetes mellitus requires identification of suitable cells that could be modified to induce regulated hormone or enzyme expression. Recent studies suggest that stem/progenitor cell populations isolated from the fetal human liver will be effective for this purpose. Of course, advances in stem cell biology raise hopes for generating alternative sources of cells in view of the limited supply of adult human organs, which should further facilitate applications of liver cell therapy.

2. GENERAL CONSIDERATIONS REGARDING THE BIOLOGY OF LIVER CELLS

The liver shares its origin with the pancreas and arises from the foregut endoderm *(1,2)*. In humans, the embryonic liver appears after 4 weeks of gestation and rapidly assumes the eventual structure of the adult organ, such that by 14 weeks of gestation, the acinar structure becomes established and bile is produced. Studies in mice indicate that the embryonic liver and pancreas develop through discrete phases, including a period in which primitive cells are first "specified" via the activation of master transcription factors, such as hepatocyte nuclear factor (HNF)-3, and then undergo "differentiation" along various cell lineages *(2)*. In parallel, the development of stromal cells, which arise from primitive cardiac mesoderm (liver) or notochord (pancreas) and, especially of endothelial cells originating from the septum transversum (liver) or dorsal aorta (pancreas), is critical during this stage *(3)*. A variety of soluble extracellular signals, including vascular endothelial growth factor, hepatocyte growth factor, and bone morphogenic protein, which emanate from primitive endothelial cells, play major roles in liver and pancreas development during this stage *(1,2)*. Activation of intracellular transcription factor signals helps complete cell lineage advancement (e.g., coordinate activity of HNF-4) and HNF-1α promotes hepatocytic differentiation, whereas HNF-6 activation promotes ductal cell differentiation *(4)*. Ways have been developed to expand hepatic stem cells from cultures of embryonic liver explants *(5)*. Such efforts could potentially lead to the expansion of relevant human cell populations for cell therapy.

A significant feature of the developing liver concerns its major role in extramedullary hematopoiesis until birth. This requires the active coexistence of stem/progenitor cell populations that simultaneously generate hepatoblasts and hematopoietic cells *(6)*. Immature fetal liver cells exhibit unique gene expression profiles, including expression of the oncofetal marker, α-fetoprotein, which is rapidly replaced by albumin expression following birth *(7,8)*. Moreover, the prevalence of hepatic stem/progenitor cells shows a remarkable decline after birth and declines further as an individual becomes older, which is relevant for choosing donor organs *(9)*.

In the adult liver, hepatocytes constitute approximately 60% of liver cells, followed by sinusoidal endothelial cells, which constitute approximately 25% of liver cells. Less prevalent liver cell types include bile duct cells, hepatic stellate cells—which store vitamin A and possess neuroregulatory functions—and Kupffer cells, which are resident macrophages *(10)*. The liver acinus is arranged in a complex fashion, in which hepatocytes in single cell-thick plates are separated from sinusoidal blood by endothelial cells. Hepatic stellate cells exist in the space of Disse (between hepatocytes and endothelial cells), whereas Kupffer cells are situated within the hepatic sinusoids adjacent to endothelial cells. The cross-talk between these cell types helps maintain liver function and appropriate responses to infections, toxins, and injuries.

The regenerative response of the liver after partial hepatectomy has been highly studied *(11,12)*. During this process, hepatocytes represent the major cell compartment that is recruited to replenish the liver mass. In the normal liver, hepatocytes exhibit little or no proliferative activity with evidence of DNA synthesis in less than 1 per 1000 cells. On the other hand, after partial hepatectomy in rodents, most hepatocytes undergo one to three rounds of DNA synthesis within 3 days. Furthermore, under suitable conditions, hepatocytes isolated from adult rodent livers are capable of undergoing more than 80 cell divisions after cell transplantation, which represents a stem cell-like property *(13)*. However, in contrast with this property in vivo, mature hepatocytes are exceedingly difficult to propagate in vitro. Recently, the telomere hypothesis has been invoked in an effort to understand the regulation of liver growth control *(14)*. The concept implies that with cell division, telomere length shortens progressively, until a critical point is reached, beyond which replicative senescence occurs. Analysis of the consequences of telomere shortening in mutant animals and humans established that hepatocytes with shortened telomeres are unable to proliferate effectively and this increases susceptibility to liver injury *(15,16)*. On the other hand, reconstitution of telomerase activity in progenitor human liver cells imparted an indefinite replication capacity to the cells *(17)*.

The adult liver harbors stem/progenitor cells that are not obvious in the normal liver but become activated under certain types of carcinogenic, toxic, or viral liver injuries *(18)*. A prototype of such cells was designated "oval cells" because of the oval shape of cell nuclei *(12,19)*. Similar types of cells have been isolated from the ductal regions of the adult pancreas *(20,21)*. Oval cells can exhibit multilineage gene expression, including genes expressed in hepatocytes, bile duct cells, and hematopoietic cells, and possess the capacity to differentiate along both hepatocytic and biliary lineages *(22–24)*. Moreover, oval cells differentiate along even nonhepatic lineages (e.g., cardiomyocytes) and begin to express insulin under suitable context *(25)*. Whether oval cells in the adult liver represent remnants of stem/progenitor cells in the fetal liver is unknown. Nonetheless, the fetal mouse liver contains cell populations characterized by specific antigen expression (e.g., CD49 and CD29), and these cells form colonies in culture and differentiate into mature hepatocytes, as do other cell types (e.g., intestinal cells) after transplantation in animals *(26,27)*.

Finally, considerable interest has recently been generated by studies of extrahepatic stem cells. These include hematopoietic and mesenchymal stem cells derived from the bone marrow, peripheral blood or umbilical cord blood, and embryonic stem (ES) cells *(18)*. Whether hematopoietic stem cells could generate liver and pancreatic cells has excited considerable interest because such cells can be readily obtained. Petersen et al. initially demonstrated that cells derived from the bone marrow differentiated into hepatocytes *(28)*. These observations were extended by studies in the mouse and humans, where evidence was obtained for the origin of liver cells from donor hematopoietic cells *(29–34)*. On the other hand, hematopoietic stem cells did not show the capacity to generate oval cells *(35)*. Also, the overall efficiency by which hematopoietic stem cells generated hepatocytes was extremely low, such that less than 10 hepatocytes in an entire mouse liver were thought to originate from donor hematopoietic cells *(36)*, although such cells could repopulate most of the liver in the presence of suitable chronic injury *(32)*. In additional studies, bone marrow-derived mouse stem cells were found to produce hepatocytes by fusing with existing liver cells, including development of aneuploid cells, which raises the possibility of oncogenic perturbations *(37,38)*. Similar findings of cell fusion have not been observed in studies of human hematopoietic stem cells transplanted into mice *(39)*, so the overall potential of hematopoietic stem cells in liver-directed cell therapy is quite uncertain.

Insights into how human ES cells could be differentiating along hepatic lineages are limited, although some success has been achieved in generating hepatocyte-like cells by manipulating cultured ES cells both in vitro and in vivo *(40–44)*. Embryoid bodies derived from ES cells showed albumin and α-fetoprotein expression and capacity to synthesize urea, which represent properties of hepatocytes. Also, transplantation of hepatocytes derived from ES cells into chemically damaged mouse liver showed that the cells could engraft in the liver. Therefore, in principle, ES cells provide opportunities for liver-directed cell therapy.

3. MECHANISMS OF CELL ENGRAFTMENT AND PROLIFERATION IN THE LIVER

The requirements for cell therapy include an ability to demonstrate that transplanted cells can engraft and create a therapeutic mass in the liver. In principle, cells could be transplanted into the liver by injection into the portal vein or its tributaries, including by intrasplenic puncture, which leads to the deposition of cells into hepatic sinusoids *(45)*. Injection of cells into the hepatic artery or splenic artery is not as effective and may produce infarcts in organs because of vascular occlusions by cells *(46)*. Similarly, injection of cells directly into the liver parenchyma is ineffective and could be hazardous with embolic complications if cells enter the hepatic veins and thus pulmonary capillaries. Also, liver cells do not survive well in arterial beds compared with low-flow beds, such as in hepatic or splenic sinusoids.

When cells do enter hepatic sinusoids, a cascade of events occurs, which eventually leads to the integration of transplanted cells in the liver parenchyma. These cell engraftment events have been summarized in working models and offer multiple ways to manipulate the process *(47)* (Fig. 1). An initial process concerns entrapment of transplanted cells in hepatic sinusoids if cells are larger in size than sinusoids, which are 6–9 μm in diameter. Although deposition of transplanted cells in hepatic sinusoids causes microcirculatory perturbations and portal hypertension, these abnormalities are transient and resolve within a few hours *(48,49)*. However, these changes are sufficient for inducing hepatic ischemia and activating Kupffer cell responses, which are extremely sensitive to such perturbations *(49,50)*. Kupffer cells are known to release multiple cytokines and chemokines capable of affecting several cell types, including transplanted hepatocytes themselves. For instance, activated Kupffer cells and phagocytes clear a significant fraction of transplanted hepatocytes *(50)*. On the other hand, Kupffer cells help permeabilize hepatic endothelial cells, which assists the entry of transplanted cells into the liver parenchyma *(51)*. The deleterious Kupffer cell response can be inhibited with suitable chemicals and this leads to significant improvement in transplanted cell engraftment *(50)*. Also, use of antagonists to block specific cytokines released by Kupffer cells is helpful in decreasing the initial loss of transplanted cells. Moreover, treatment of animals with vasodilatory drugs, such as nitroglycerin, can prevent hepatic sinusoidal ischemia and improve cell engraftment *(49)*.

The endothelial cell plays a central role in directing engraftment of transplanted cells. Adherence of transplanted hepatocytes to the hepatic endothelium requires adhesion molecules, which helps in the "homing" of cells into the liver parenchyma. Similar cell adhesion mechanisms appear relevant in the homing of stem cells in the liver and other organs. Modulation of cell surface-associated extracellular matrix receptors, particularly hepatic integrins and their fibronectin receptor ligands on endothelial cells, play significant roles in directing cell engraftment in the liver *(52)*. The process of cell entry into the space of Disse requires physical disruption of the endothelial barrier *(51)*. This process is facilitated by early activation of hepatic stellate cells, which are capable of releasing multiple soluble factors, including vascular endothelial growth factor, which permeabilizes

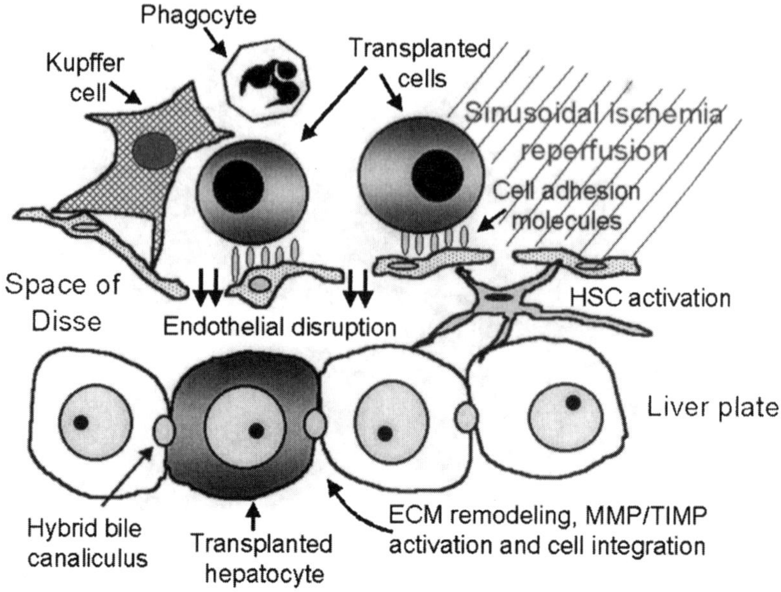

Fig. 1. Mechanisms regulating cell engraftment and proliferation in the liver. The working model depicts how deposition of transplanted cells activates multiple events in the liver. Among the earliest events is the onset of sinusoidal ischemia-reperfusion resulting from occlusion of blood flow in proximal sinusoids by cell emboli. Simultaneously, transplanted cells adhere to endothelial cells by incorporating specific adhesion molecules. Kupffer cells, phagocytes, and hepatic stellate cells are activated within several hours after cell transplantation. This results in the expression of multiple regulatory cytokines, chemokines, and growth factors. Disruption of the endothelium leads to translocation of transplanted cells into liver plates. Finally, transplanted cells become incorporated in the liver parenchyma with reconstitution of plasma membrane structures, including bile canaliculi and gap junctions. The coordinated expression of matrix metalloproteinases (MMP-2, MMP-3, MMP-9, MMP-13, and MMP-14) and tissue inhibitors of matrix metalloproteinases (TIMP-1 and TIMP-2) facilitates extracellular matrix remodeling. Although transplanted cells do not proliferate in the normal liver, damage to native hepatocytes without injury in transplanted cells is most effective in inducing transplanted cell proliferation.

endothelial cells, as well as trophic factors, such as hepatocyte growth factor and basic fibroblast growth factor. Vascular endothelial growth factor is additionally produced by transplanted and native hepatocytes before the entry of transplanted cells into the liver parenchyma *(47)*. Moreover, a variety of matrix metalloproteinases (e.g., MMP-2, MMP-3, MMP-9, MMP-13, MMP-14), as well as the tissue inhibitor of matrix metalloproteinase-1, are expressed shortly after cell transplantation to assist in endothelial disruption and tissue remodeling. These molecules are largely produced in hepatic stellate cells.

Eventually, the endothelial cell layer is disrupted in proximity with transplanted cells 16–20 hours after cell transplantation *(47)*. This permits transplanted cells to physically translocate into the liver plate and transplanted cells begin to integrate in the parenchyma. During this process, plasma membranes are reorganized with development of hybrid gap junctions and bile canaliculi between transplanted cells and adjacent native cells, a process that is completed during 3–7 days after cell transplantation. This restoration of cell polarity is another critical element in transplanted cell engraftment and provides transplanted cells the ability to secrete bile and excrete biliary toxins *(53)*. Manipulation of the endothelial cell barrier offers another way to improve cell engraftment. For instance, prior disruption of the hepatic endothelium by drugs or chemicals, such as cyclophosphamide, monocrotaline, or doxorubicin, improves transplanted cell engraftment in the liver *(51)*.

After integrating in the liver parenchyma, transplanted hepatocytes survive and exhibit normal function throughout the life span of rodents *(54)*. Overall, 1–2% of the liver mass can be replaced by transplanted hepatocytes after a single session of cell transplantation and this can be increased to 5–7% by three sessions of cell transplantation *(55)*. However, transplanted cells do not proliferate in the normal liver and replacement of less than 10% liver with transplanted cells may not provide significant therapeutic benefit under most circumstances *(54)*. Therefore, further manipulations have been necessary to determine whether transplanted cells could be induced to proliferate in the liver. These manipulations have included subversion of cell cycle controls in transplanted cells or induction of injury in native hepatocytes without causing damage to transplanted cells.

Manipulating liver growth controls to drive proliferation in transplanted cells is an attractive concept. For instance, one could use specific growth factors to accomplish this goal. However, infusion of hepatocyte growth factor in rodents was unsuccessful in inducing proliferation in transplanted cells *(56)*. Whether alternative approaches could be successful (e.g., manipulation of growth factor receptor expression in transplanted cells) is unknown. Another approach concerns removal of cell-cycle checkpoint controls by abrogating suppressor gene activity. This principle has been effective in studies with mutant hepatocytes deficient in the cell cycle suppressor gene, $p27^{c\text{-}kip}$ *(57)*. However, manipulation of cell cycle controls raises issues with the undefined potential for oncogenic perturbations in the long term.

Induction of hepatocyte injury in the native liver has by far been most successful for liver repopulation. Studies of chemical hepatotoxins, as well as toxic transgenes, established this principle. For instance, use of carbon tetrachloride, which damages native hepatocytes and spares transplanted hepatocytes, led to proliferation in transplanted cells *(58)*. Similarly, transplanted cells were shown to proliferate extensively in alb-uPA transgenic mice, which undergo extensive hepatic damage by a toxic transgene driven by the albumin promoter *(59)*. Several additional animal models have verified these principles, including the FAH mutant mouse, in which accumulation of toxic intermediates in the tyrosine metabolic pathway provides the stimulus for proliferation of wild-type cells *(13)*. Induction of apoptosis in mice susceptible to Fas ligand-mediated apoptosis *(60)* was also highly effective. The FAH mouse has been extraordinarily helpful in issues concerning the stem cell potential of hepatocytes and other liver or pancreatic cells, stem cell plasticity, and correction of tyrosinemia *(13,21,32,35, 37,38,57)*. Similarly, Fas ligand-induced apoptosis has been effective in mouse studies of liver repopulation, stem cell biology, and therapeutic manipulations *(61,62)*. The alb-uPA transgene-based mouse strains have been helpful in studies of xenotransplantation, including human hepatocytes to develop viral hepatitis models *(63–65)*.

Finally, hepatic injury with cytotoxic or genotoxic perturbations with chemicals and radiation has also been effective in promoting transplanted cell proliferation. For instance, treatment of animals with retrorsine, a DNA-binding alkaloid, in combination with partial hepatectomy or thyroid hormone inhibits hepatocellular proliferation and survival *(66–68)*. The combination of radiation and partial hepatectomy or ischemia-reperfusion injury in the liver also produces the right microenvironment for inducing proliferation in transplanted hepatocytes *(69–72)*. Altogether, these studies showed that the liver of rats preconditioned with retrorsine or radiation could be repopulated virtually completely with transplanted cells.

4. LIVER-DIRECTED CELL THERAPY FOR SPECIFIC DISORDERS

Many conditions will be amenable to liver-directed cell therapy (Table 1). In general, establishing therapeutic efficacy in an unequivocal manner will be highly important for defining the benefits of cell therapy. This should require demonstrations of causality between the magnitude of liver repopulation and therapeutic effects. Monogenetic disorders that affect the liver or manifest with extrahepatic consequences are particularly prominent targets for such efforts, in part because disease correction can be monitored simply and effectively in such situations. On the other hand, identification of liver repopulation requires tissue sampling and morphological analysis of transplanted cells by unique genetic markers (e.g., sex chromosomes, DNA polymorphisms). Preclinical studies in authentic animal models are necessary to first define what types of cells will be suitable for liver-directed cell therapy, to demonstrate the magnitude of liver repopulation needed for therapeutic effect, and to establish whether the natural history of diseases can be altered by cell therapy.

Table 1
Partial List of Potentially Suitable Conditions for Liver-Directed Cell Therapy[a]

Liver is target of disease	*Nonhepatic organs manifest disease*
Genetic Disorder	**Deficiency states**
• α-1 antitrypsin deficiency	• Congenital hyperbilirubinemia (e.g., Crigler-Najjar syndrome)
• Erythropoietic protoporphyria	• Familial hypercholesterolemia
• Lipidoses (e.g., Niemann-Pick disease)	• Sporadic hypercholesterolemia
• Progressive familial intrahepatic cholestasis	• Hyperammonemia syndromes
• Refsum's disease	• Defects of carbohydrate metabolism
• Tyrosinemia, type 1	• Oxalosis
• Wilson's disease	• Diabetes mellitus, type 1
Acquired disorders	**Coagulation defects**
• Acute liver failure	• Hemophilia A
• Chronic viral hepatitis	• Factor IX deficiency
• Cirrhosis and liver failure	**Immune disorders**
• Fatty degeneration of liver	• Hereditary angioedema
• Hepatic cancer	

[a]Includes hepatocytes and other cell types.

4.1. Liver-Directed Cell Therapy for Inborn Errors of Metabolism

Several excellent animal models are available to establish the principles of liver cell therapy. These animal models include: the Gunn rat model of Crigler-Najjar Syndrome type 1 *(73)*, in which bilirubin-UDP-glucuronosyltransferase (UGT1A1) activity is deficient and unconjugated bilirubin accumulates producing neurotoxicity; Nagase analbuminemic rats (NAR), which exhibit extremely low levels of serum albumin resulting from defective albumin mRNA processing; the Watanabe heritable hyperlipidemic rabbit, which lack cell surface receptors for low-density lipoproteins and models familial hypercholesterolemia *(74)*; the Long-Evans Cinnamon (LEC) rat, an animal model for Wilson's disease *(75)*; the FAH mouse, which models hereditary tyrosinemia type-1 *(13,21)*; and the mdr-2 knockout mice, which model progressive familial intrahepatic cholestasis *(76)*. Mutant animals with diseases of the urea cycle, porphyria, lipidoses, and coagulation disorders are also available *(77–80)*. Similarly, animal models have been identified to study acute or chronic liver failure, cirrhosis and viral hepatitis *(63–65,81–83)*. Of course, type 1 diabetes mellitus can be induced in animals by depleting pancreatic β-cell mass in various ways, including with streptozotocin toxicity.

Transplantation of normal hepatocytes with adequate amounts of liver repopulation can markedly ameliorate metabolic abnormalities in Gunn rats and NAR *(73)*, Watanabe rabbits *(74)*, LEC rats *(75)*, FAH mice *(21)*, mdr-2 mice *(76)*, and lipoproteinemic mice *(61)*. Similarly, primary oval cells isolated from the normal rat liver can differentiate into mature hepatocytes after transplantation into NAR or LEC rats and correct diseases in these animals *(84)*. Of course, these studies indicate that the liver of animals needs to be perturbed for transplanted cells to proliferate, with the exception of animals with chronic ongoing liver damage, as encountered in FAH mice and LEC rats. Early studies in patients have begun to bear out these results in animals. For example, transplantation of genetically modified autologous hepatocytes in patients with familial hypercholesterolemia *(85)* and of allogeneic hepatocytes in patients with ornithine transcarbamylase (OTC) deficiency, α-1-antitrypsin deficiency, or Crigler-Najjar syndrome type 1 *(86–88)* led to limited therapeutic efficacy but not cures. These results are likely the result of limited liver repopulation.

4.2. Liver-Directed Cell Therapy for Acute and Chronic Liver Failure

Results of hepatocytes transplantation in animal models of acute liver failure and chronic liver disease have been mixed. These animal models often pose difficulties because of variable susceptibilities of individual animals to disease and the possibility of improved outcomes unrelated to hepatocyte regeneration *(89)*. Nonetheless, more recent studies in better defined genetic animals models have begun to demonstrate that cell therapy could have therapeutic potential in acute liver failure *(81,82)*. Clinical studies of hepatocyte transplantation in acute liver failure are limited *(86,90,91)*. It is difficult to conduct controlled cell transplantation studies in acute liver failure because of emergency settings, the need to perform orthotopic liver transplantation whenever a donor liver becomes available, and a lack of unequivocal markers to assess metabolic and synthetic contributions of transplanted cells.

End-stage liver disease with complications, such as hepatic encephalopathy and coagulopathy, represents another challenging condition for cell therapy. Many patients with chronic liver failure are candidates for orthotopic liver transplantation. However, the current organ supply is insufficient and fourfold or greater disproportionality exists in the United States between people on waiting lists versus recipients of liver transplants. Many liver recipients develop recurrent disease in the transplanted organ (e.g., hepatitis C). These individuals often show rapid advancement toward liver failure and have no further therapeutic prospects. Moreover, in many parts of the world, liver transplantation is not available either because of prohibitive costs or lack of donor organs. Therefore, cell transplantation could have a potential role to play in this situation, especially if transplanted cells could be made to resist viral hepatitis or other ongoing disease processes in the recipient. Hepatocyte transplantation in rats with hepatic encephalopathy has been shown to improve encephalopathy scores and partially correct changes in serum amino acid levels *(83,92,93)*. Studies in animals with cirrhosis showed that transplanted hepatocytes could integrate in the liver parenchyma despite extensive fibrosis *(94)*. Moreover, intrasplenic cell transplantation in extremely sick cirrhotic rats improved liver tests, coagulation abnormality, and mortality *(83)*. These findings suggest that creation of additional reservoirs of hepatocytes could prolong survival in end-stage liver disease. The clinical experience of cell transplantation in chronic liver disease is limited. In an early study of 10 patients with cirrhosis, transplantation of autologous hepatocytes in spleen may have improved the condition of 1 patient *(95)*. In several patients with chronic liver disease, it was unclear whether transplantation of allogeneic hepatocytes via the splenic artery *(86)* was responsible for improving liver function. Therefore, further studies of cell transplantation are necessary in such situations.

4.3. Liver-Directed Cell Therapy for Type 1 Diabetes Mellitus

It is reasonable to conclude that liver-directed cell therapy has prospects for type 1 diabetes mellitus. Besides the developmental relationships between liver and pancreas, additional evidence indicates that hepatocyte-like cells can emerge in the pancreas. Such evidence includes studies in hamsters or rats treated with carcinogens or peroxisome proliferators *(96,97)*, dietary copper depletion and repletion in rats *(20,98)*, transgenic mice expressing keratinocyte growth factor under insulin promoter *(99)*, and transplantation of murine pancreatic oval cells in FAH mice *(21)*. On the other hand, some liver tumors display typical pancreatic markers (e.g., amylase and lipase) *(100)*. Pancreatic genes are expressed in sorted fetal mouse liver cells, including the β-cell transcription factor, Pdx-1, as well as amylase and lipase *(27)*. Moreover, expression of transgenes, such as Pdx-1 or neuroD-β cellulin in liver cells induces insulin expression in rodent and human cells *(101–104)*. This particular finding should be of much interest because certain progenitor cell populations in the fetal or adult liver, including those with oval cell properties, are thought to be amenable to such genetic manipulation. Because insulin expression in pancreatic β cells is driven in a hierarchical manner, including HNF-3β-mediated transcriptional regulation of Pdx-1 gene expression followed by additional contributions from neuroD and several other transcription factors, it stands to reason that the transcriptional machinery in some cells will be amenable to genetic modulation. If these manipulations could be combined with effective cell populations that could be transplanted, one would begin to advance cell therapy for diabetes mellitus. For instance, reconstitution of telomerase activity in fetal human liver stem/progenitor cells was associated with extensive replication and immortalization of cells without evidence for oncogenic perturbations *(17)*. These cells expressed a variety of transcription factors observed in liver cells. Moreover, in response to Pdx-1 transgene expression, cells began to express insulin in a regulated fashion, although all elements of β-cell phenotype were not reproduced *(103)*. Nonetheless, transplantation of Pdx-1-expressing immortalized fetal human liver cells in diabetic immunotolerant mice resulted in correction of hyperglycemia.

5. SUMMARY

Further analysis of liver progenitor cells offers hope that it will be possible to combine insights into regulation of insulin expression, stem cell biology to obtain optimal cell types, and liver repopulation mechanisms to achieve the requisite amount of transplanted cell mass. These advances should provide ways to optimize utilization of the limited supply of adult human islets and to develop strategies for overcoming organ shortages for treatment of genetic or acquired liver disease.

ACKNOWLEDGMENTS

Supported in part by NIH grants R01 DK46952, P30 DK41296 and P01 DK-052956.

REFERENCES

1. Slack JM. Developmental biology of the pancreas. Development 2002;121:1569–1580.
2. Zaret KS. Regulatory phases of early liver development: paradigms of organogenesis. Nat Rev Genet 2002;3:499–512.
3. Lammert E, Cleaver O, Melton D. Role of endothelial cells in early pancreas and liver development. Mech Dev 2003;120:59–64.
4. Parviz F, Matullo C, Garrison WD, et al. Hepatocyte nuclear factor 4alpha controls the development of a hepatic epithelium and liver morphogenesis. Nat Genet 2003;34:292–296.
5. Monga SP, Tang Y, Candotti F, et al. Expansion of hepatic and hematopoietic stem cells utilizing mouse embryonic liver explants. Cell Transplantation 2001;10:81–89.
6. Hartner JC, Schmittwolf C, Kispert A, Muller AM, Higuchi M, Seeburg PH. Liver disintegration in the mouse embryo caused by deficiency in the RNA-editing enzyme ADAR1. J Biol Chem 2004;279:4894–4902.
7. Badve S, Logdberg L, Sokhi R, et al. An antigen reacting with Das-1 monoclonal antibody is ontogenically regulated in diverse organs including liver and indicates sharing of developmental mechanisms among cell lineages. Pathobiology 2000;68:76–86.
8. Malhi H, Irani AN, Gagandeep S, Gupta S. Isolation of human progenitor liver epithelial cells with extensive replication capacity and differentiation into mature hepatocytes. J Cell Sci 2002;115:2679–2688.
9. Sigal S, Gupta S, Gebhard DF Jr, Holst P, Neufeld D, Reid LM. Evidence for a terminal differentiation process in the liver. Differentiation 1995;59:35–42.
10. Riccalton-Banks L, Bhandari R, Fry J, Shakesheff KM. A simple method for the simultaneous isolation of stellate cells and hepatocytes from rat liver tissue. Mol Cell Biochem 2003;248:97–102.

11. Michalopoulos GK, DeFrances MC. Liver regeneration. Science 1997;276:60–66.
12. Fausto N, Campbell JS. The role of hepatocytes and oval cells in liver regeneration and repopulation. Mech Dev 2003;120:117–130.
13. Overturf K, Al-Dhalimy M, Ou C-N, Finegold M, Grompe M. Serial transplantation reveals the stem-cell-like regenerative potential of adult mouse hepatocytes. Am J Pathol 1997;151: 1273–1280.
14. Sharpless NE, DePinho RA. Telomeres, stem cells, senescence, and cancer. J Clin Invest 2004;113:160–168.
15. Rudolph KL, Chang S, Millard M, Schreiber-Agus N, DePinho RA. Inhibition of experimental liver cirrhosis in mice by telomerase gene delivery. Science 2000;287:1253–1258.
16. Wiemann SU, Satyanarayana A, Tsahuridu M, et al. Hepatocyte telomere shortening and senescence are general markers of human liver cirrhosis. FASEB J 2002;16:935–942.
17. Wege H, Le HT, Chui MS, et al. Telomerase reconstitution immortalizes human fetal hepatocytes without disrupting their differentiation potential. Gastroenterology 2003;124:432–444.
18. Alison MR, Vig P, Russo F, et al. Hepatic stem cells: from inside and outside the liver? Cell Prolif 2004;37:1–21.
19. Farber E. Similarities in the sequence of early histological changes induced in the liver of the rat by ethionine, 2-acetylaminofluorene and 3′-methyl-4-dimethyl-aminoazobenzene. Cancer Res 1956;16:142–149.
20. Dabeva MD, Hwang SG, Vasa SR, et al. Differentiation of pancreatic epithelial progenitor cells into hepatocytes following transplantation into rat liver. Proc Natl Acad Sci USA 1997;94:7356–7361.
21. Wang X, Al-Dhalimy M, Lagasse E, Finegold M, Grompe M. Liver repopulation and correction of metabolic liver disease by transplanted adult mouse pancreatic cells. Am J Pathol 2001;158:571–579.
22. Lazaro CA, Rhim JA, Yamada Y, Fausto N. Generation of hepatocytes from oval cell precursors in culture. Cancer Research 1998;58:5514–5522.
23. Petersen BE, Goff JP, Greenberger JS, Michalopoulos GK. Hepatic oval cells express the hematopoietic stem cell marker Thy-1 in the rat. Hepatology 1998;27:433–445.
24. Ott M, Rajvanshi P, Sokhi R, et al. Differentiation-specific regulation of transgene expression in a diploid epithelial cell line derived from the normal F344 rat liver. J Pathol 1999;187:365–373.
25. Malouf NN, Coleman WB, Grisham JW, et al. Adult-derived stem cells from the liver become myocytes in the heart in vivo. Am J Pathol 2001;158:1929–1935.
26. Taniguchi H, Kondo R, Suzuki A, et al. Clonogenic colony-forming ability of flow cytometrically isolated hepatic progenitor cells in the murine fetal liver. Cell Transplant 2000;9:697–700.
27. Suzuki A, Zheng Yw YW, Kaneko S, et al. Clonal identification and characterization of self-renewing pluripotent stem cells in the developing liver. J Cell Biol 2002;156:173–84.
28. Petersen BE, Bowen WC, Patrene KD, et al. Bone marrow as a potential source of hepatic oval cells. Science 1999;284:1168–1170.
29. Theise ND, Badve S, Saxena R, et al. Derivation of hepatocytes from bone marrow cells in mice after radiation-induced myeloablation. Hepatology 2000;31:235–240.
30. Theise ND, Nimmakayalu M, Gardner R, Illei PB, Morgan G, Teperman L, Henegariu O, Krause DS 2000;Liver from bone marrow in humans. Hepatology 32:11–16
31. Alison MR, Poulson R, Jeffrey R, et al. Hepatocytes from non-hepatic adult stem cells. Nature 2000;406:257.
32. Lagasse E, Connors H, Al Dhalimy M, et al. Purified hematopoietic stem cells can differentiate into hepatocytes in vivo. Nat Med 2000;6:1229–1234.

33. Korbling M, Katz RL, Khanna A, et al. Hepatocytes and epithelial cells of donor origin in recipients of peripheral-blood stem cells. N Engl J Med 2002;346:738–746.
34. Wang X, Ge S, McNamara G, Hao QL, Crooks GM, Nolta JA. Albumin-expressing hepatocyte-like cells develop in the livers of immune-deficient mice that received transplants of highly purified human hematopoietic stem cells. Blood 2003;101:4201–4208
35. Wang X, Foster M, Al-Dhalimy M, Lagasse E, Finegold M, Grompe M. The origin and liver repopulating capacity of murine oval cells. Proc Natl Acad Sci USA 2003;100(Suppl. 1): 11881–11888.
36. Wagers AJ, Sherwood RI, Christensen JL, Weissman IL. Little evidence for developmental plasticity of adult hematopoietic stem cells. Science 2002;297:2256–1159.
37. Terada N, Hamazaki T, Oka M, et al. Bone marrow cells adopt the phenotype of other cells by spontaneous cell fusion. Nature 2002;416:542–545.
38. Wang X, Willenbring H, Akkari Y, et al. Cell fusion is the principal source of bone-marrow-derived hepatocytes. Nature 2003;422:897–901.
39. Newsome PN, Johannessen I, Boyle S, et al. Human cord blood-derived cells can differentiate into hepatocytes in the mouse liver with no evidence of cellular fusion. Gastroenterology 2003;124:1891–1900.
40. Odorico JS, Kaufman DS, Thomson JA. Multilineage differentiation from human embryonic stem cell lines. Stem Cells 2001;19:193–204.
41. Yamada T, Yoshikawa M, Kanda S, et al. In vitro differentiation of embryonic stem cells into hepatocyte-like cells identified by cellular uptake of indocyanine green. Stem Cells 2002;20:146–154.
42. Chinzei R, Tanaka Y, Shimizu-Saito K, et al. Embryoid-body cells derived from a mouse embryonic stem cell line show differentiation into functional hepatocytes. Hepatology 2002;36:22–29.
43. Fair JH, Cairns BA, Lapaglia M, et al. Induction of hepatic differentiation in embryonic stem cells by co-culture with embryonic cardiac mesoderm. Surgery 2003;134:189–196.
44. Yamamoto H, Quinn G, Asari A, et al. Differentiation of embryonic stem cells into hepatocytes: biological functions and therapeutic application. Hepatology 2003;37:983–993.
45. Gupta S, Lee C-D, Vemuru RP, Bhargava KK. ^{111}Indium-labeling of hepatocytes for ana¬≠lyzing biodistribution of transplanted cells. Hepatology 1994;19:750–757.
46. Nagata H, Ito M, Shirota C, Edge A, McCowan TC, Fox IJ. Route of hepatocyte delivery affects hepatocyte engraftment in the spleen. Transplantation 2003;76:732–734.
47. Gupta S, Rajvanshi P, Sokhi RP, et al. Entry and integration of transplanted hepatocytes in liver plates occur by disruption of hepatic sinusoidal endothelium. Hepatology 1999;29:509–519.
48. Gupta S, Rajvanshi P, Malhi H, et al. Cell transplantation causes loss of gap junctions and activates GGT expression permanently in host liver. Am J Physiol Gastroint Liver Physiol 2000;279:G815–G826.
49. Slehria S, Rajvanshi P, Ito Y, et al. Hepatic sinusoidal vasodilators improve transplanted cell engraftment and ameliorate microcirculatory perturbations in the liver. Hepatology 2002;35:1320–1328.
50. Joseph B, Malhi H, Bhargava KK, Palestro CJ, McCuskey RS, Gupta S. Kupffer cells participate in early clearance of syngeneic hepatocytes transplanted in the rat liver. Gastroenterology 2002;123:1677–1685.
51. Malhi H, Annamaneni P, Slehria S, et al. Cyclophosphamide disrupts hepatic sinusoidal endothelium and improves transplanted cell engraftment in rat liver. Hepatology 2002;36:112–121.
52. Kumaran V, Joseph B, Benten D, Gupta S. Hepatic integrin-dependent extracellular matrix (ECM) component interactions regulate hepatocyte engraftment in the liver. Hepatology 2003;38:216A.

53. Gupta S, Rajvanshi P, Lee C-D. Integration of transplanted hepatocytes in host liver plates demonstrated with dipeptidyl peptidase IV deficient rats. Proc Natl Acad Sci USA 1995;92:5860–5864.
54. Sokhi RP, Rajvanshi P, Gupta S. Transplanted reporter cells help in defining onset of hepatocyte proliferation during the life of F344 rats. Am J Physiol Gastroint Liver Physiol 2000;279:G631–G640
55. Rajvanshi P, Kerr A, Bhargava KK, Burk RD, Gupta S. Efficacy and safety of repeated hepatocyte transplantation for significant liver repopulation in rodents. Gastroenterology 1996;111:1092–1102.
56. Gupta S, Rajvanshi P, Aragona E, Yerneni PR, Lee C-D, Burk RD. Transplanted hepatocytes proliferate differently after CCl4 treatment and hepatocyte growth factor infusion. Am J Physiol 1996;276:G629–G638.
57. Karnezis AN, Dorokhov M, Grompe M, Zhu L. Loss of p27(Kip1) enhances the transplantation efficiency of hepatocytes transferred into diseased livers. J Clin Invest 2001;108:383–90.
58. Gupta S, Rajvanshi P, Sokhi R, Vaidya S, Irani AN, Gorla GR. Position-specific gene expression in the liver lobule is directed by the microenvironment and not by the previous cell differentiation state. J Biol Chem 1999;274:2157–2165.
59. Rhim JA, Sandgren EP, Degen JL, Palmiter RD, Brinster RL. Replacement of diseased mouse liver by hepatic cell transplantation. Science 1994;263:1149–1152.
60. Mignon A, Guidotti JE, Mitchell C, et al. Selective repopulation of normal mouse liver by Fas/CD95-resistant hepatocytes. Nat Med 1998;10:1185–1188.
61. Mitchell C, Mignon A, Guidotti JE, et al. Therapeutic liver repopulation in a mouse model of hypercholesterolemia. Hum Mol Genet 2000;9:1597–1602.
62. Mallet VO, Mitchell C, Mezey E, et al. Bone marrow transplantation in mice leads to a minor population of hepatocytes that can be selectively amplified in vivo. Hepatology 2002;35:799–804.
63. Petersen J. Dandri M, Gupta S, Rogler CE. Liver repopulation with xenogenic hepatocytes in B and T cell-deficient mice leads to chronic hepadnavirus infection and clonal growth of hepatocellular carcinoma. Proc Natl Acad Sci USA 1998;95:310–315.
64. Dandri M, Burda MR, Török E, et al. Repopulation of mouse liver with human hepatocytes and in vivo infection with hepatitis B virus. Hepatology 2001;33:981–988.
65. Mercer DF, Schiller DE, Elliott JF, et al. Hepatitis C virus replication in mice with chimeric human livers. Nat Med 2001;7:927–933.
66. Laconi E, Oren R, Mukhopadhyay DK, et al. Long-term, near-total liver replacement by transplantation of isolated hepatocytes in rats treated with retrorsine. Am J Pathol 1998;153:319–329.
67. Oren R, Dabeva MD, Karnezis AN, et al. Role of thyroid hormone in stimulating liver repopulation in the rat by transplanted hepatocytes. Hepatology 1999;30:903–913.
68. Guo D, Fu T, Nelson JA, Superina RA, Soriano HE. Liver repopulation after cell transplantation in mice treated with retrorsine and carbon tetrachloride. Transplantation 2002;73:1818–1824.
69. Guha C, Sharma A, Gupta S, et al. Amelioration of radiation-induced liver damage in partially hepatectomized rats by hepatocyte transplantation. Cancer Res 1999;59:5871–5874.
70. Guha C, Parashar B, Deb NJ, et al. Normal hepatocytes correct serum bilirubin after repopulation of Gunn rat liver subjected to irradiation/partial resection. Hepatology 2002;36:354–362.
71. Gorla GR, Malhi H, Gupta S. Polyploidy associated with oxidative DNA injury attenuates proliferative potential of cells. J Cell Sci 2001;114:2943–2951.
72. Malhi H, Gorla GR, Irani AN, Annamaneni P, Gupta S. Cell transplantation after oxidative hepatic preconditioning with radiation and ischemia-reperfusion leads to extensive liver repopulation. Proc Natl Acad Sci USA 2002;99:13114–13119.

73. Demetriou AA, Levenson SM, Novikoff PM, et al. Survival, organization and function of microcarrier-attached hepatocytes transplanted in rats. Proc Natl Acad Sci USA 1986;83: 7475–7479.
74. Gunsalus JR, Brady DA, Coulter SM, Gray BM, Edge ASB. Reduction of serum cholesterol in Watanabe rabbits by xenogeneic hepatocellular transplantation. Nat Med 1997;3:48–49.
75. Malhi H, Irani AN, Volenberg I, Schilsky ML, Gupta S. Early cell transplantation in LEC rats modeling Wilson's disease eliminates hepatic copper with reversal of liver disease. Gastroenterology 2002;122:438–447.
76. De Vree JM, Ottenhoff R, Bosma PJ, Smith AJ, Aten J, Oude Elferink RP. Correction of liver disease by hepatocyte transplantation in a mouse model of progressive familial intrahepatic cholestasis. Gastroenterology 2000;119:1720–1730.
77. Batshaw ML, Robinson MB, Ye X, et al. Correction of ureagenesis after gene transfer in an animal model and after liver transplantation in humans with ornithine transcarbamylase deficiency. Pediatr Res 1999;46:588–593.
78. Libbrecht L, Meerman L, Kuipers F, Roskams T, Desmet V, Jansen P. Liver pathology and hepatocarcinogenesis in a long-term mouse model of erythropoietic protoporphyria. J Pathol 2003;199:191–200.
79. Jin HK, Schuchman EH. Ex vivo gene therapy using bone marrow-derived cells: combined effects of intracerebral and intravenous transplantation in a mouse model of Niemann-Pick disease. Mol Ther 2003;8:876–885.
80. Sarkar R, Tetreault R, Gao G, et al. Total correction of hemophilia A mice with canine FVIII using an AAV 8 serotype. Blood 2004;103:1253–1260.
81. Gagandeep S, Sokhi R, Slehria S, et al. Hepatocyte transplantation improves survival in mice with liver toxicity induced by hepatic overexpression of Mad1 transcription factor. Molec Ther 2000;1:358–365.
82. Braun KM, Degen JL, Sandgren EP. Hepatocyte transplantation in a model of toxin-induced liver disease: variable therapeutic effect during replacement of damaged parenchyma by donor cells. Nat Med 2000;6:320–326.
83. Nagata H, Ito M, Cai J, Edge AS, Platt JL, Fox IJ. Treatment of cirrhosis and liver failure in rats by hepatocyte xenotransplantation. Gastroenterology 2003;124:422–431.
84. Yasui O, Miura N, Terada K, Kawarada Y, Koyama K, Sugiyama T. Isolation of oval cells from Long-Evans Cinnamon rats and their transformation into hepatocytes in vivo in the rat liver. Hepatology 1997;25:329–334.
85. Grossman M, Rader DJ, Muller DWM, et al. A pilot study of ex vivo gene therapy for homozygous familiar hypercholesterolaemia. Nat Med 1995;1:1148–1154.
86. Strom SC, Fisher RA, Rubinstein WS, et al. Transplantation of human hepatocytes. Transplant Proc 1997;29:2103–2106.
87. Strom SC, Fisher RA, Thompson MT, et al. Hepatocyte transplantation as a bridge to orthotopic liver transplantation in terminal liver failure. Transplantation 1997;63:559–569.
88. Fox IJ, Chowdhury JR, Kaufman SS, et al. Treatment of the Crigler-Najjar syndrome type I with hepatocyte transplantation. New Engl J Med 1998;338:1422–1426.
89. Chamuleau RAFM. Hepatocyte transplantation for acute hepatic failure. In: Mito M, Sawa M, eds. Hepatocyte Transplantation. Basel: Karger Landes Systems, 1999, pp. 159–167.
90. Habibullah CM. Hepatocyte transplantation: need for liver cell bank. Trop Gastroenterol 1992;13:129–131.
91. Bilir BM, Guinette D, Karrer F, et al. Hepatocyte transplantation in acute liver failure. Liver Transpl 2000;6:32–40.

92. Ribiero J, Nordlinger B, Ballet F, et al. Intrasplenic hepatocellular transplantation corrects hepatic encephalopathy in portacaval shunted rats. Hepatology 1992;15;12–18.
93. Schumacher IK, Okamoto T, Kim BH, Chowdhury NR, Chowdhury JR, Fox IJ. Transplantation of conditionally immortalized hepatocytes to treat hepatic encephalopathy. Hepatology 1996;24:337–343.
94. Gagandeep S, Rajvanshi P, Sokhi R, et al. Transplanted hepatocytes engraft, survive and proliferate in the liver of rats with carbon tetrachloride-induced cirrhosis. J Pathol 2000;191:78–85.
95. Mito M, Kusano M, Kauwara Y. Hepatocyte transplantation in man. Transpl Proc 1992;24:3052–3053.
96. Scarpelli DG, Rao MS. Differentiation of regenerating pancreatic cells into hepatocyte-like cells. Proc Natl Acad Sci USA 1981;78:2577–2581.
97. Hoover KL, Poirier LA. Hepatocyte-like cells within the pancreas of rats fed methyl-deficient diets. J Nutr 1986;116:1569–1575.
98. Rao MS, Yukawa M, Omori M, Thorgeirsson SS, Reddy JK. Expression of transcription factors and stem cell factor precedes hepatocyte differentiation in rat pancreas. Gene Expr 1996;6:15–22.
99. Krakowski ML, Kritzik MR, Jones EM, et al. Pancreatic expression of keratinocyte growth factor leads to differentiation of islet hepatocytes and proliferation of duct cells. Am J Pathol 1999;154:683–691.
100. Hruban RH, Molina JM, Reddy MN, Boitnott JK. A neoplasm with pancreatic and hepatocellular differentiation presenting with subcutaneous fat necrosis. Am J Clin Pathol 1987;88:639–645.
101. Yang L, Li S, Hatch H, et al. In vitro trans-differentiation of adult hepatic stem cells into pancreatic endocrine hormone-producing cells. Proc Natl Acad Sci USA 2002;99:8078–8083.
102. Ber I, Shternhall K, Perl S, et al. Functional, persistent, and extended liver to pancreas transdifferentiation. J Biol Chem 2003;278:31950–1957.
103. Zalzman M, Gupta S, Giri RK, et al. Reversal of hyperglycemia in mice using human expandable insulin-producing cells differentiated from fetal liver progenitor cells. Proc Natl Acad Sci USA 2003;100:7253–7258.
104. Kojima H, Fujimiya M, Matsumura K, et al. NeuroD-betacellulin gene therapy induces islet neogenesis in the liver and reverses diabetes in mice. Nat Med 2003;9:596–603.

10 The Manipulation of Mesenchymal Stem Cells for Bone Repair

Shelley R. Winn

CONTENTS

1. INTRODUCTION

Bone homeostasis is a dynamic process consisting of mutually dependent interactions between cells, substrates, and molecular signals that are, in turn, influenced by hormones, mitogens and differentiation factors. In general, when this environment is perturbed as a consequence of disease, including osteoporosis or injury, cell and molecular signals initiate a cascade of genetically programmed repair processes. Depending on the molecular signals and responding cells, the response to injury typically promotes regeneration to a form and function virtually indistinguishable from the preinjured state. However, if the injury becomes too extensive (i.e., becomes of a critical size), these regenerative processes are insufficient for meaningful repair. In these cases, a variety of therapeutic interventions including autografting, grafting from banked bone, or grafts of supplemental bone graft substitute materials are used. For numerous reasons, each of these therapies is associated with an unacceptably high failure rate *(1)*.

Surgeons have used autogenous and allogeneic bone grafts to augment fracture healing and provide continuity defect regeneration (reviewed in ref. *2*). Contemporary treatments include bone grafts, alloplastics, electrical stimulation, distraction osteogenesis, guided bone regeneration, and local growth factor administration. Most recently, early clinical trials have been initiated to evaluate

From: *Contemporary Endocrinology: Stem Cells in Endocrinology*
Edited by: L. B. Lester © Humana Press Inc., Totowa, NJ

the potential of stem cell and gene therapy (reviewed in refs. *3–7*). Despite the likelihood that new therapies on the clinical horizon will supersede autograft supremacy, it remains the gold standard for restoring form and function and promoting bone regeneration of critical-sized defects and recalcitrant fractures *(5,6)*. The widespread applicability of autogenous grafting is limited by a finite supply of donor tissue, increased donor site morbidity, protracted hospitalization, and increased costs.

The overall objective for this chapter is to provide a brief review of the biology of fracture healing and present some of the strategies involved with the use of mesenchymal stem cells (MSCs) for bone regenerative therapies including novel therapies for osteoporosis. Mesenchymal stem cells or human bone marrow stromal stem cells are pluripotent progenitor cells that can generate cartilage, bone, muscle, tendon, ligament, and fat. These progenitors exist postnatally with low incidence and extensive renewal potential. When combined with their inherent developmental plasticity they seem well suited to replace damaged tissues. In essence, mesenchymal stem cells can be cultured to expand their numbers then transplanted to the injured site or after seeding in or on shaped biomimetic scaffolds. Thus, alternative approaches for skeletal repair is enabled including the selection, expansion, and modulation of osteoprogenitor cells in combination with conductive or inductive scaffolds to support and guide regeneration together with judicious selection of osteotropic growth factors. In addition to bone regenerative therapies, MSCs, or stromal progenitors from bone marrow, have been used in a variety of animal models. These include, but are not limited to, cardiac disorders *(8–11)*, lung diseases *(12,13)*, myelin deficiencies *(14)*, osteogenesis imperfecta *(15,16)*, parkinsonism *(17,18)*, spinal cord injury *(19–22)*, and stroke *(23)*. Clinical trials have been reported using MSCs for Hurler's syndrome and metachromatic leukodystrophy *(24)*, osteogenesis imperfecta *(16,25,26)*, and to enhance engraftment of heterologous bone marrow transplants *(27)*.

2. FRACTURE HEALING

Restoring form and function to the prefractured condition is the ultimate desired clinical outcome from treatments for bone fractures. The ability of bone to regenerate is self-limiting, thus, supplementation is required when bony deficits exceed a critical size. A critical-sized defect is defined as an intraosseous deficiency that will not heal with more than 10% new bone formation within the life expectancy of the patient *(28)*.

Fracture healing has been extensively studied in nongeriatric, nonosteoporotic models to identify the cells and molecular factors that underlie the regenerative process. An overview of fracture healing is presented but it is worth noting that other comprehensive reports describing the fracture healing model are also available *(29–35)*.

2.1. The Acute Injury Phase

A bone fracture incites an inflammatory response coupled with complement activation, and extravasation secondary to damage to blood vessels. Proximal to the fracture site, an acidotic state ensues with a decrease in pH *(4,5)*. The proteolytic degradation of extracellular matrix produces chemotactic remnants that attract monocytes and macrophages to the wound bed *(36)*. Activated macrophages release fibroblast growth factor (FGF) and vascular endothelial growth factor (VEGF), stimulating endothelial cells to express plasminogen activator and procollagenase *(36)*. Chemokines at the fracture site attract polymorphonuclear leukocytes (PMNs) and growth factors released from the α granules of degranulating platelets attract additional PMNs, as well as lymphocytes, monocytes, and macrophages.

The extravasated blood collects, clots, and forms a hematoma. The resulting hemostatic plug further inhibits blood volume depletion. Platelets mediate the clotting cascade by providing hemostasis control and modulate signaling elements through isoforms of platelet derived growth factor (PDGF), transforming growth factor-β (TGF-β), insulin-like growth factors, epidermal growth factor, and FGFs (Fig. 1A).

The injury environment within the initial 24–48 hours is further characterized by a diminished oxygen tension and pH; conditions needed for normal housekeeping activities of PMNs and macrophages. The PMNs remove microbes and microdebris, whereas the macrophages cleanse the region of larger sized materials. Macrophages can develop into polykaryon, multinucleated giant cells when it is necessary to manage a protracted invasion of foreign material/cells. Macrophages also provide a sustained source of cytokines, interleukins (e.g., IL-1, IL-6), tumor necrosis factor, macrophage colony stimulating factor, PDGF, and TGFβ isoforms important for cell activity, recruiting cells, and provoking mitogenesis and chemotaxis.

2.2. The Proliferative Stage

By 3–5 days after the initial fracture, a repair blastema (granulation tissue) develops, consisting of new blood vessels, soluble signaling molecules, and a variety of collagen isotypes that localizes, protects, and temporally positions growth or morphogenetic factors to optimize cell-factor interactions *(37)* (Fig. 1B). Blastema-rich collagen provides a solid-state matrix for differential cell attachment and promotion of cell transductive mechanisms. For example, undifferentiated cells interacting with neovasculature and osteoprogenitor cells within the periosteum and endosteum are attracted to the fracture site by chemotactic signals (e.g., TGF-β, bone morphogenetic protein [BMP]), where they anchor to the granulation tissue collagen and differentiate into chondrocytes and osteoblasts in the presence of BMPs. As such, this program combines cell anchorage,

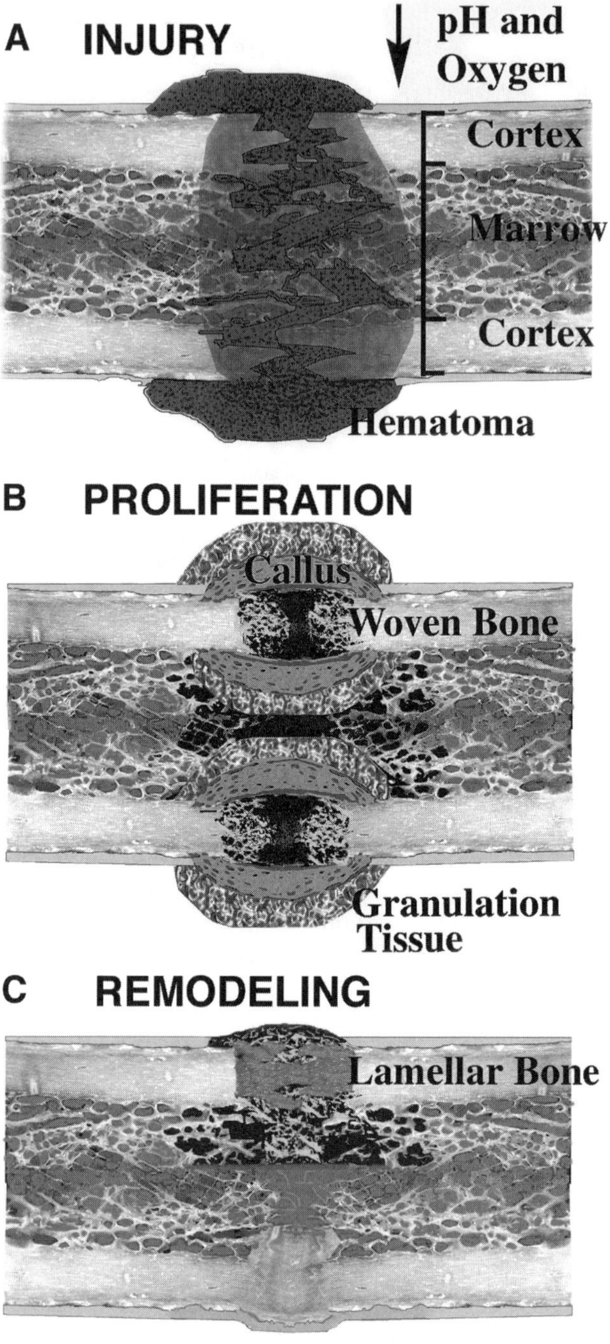
A INJURY
pH and
Oxygen
Cortex
Marrow
Cortex
Hematoma
B PROLIFERATION
Callus
Woven Bone
Granulation
Tissue
C REMODELING
Lamellar Bone

mechanotransduction, and cell-factor interactions to promote cell differentiation to specific phenotypes allowing the fracture healing cascade to repair the wound.

Callus formation (i.e., the initial repair component) results from cell differentiation, an accumulation of cell expression products, and the maturation of the extracellular matrix over several weeks. Components of the callus include vascular elements, stromal products, cells (such as, chondrocytes, chondroclasts, fibroblasts, endothelial cells, smooth muscle cells, preosteoblasts, and pluripotential cells), cartilage, and very immature bone. Cartilage is subsequently replaced by woven bone, defined as cellular, randomly oriented spicules of immature bone. Woven bone will mature into lamellar bone, which is less cellular than woven bone, and consists of thin sheets of bone (approximately 100 μm thick) oriented to support fracture fragments. Although some lamellar bone will remain, most will remodel to Haversian bone (Fig. 1C). Teams of cells and a variety of growth factors and hormones (e.g., parathyroid hormone, TGF-β, FGFs, VEGFs, BMPs, PDGFs, insulin-like growth factors *[38]*) are critical components to this dynamic process (Fig. 1C). In general, fracture healing is completed by about 6–8 weeks postinjury, provided the injured site doesn't exhibit fracture segment instability (see the following section).

In the endochondrally derived appendicular skeleton, cartilage predominates during fracture healing. However, in the intramembranous bones of the craniofacial complex, cartilage formation during fracture healing is associated with fracture segment instability. If fragments are unstable (mobile), cartilage will prevail. Cell-shape alterations in unstable bone impede neovascularization producing an environment conducive for chondrogenesis. In a stable environment

---

Fig. 1. (*opposite page*) The major sequence of events observed during fracture healing. **(A)** The extravasated blood will clot, forming a hematoma (a hemostatic plug), and inhibit additional blood volume depletion. Platelets function both as providing hemostatic control and secreting mediators, such as isoforms of platelet derived growth factor (PDGF), transforming growth factor-β (TGF-β), insulin-like growth factors (IGFs), epidermal growth factor (EGF), and fibroblast growth factors (FGFs). **(B)** By 3–5 days after the initial fracture, a repair blastema (granulation tissue) develops, composed of new blood vessels, soluble signaling molecules, and a variety of collagen isotypes. The collagenous components localize, protect and temporally positions growth factors (e.g., PDGF, TGF-β, IGFs, EGF, FGFs, and vascular endothelial growth factor [VEGF]), or bone morphogenetic factors to optimize cell-factor interactions with receptive cells. **(C)** Woven bone is replaced with lamellar bone during remodeling. Hormones and growth factors modulate osteoblastic and osteoclastic activities to re-form haversian bone and restore contour and function. (Adapted from Hollinger and Wong *[34]*.)

in which the neovasculature within the craniofacial complex can be stimulated by proangiogenic modulators (FGF-1, VEGFs) to discourage chondrogenesis, fracture healing progresses by direct bone formation. Stability of the fragments typically results in bone regeneration and reestablishment of normal form and functional status in the same 6- to 8-week time frame.

Regenerating a structure indistinguishable from the preinjured tissue is dependent on activities of red blood cells, leukocytes, fibroblasts, endothelial cells, committed pluripotential cells, and stem cells. Downstream, the more mature osteoblasts and osteoclasts constitute the community of cells that form bone. A basal level activity of these cells is inadequate to address the acute challenge of fracture healing so these cells must be primed for the task of healing. Cells must be recruited, expanded in number, and primed by the proper combination of growth factors. Additional cell renewal is crucial for bone regeneration and homeostasis.

Osteoblast-osteoclast renewal is essential to sustain the dynamics of bone wound healing over an 8- to 10-week period. Neither osteoblasts nor osteoclasts are immortal. Osteoclasts have a life expectancy of about 2 weeks. After approximately 4 weeks, most osteoblasts undergo apoptosis (cell death), although a small percentage become cells that line the trabeculae and others become embedded within the calcified matrix to become osteocytes. The continual cell source for osteoblasts has been localized to bone marrow stromal cells and blood vessel pericytes. The former have adipogenic and chondrogenic potential, the lineage being determined by the quantitative availability of specific BMPs *(39,40)*. Molecular lures for pericytes, preosteoblast cells from endosteum, periosteum, and marrow may include fragments of collagen and breakdown products at the fracture. Additional molecules providing chemotactic signals for cells to the fracture site include osteocalcin, bone sialoprotein, and γ-carboxyglutamic acid *(41)*, as well as FGF and PDGF. For osteoclasts, signals to attract monocytes to the healing wound include fragments of fibronectin (a ubiquitous attachment factor) and extracellular degradation products. Moreover, local preosteoblasts secrete TRANCE (a member of the tumor necrosis factor family), that activates preosteoclast-like cells through the receptor RANK *(41,42)*. Differentiated osteoblasts express IL-1, IL-6, and IL-11 that push osteoclast differentiation *(43)*.

After cell recruitment to the fracture site, additional cells are created via mitogenesis and differentiation. The responding cell population is sufficiently versatile to permit differentiation pathways that include adipogenesis, fibrogenesis, myogenesis, neurogenesis, chondrogenesis, and osteogenesis *(39,40,42, 44–48)*. Determinants for cell fate (i.e., differentiation) may include extracellular signals, the BMPs and TGF-β isoforms. In addition, intracellular signaling molecules have been described that either sustain the action of extracellular cues or induce differentiation themselves *(35,49–51)*.

2.3. Remodeling

Remodeling is the final component to the fracture healing process. The term *remodeling* describes the dynamic events associated with bone regeneration and homeostasis in the mature skeleton. Modeling involves processes similar to the sculpting of bone before the closure of the epiphyseal plates. Homeostatic remodeling can be envisioned as an activation-resorption-formation process. Activation occurs by stimulating osteoblasts with signaling factors such as parathyroid hormone to vacate an area of bone. After the bone is vacated, osteoclasts take residence, become stimulated, attach, resorb, and eventually cease resorbing and deattach. Other signals are present in Howship's lacunae (osteoclastic resorptive pits) that attract osteoblasts that secrete osteoid, which, on calcification, restores bone. This dynamic alternating interaction between osteoblasts and osteoclasts has been described as the basic multicellular bone unit and the resulting bone is the basic structural unit *(34)*. This activation-resorption-formation process occurs over a 4- to 6-month time frame.

2.4. Fracture Healing: Mechanisms to Direct the Development of New Technologies

The knowledge gained in deciphering the mechanisms and time course of fracture healing provides the physiologic directive for developing rational therapeutics. For a successful regenerative process, cells, extracellular matrix, blood vessels, and signaling molecules (extracellular and intracellular) must be systematically arranged in space and time to ensure and sustain the delicate balance needed for bone regeneration. For most regenerative applications, the autogenous graft is the benchmark that alternatives should be judged against. Autografts and allogeneic banked bone provide patients with bone deficiencies the greatest chance for regeneration. Successful clinical outcome from autografts can exceed 80%, whereas allogeneic preparations are generally less successful *(52,53)*. Reasons for these clinical observations have been reviewed extensively *(1,52–59)*, but the most obvious benefit of transplanting autogenous cells is the ability to avoid rejection by the recipients immune system.

New grafting strategies from both clinicians and basic scientists are designed to develop options for surgeons that will rival the autograft. One of the most promising developments is embedded within an evolving field known as tissue engineering *(60)*. Individuals engaged in this field have diverse backgrounds with expertise in developmental biology, cell and molecular biology, materials science, polymer chemistry, and engineering. The goal of tissue engineering is to develop tissue equivalents to replace or repair defective parts. Cell sourcing represents a major component of the tissue-engineered equivalent, and recent advances in the purification and expansion of MSCs has generated a renewed enthusiasm for their study *(61)*.

3. COMPONENTS OF BONE REGENERATIVE THERAPEUTICS

3.1. Background: Adult Stem Cells

Within the adult organism, an organized and strictly regulated process involving mitogenesis, migration, differentiation, and maturation guides the production and maintenance of the vast majority of cell lineages. Stem cells are the earliest cells in this sequence and can give rise to diversely differentiated cell types and tissues. Traditionally, stem cells are divided into two groups: embryonic stem cells capable of generating all differentiated cell types (pluripotent); these cells generate the second group, which are tissue- or organ-specific stem cells (multipotent). The hematopoietic stem cell, which gives rise to all the cell types of the blood and immune system, and the mesenchymal stem cell, which produce the connective tissues of the body are examples of multipotent stem cells.

The tissue- and organ-specific multipotent stem cell has traditionally been believed to be restricted to a committed pathway specific for the tissue that it resides in. However, several reports have challenged this concept of restriction indicating that adult stem cells from a particular tissue or organ can be induced to differentiate into cells of a distinctly different tissue or organ (i.e., transdifferentiation). Examples include brain into blood *(62)*, marrow into brain *(63–66)*, marrow into liver *(67,68)*, marrow into muscle *(69,70)*, muscle into marrow *(71)*, and marrow to skin *(72,73)*. In addition to their near limitless capability for expansion and multipotent capabilities, adult stem cells may actually exhibit greater plasticity toward a pluripotent modality. However, the data have not clearly demonstrated that a transdifferentiated cell can fulfill the normal functions of its new and unique home.

3.2. Mesenchymal Stem Cells

MSCs or marrow stromal cells, as with hematopoietic stem cells, reside in the bone marrow and are critical for repairing injured tissues. MSCs are found to a lesser extent around blood vessels (pericytes), in fat, muscle, skin, and other locations *(74)*. These progenitor cells are not only capable of providing a rich and abundant source of transplant material, but *in situ*, also give rise to daughter cells with a more restricted developmental path. The lineage committed cells within MSCs can form specialized connective tissues including bone, cartilage, fat, ligament, marrow stroma, muscle, muscle, and a host of others *(75)* (Fig. 2).

The existence of precursor cells residing in human postnatal bone marrow with the potential to form multiple mesenchymal lineages was proposed by Friedenstein et al. in the late 1960s *(76)*. Friedenstein coined the phrase *colony-forming units fibroblastic* to describe bone marrow stromal cell isolates that were adherent, nonphagocytic, fibroblastic, and clonogenic in nature *(77)*. Under well-

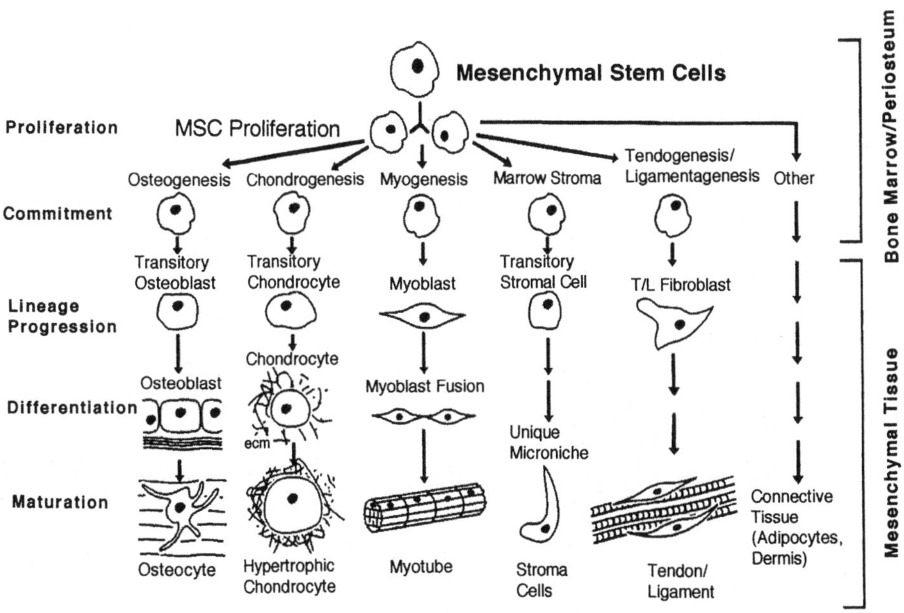

Fig. 2. The mesengenic process. Mesenchymal stem cells (MSCs) exhibit a potential for differentiating into a variety of mesenchymal tissues, for example, bone, cartilage, muscle, marrow stroma, tendons, ligaments, fat, and dermis. Commitment of the MSCs, as well as the next phase in which lineage-committed cells evolve through several transitory stages during lineage progression, is directed by the action of specific growth factors or cytokines. Terminal differentiation is associated with cessation of proliferation and the secretion of highly site-specific extracellular matrices. In maturation, the differentiated cells acquire the ability to function in tissue homeostasis. The cells in the end-stage differentiation processes exhibit fixed half-lives and can be expected to die, being replaced by newly differentiated cells arising from the continuous transition phases down the lineage pathway. (Reprinted with permission from ref. *75*.)

defined conditions, colony-forming units fibroblastics formed multiple mesenchymal tissues including bone, cartilage, fat, myelosupportive stroma, smooth muscle, cardiomyocytes, and tendon. The term *mesenchymal stem cells* was coined to describe a uniform population of stromal cells with a rapid ability to adhere to tissue culture plastic. The MSCs exhibited an extensive proliferative capacity and demonstrated the ability to differentiate into bone, cartilage and fat lineages *(78)*. This MSC population may represent a subset of putative pluripotent stem cells selected based on their rapid adhesion to plastic and their high mitotic index when cultured with 10% fetal bovine serum. They also express a unique set of surface protein markers (SH2, SH3, and SH4) not localized on hematopoietic precursors *(61,79)*.

MSCs lack the expression of surface markers CD1(a), CD11(b), CD14, CD34, CD45, and CD133 found on hematopoietic stem cells. They do, however, constitutively secrete IL-6, -7, -8, -11, -12, -14, and -15; macrophage colony stimulating factor (M-CSF); leukemia inhibitory factor (LIF); Flt-3 ligand; and SCF and can be induced with IL-1 α to produce IL-1 α, LIF, granulocyte colony stimulating factor (G-CSF), and granulocyte macrophage colony stimulating factor (GM-CSF) *(80–82)*. MSCs express several IL receptors, such as IL-1R (CD121), IL-3R (CD123), IL-6R (CD126), and IL-7R (CD127). They also express the transferrin receptor (CD71) and a variety of adhesion molecules, including activated leukocyte cell adhesion molecule (ALCAM) (CD166), intracellular adhesion molecule ICAM-2 (ICAM)-1 (CD54), (CD102), ICAM-3 (CD50), platelet-endothelial cell adhesion molecule (PECAM) (CD31), E-selectin (CD62E), L-selectin (CD62L), vascular cell adhesion molecule (VCAM) (CD31), the hyaluronate receptor (CD44) and several integrins, including very late activation antigen (VLA)-β (CD29), VLA-α (CD49), and a variety of α subunits (Table 1), and β 4 integrin (CD104). Table 1 offers a list of many of the surface markers used to characterize MSCs *(61,63,82,83)*.

Certain subfractions of marrow-derived stromal cells have enhanced multipotential capabilities. For example, Verfaillie and associates isolated and described a marrow cell population they defined as multipotential adult progenitor cells (MAPCs) *(84–87)*. The MAPCs appear to be more multipotential than MSCs because they can differentiate into hematopoietic cells. While the MAPCs and MSCs initially cohabitate in adherent cultures the MAPCs can be easily selected by exposure to a low nutrient medium containing low concentrations of serum and a specific growth factor cocktail. These cells express telomerase, and the telomerase length is maintained after many cell doublings. To date, the MAPCs are apparently immortal in tissue culture. As research in this field continues, a likely transplant scenario will unfold that certain subfractions of tissue-derived stem cells will be maximally effective in repairing a specific tissue injury.

3.3. Mesenchymal Stem Cell Use in Bone Regeneration

MSCs have been tested in a variety of animal models for their potential to regenerate skeletal tissues. Species and implant site differences, both with regard to the chemical microenvironment, architecture and mechanical loads, and variable MSC lineage responses, have resulted in novel and unexpected outcomes. In tissue culture studies, exposure of human MSCs to dexamethasone results in an osteogenic lineage *(88)*, whereas the same treatment elicits an adipogenic lineage in mouse MSCs *(89)*. Low-dose exposure of mouse MSCs to human recombinant BMP-2 elicits an osteogenic lineage *(90)*. In contrast, high doses of BMP-2 are required for a similar effect on human MSCs *(91)*. However, downstream pathways of transcription factors (e.g., Cbfa 1) appear to be similar for osteogenic differentiation across phylogeny. Caution should be exercised when

Table 1
Surface Marker Characteristics of Human MSCs

Surface marker type	*Designation*
Adhesion molecules	
Integrins	αvβ3
	αvβ5
	VLA-α1 (DC49a)
	VLA-α2 (CD49b)
	VLA-α3 (CD49c)
	VLA-α5 (CD49e)
	VLA-α6 (CD49f)
	VLA-β (CD29)
	VLA-β4 (CD104)
Others	ALCAM (CD166)
	ICAM-1 (CD54)
	ICAM-2 (CD102)
	ICAM-3 (CD50)
	NCAM (CD56)
	PECAM (CD31)
	VCAM (CD106)
	Endoglin (CD105)
	E-selectin (CD62E)
	Hyaluronate (CD44)
Growth factor Receptor	
	IL-1R (CD121)
	IL-2R (CD25)
	IL-3R (CD123)
	IL-4R (CD124)
	IL-6R (CD126)
	IL-7R (CD127)
	EGFR
	FGFR
	IFN-ψR (CDw119)
	PDGFR (CD140a)
	SCFR
	TGF-βR
	TNFR (CD120)
	Transferrin (CD71)
Other Markers	
	SH-2 (CD105)
	SH-3
	SH-4
	STRO-1
	Thy-1 (CD90)

VLA, very late activation antigen; ALCAM, activated leukocyte cell adhesion molecule; ICAM, intracellular adhesion molecule; NCAM, neural cell adhesion molecule; PECAM, platelet-endothelial cell adhesion molecule; VCAM, vascular cell adhesion molecule; IL, interleukin; EGFR, epidermal growth factor receptor; FGFR, fibroblast growth factor receptor; IFN, interferon; PDGFR, platelet-derived growth factor receptor; SCFR, stem cell factor receptor; TGF, transforming growth factor; TNFR, tumor necrosis factor receptor; SH, surface marker; STRO, stromal cell surface marker.

interpreting data from animal MSCs and implying human MSCs will respond similarly for regenerating skeletal tissues.

MSCs are generally accepted as the source of precursor cells for osteoblast turnover in normal bone homeostasis and they are also recruited for bone healing in fracture repair *(92)*. Because autografts and allogeneic banked bone have their limitations, alternative strategies have been sought for the repair of clinically significant bone defects, including porous scaffolds loaded with MSCs. Effective scaffolds for bone regeneration must exhibit the trait of osteoconduction (i.e., templates for the regeneration and ingrowth of bone tissue at osseous sites) *(93–95)*, but their lack of an osteoinductive potential has limited most of the bone substitute material field as a stand alone technology for repairing critical-sized defects. Osteoinductive agents (i.e., autoinduction) *(96)* induce the formation of bone at an ectopic (nonbone) site.

3.4. Bone Morphogenetic Proteins

The most well understood and characterized osteoinductive substances are BMPs. Since Professor Marshall Urist's initial description of BMP as a molecule capable of inducing an osteogenic response in a nonbony site (autoin-duction) *(96)*, that was later adapted to osteoinduction *(97)*, at least 16 BMPs have been described, cloned, and characterized (reviewed in refs. *2,98*). BMPs are members of the TGF-β superfamily of factors and are signaling molecules that have attracted considerable attention for bone regeneration *(99–103)*. However, not all BMPs are osteoinductive, and furthermore, BMPs do more than prompt bone regeneration. BMPs are involved in the developmental and functional organization of limbs, digits, liver, brain, kidney, muscle, and spleen *(104–112)*. Recombinant human BMP-2, -3, -4, and -7 are osteoinductive and have been used initially as a purified or recombinant protein soaked in a scaffold and applied to a bone defect, and more recently delivered via gene therapy vectors in bone regenerative strategies (reviewed in refs. *7,95,98,113*).

The clinical appeal of the osteoinductive BMPs lies in their capacity to promote bone regeneration. However, preclinical tests clearly indicate that significant dose-response differences exist across species with a significant dose escalation required for BMPs to work successfully as the phylogenetic ladder is ascended. For example, when progressing from rat to rabbit, a 3× dose was needed and from rabbit to dog, a 10× increase was needed to achieve comparable results. Similarly, when scaling from dogs to nonhuman primates and clinical studies in patients, a 3× to 5× increase in BMP dosing is required for similar bone regeneration *(53,114–117)*. The limited clinical data have evaluated superphysiologic BMP doses ranging from 1.7 to 3.4 mg *(116,118,119)*. A legitimate concern is whether the BMP that is removed or diffuses away from the local osseous wound to other tissues may induce either unwanted bone formation or contribute to an unexpected outcome. BMPs are *morphogens,* and morphogens exert profound cellular effects that are dose- and cell phenotype–dependent. Technologies that deliver sustained, physiological levels of local, time-dependent BMPs or other important signaling molecules would be welcomed.

3.5. MSCs Applied to Small Animal Models

A series of preclinical studies has been performed to evaluate the clinical potential of MSCs to repair bone defects *(120,121).* Culture expanded, marrow-derived syngeneic MSCs were used to repair a femur segmental defect in rats. A porous hydroxyapatite/β-tricalcium phosphate ceramic cylinder was seeded with syngeneic MSCs and implanted in an 8-mm long diaphyseal defect. In contrast to the ceramic cylinder only implants, the defects treated with the MSC-loaded implants produced continuous bone across the defect. In a similar animal model, human MSCs were loaded into the ceramic cylinders described previously, and implanted in identical femoral defects created in athymic, immunologically incompetent (T cell-deficient) rats. Complete union between regenerating bone and the cell-loaded ceramic implants was observed at 12 weeks. Biomechanical testing confirmed that the MSC-loaded ceramic cylinders were significantly stronger, with regard to stiffness and torque, as compared with the cell-free control cylinders. A recent report described a study to determine whether ex vivo BMP-9 transduced human MSCs could induce endochondral bone formation in athymic nude rats *(122).* Computed tomography and histological analysis demonstrated ectopic bone formation in the thigh muscle injection sites. The use of ex vivo gene therapy to generate MSCs capable of secreting potent bone-inducing soluble factors may be an effective method for repairing bony defects.

Another class of cells, the muscle-derived stem cells, has also been evaluated for their potential in repairing bone defects. Many reports have suggested that within skeletal muscle there are inducible osteoprogenitor cells that can be stimulated to produce bone. The previously described report by Urist demonstrated that implanted cancellous bone can induce ectopic bone in skeletal muscle *(96).* Khouri et al. evaluated the ability of BMP-3 to induce bone in a variety of body tissues, including Achilles tendon, adductor muscle, epididymal fat, kidney, liver, sciatic nerve, and spleen *(123).* BMP-3 induced the most bone when injected into skeletal muscle. The bone regenerative capabilities were further evaluated by implanting a muscle flap injected with BMP-3 protein into a calvarial defect. With this implant, the calvarial defect was completely healed. This pioneering study laid the foundation for future investigations evaluating skeletal muscle and muscle-derived stem cells for bone healing. Many of these studies and the current state of the art regarding muscle-based gene therapy and tissue engineering to improve bone healing has been reviewed *(124)*.

The local application of animal and human MSCs incorporating exogenous genes is an appealing option to compensate for the required high dose for effect of growth factor at an osseous wound site *(5,6)*. MSCs can be transduced with bone-enhancing signaling molecules using different vector systems without adversely affecting the normal functioning of MSCs *(125)*. The introduction of functional genes into animals to replace dysfunctional mutations has met with generally encouraging initial results *(15,16,125)*. The introduction of MSCs with a wild-type gene for type I collagen has corrected the deficits in experimental models of osteogenesis imperfecta. An autogenous ex vivo adenoviral gene transfer approach to generate BMP-2-producing stromal cell line and MSCs has produced substantial healing when implanted into a large bone defect of the femur *(127,128)*. Critical-sized defects in rats have also been successfully treated with adenoviral gene transfer of autogenous MSCs delivered by allogeneic, inactivated demineralized bone matrix *(128)*. However, the authors of the study stated concerns about safety of the adenoviral vector, specifically the immunologic sequelae (both from the vector and the allogeneic delivery system), and the fate of BMP-transfected cells.

Ex vivo forms of local gene therapy have also included cultured periosteal-derived MSCs transduced retrovirally with the BMP-7 gene and delivered with poly(glycolic) acid to restore critical-sized calvarial defects in rabbits *(129)* and retroviral transduction to re-introduce human MSCs expressing a reporter gene and IL-3 *(130)*. Mouse MSCs have also demonstrated myogenic potential by delivering a normal dystrophin gene into an *mdx* mouse, a murine model of muscular dystrophy *(131)*. In some regards, retroviral vectors are superior to adenoviral-based systems because the transfected gene becomes incorporated into the cell genome, thus prolonging expression. However, permanent incorporation into the host genome by random insertion events raises other safety issues related to insertional mutagenesis *(7)*. Work on suitable strategies for different vectors could make targeted gene therapy a rational and efficient alternative to methods that use exogenous growth factors (reviewed in ref. *7*).

3.6. MSCs Applied to Large Animal Models

The ability of MSC-loaded implants to repair gap defects in larger animals has been detailed in several reports *(132–135)*. As was described previously in the small-animal model section, the healing of a 21-mm osteoperiosteal segmental defect in dogs was enhanced using the porous hydroxyapatite/β-tricalcium phosphate ceramic cylinder loaded with autologous culture-expanded MSCs *(132)*. Radiographic examination and quantitative histomorphometry at 16 weeks confirmed that control implants did not impact the critical-sized defect gap in these animals. In contrast, the MSC-loaded ceramic implants regenerated new bone throughout the porous ceramic structure in a manner that was continuous with the contours of the adjacent bone. Recently, an allogeneic MSC preparation was evaluated in the same model system and produced qualitatively and quantitatively similar results *(133)* with new bone formed throughout the implant. Importantly, even though these animals were never exposed to systemic immunosuppression, no adverse host reaction was detected at any time point.

Recently, Chang et al. reported the use of ex vivo gene therapy for critical-size craniofacial bone defects *(134)* and for tissue-engineered maxillofacial bone regeneration *(135)* in a miniature swine model. Autologous MSCs transduced ex vivo with adenovirus-mediated human BMP-2 gene therapy and were reintroduced into 5 cm^2 cranial defects. Near-complete repair of the cranial defect was observed after 3 months in the defect sites receiving MSCs expressing BMP-2 delivered in a collagen type I construct compared to minimal regeneration in the control sites receiving MSCs containing *Lac Z* expressing MSCs. A similar strategy evaluated MSCs expressing BMP-2 delivered in a collagen type I construct implanted into 1.2 cm^2 maxillary defects *(135)*. Complete repair of the maxillary defect was observed after 3 months in the defect sites receiving MSCs expressing BMP-2 delivered in a collagen type I construct compared to minimal regeneration in the control sites receiving *Lac Z* expressing MSCs. Biomechanical testing confirmed that in the maximal compressive strength of new bone formed by the BMP-2 cell constructs was comparable to control, intact maxilla.

The clinical use of autologous MSCs has initially been reported in a feasibility and safety trial *(136)*. Rapid hematopoietic recovery after coinfusion of autologous MSCs was observed in breast cancer patients receiving high dose chemotherapy *(27)*. Allogeneic MSCs have also been evaluated to slow or halt the progression of a inborn lysosomal enzyme genetic disorder *(24)*, and osteogenesis imperfecta *(25,26)*. Several other trials for improving heme engraftment and several planned trials for heme engraftment are under way (reviewed in ref. *137*).

4. TISSUE ENGINEERING

Optimal bone regeneration, as well as the surgical reconstruction of other tissues, will require a reparative cell source, an appropriate scaffold and an effective extracellular milieu to introduce the cells to the wound environment and support tissue specific regenerative events. In addition, phenotype specific bioactive factors (e.g., cytokines, growth factors) must interact with the implanted cells in a reparative sequence analogous to fracture healing for the tissue-engineered implant to achieve regeneration of a functional tissue. The engineering of complex three-dimensional tissues complete with integrated vascular access

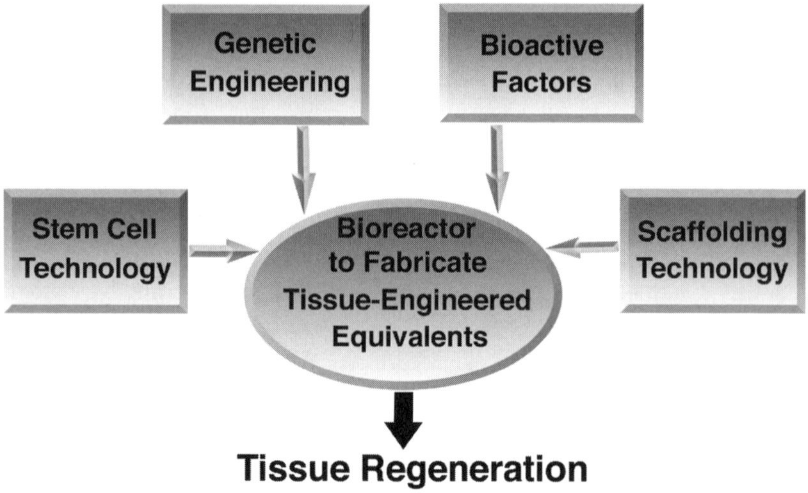

Fig. 3. The tools necessary for tissue engineering. The addition of stem cell technology, a reparative cell source, to other components of tissue engineering will advance the development of tissue-engineered equivalent structures. Genetic engineering of the reparative cells may also provide a source of bioactive factors (e.g., cytokines, growth factors, morphogens) that are released in a sustained manner at physiological levels. Complex, three-dimensional tissue-engineered equivalents will be developed and could be matured in a bioreactor to formulate tissue-engineered equivalents for the successful replacement of damaged or diseased tissues.

formulated in, for example bioreactors, should revolutionize tissue-engineered equivalents for the successful replacement of damaged or diseased tissues (Fig. 3).

5. FUTURE DIRECTIONS

Transplantation of MSCs represents a new avenue for improved cellular therapy with potential clinical applications in hematopoietic engraftment, gene therapy, and regenerative strategies. Preliminary clinical observations of MSC cotransplants may accelerate hematopoietic reconstitution after cord-blood-derived and autologous stem cell transplantation. Transplants of MSCs expressing an intact or amplified gene for type I collagen may provide a therapeutic role in overcoming the genetic disorder in patients with osteogenesis imperfecta. Genetically modified MSCs may also provide an effective means to correct other inborn errors of metabolism. With respect to allografts, cotransplants of donor-derived MSCs may ameliorate graft-vs-host disease by their immunosuppressive effect *(138)*. MSC therapy could also be an important bone engineering consideration for elderly patients (i.e., osteoporosis) *(139)*. As for any clinical therapeutic with promising preliminary results, randomized trials are absolutely necessary to clearly delineate a beneficial therapeutic outcome.

6. CONCLUSIONS

The autogenous graft, allogeneic banked bone, and various alloplastics, as well as technical improvements in distraction osteogenesis and electrical stimulation, will continue to provide beneficial clinical treatments to correct osseous deficiencies. However, the greatest challenges, excitement, and opportunities for bone regeneration lie in the field of tissue engineering. Improvements in tissue-engineered products will guarantee efficiency, effectiveness, and predictability required to promote regeneration. Advancing MSC technology is one of the critical features to arriving at a successful tissue-engineered product. Tissue-engineered bone regeneration products will emerge as rational therapies that will eventually supersede the autograft as the therapy of choice for regenerating osseous defects.

REFERENCES

1. Enneking WF, Mindell ER. Observations on massive retrieved human allografts. J Bone Joint Surg 1991;73-A:1123–1142.
2. Reddi AH. Initiation of fracture repair by bone morphogenetic proteins. Clin Orthop Rel Res 1998;355S:S66–S72.
3. Burgess EA, Hollinger JO. Options for engineering bone. In: Patrick CW Jr, Mikos AG, McIntire LV, eds. Frontiers in Tissue Engineering. New York, Pergamon, 1998, pp. 383–399.
4. Hollinger JO, Mayer MH. Bone regeneration: concepts and update. In: McCarthy J, ed. Distraction of the Craniofacial Skeleton. New York, Springer-Verlag, 2001.
5. Bonadio J, Goldstein SA, Levy RJ. Gene therapy for tissue repair and regeneration. Adv Drug Deliv Rev 1998; 33:53–69.
6. Bonadio J, Smiley E, Patil P, Goldstein S. Localized, direct plasmid gene therapy *in vivo*: prolonged therapy results in reproducible tissue regeneration. Nat Med 1999;5:753–759.
7. Winn SR, Hu Y, Sfeir C, Hollinger JO. Gene therapy approaches for modulating bone regeneration. Adv Drug Deliv Rev 2000;42:121–138.
8. Wang J-S, Shum-Tim D, Galipeau J, Chedrawy E, Eliopoulos N, Chiu RC-J. Marrow stromal cells for cellular cardiomyoplasty: feasibility and potential clinical advantages. J Thor Cardiovasc Surg 2000;120:999–1006.
9. Toma C, Pittenger MF, Cahill KS, Byrne BJ, Kessler PD. Human mesenchymal stem cells differentiate to a cardiomyocyte phenotype in the adult murine heart. Circulation 2002;1015: 93–98.
10. Tomita S, Mickle DAG, Weisel RD, et al. Improved heart function with myogenesis and angiogenesis after autologous porcine bone marrow stromal cell transplantation. J Thorac Cardiovasc Surg 2002;123:1132–1140.
11. Shake JG, Gruber PJ, Baumgartner WA, et al. Mesenchymal stem cell implantation in a swine myocardial infarct model: engraftment and functional effects. Ann Thoracic Surg 2002;73: 1919–1926.
12. Kotton DN, Ma BY, Cardoso WV, et al. Bone marrow-derived cells as progenitors of lung alveolar epithelium. Dev Dis 2001;128:5181–5188.

13. Ortiz LA, Gambelli F, McBride C, et al. Mesenchymal stem cell engraftment in lung is enhanced in response to bleomycin exposure and ameliorates its fibrotic effects. Proc Natl Acad Sci USA 2003;100:8407–8411.
14. Jin HK, Carter JE, Huntley GW, Schuchman EH. Intracerebral transplantation of mesenchymal stem cells into acid sphingomyelinase-deficient mice delays the onset of neurological abnormalities and extends their life span. J Clin Invest 2002;109:1183–1191.
15. Pereira RF, Oh MD, Laptev AV, et al. Marrow stromal cells as a source of progenitor cells for nonhematopoietic tissues in transgenic mice with a phenotype of osteogenesis imperfecta. Genetics 1998;95:1142–1147.
16. Horwitz EM, Prockop DJ, Fitzpatrick LA, et al. Transplantability and therapeutic effects of bone marrow-derived mesenchymal cells in children with osteogenesis imperfecta. Nat Med 1999;5:309–313.
17. Schwarz EJ, Alexander GM, Prockop DJ, Azizi SA. Multipotential marrow stromal cells transduced to produce L-DOPA: engraftment in a rat model of parkinson disease. Human Gene Ther 1999;10:2539–2549.
18. Li Y, Chen J, Want L, Zhang LJ, Lu M, Chopp M. Intracerebral transplantation of bone marrow stromal cells in a 1-methyl-4-phenyl-1,2,3,6-tetrahydropyridine mouse model of Parkinson's disease. Neurosci Lett 2001; 316:67–70.
19. Chopp M, Zhang XH, Li Y, et al. Spinal cord injury in rat: treatment with bone marrow stromal cell transplantation. Neuro Rep 2000;11:3001–3005.
20. Hofstetter CP, Schwarz E, Hess D, et al. Marrow stromal cells form guiding strands in the injured spinal cord and promote recovery. Proc Natl Acad Sci USA 2002;99:2199–2204.
21. Akiyama Y, Radtke C, Kocsis JD. Remyelination of the Rat Spinal Cord by Transplantation of Identified Bone Marrow Stromal Cells. Journal of Neuroscience 2002; 22:6623–6630.
22. Wu S, Suzuki Y, Ejiri Y, et al. Bone marrow stromal cells enhance differentiation of cocultured neurosphere cells and promote regeneration of injured spinal cord. J Neurosci Res 2003;72:343–351.
23. Li Y, Chen J, Chen XG, et al. Human marrow stromal cell therapy for stroke in rat: neurotrophins and functional recovery. Neurology 2002;59:514–523.
24. Koc ON, Day J, Nieder M, Gerson SL, Lazarus HM, Krivit W. Allogenic mesenchymal stem cell infusion for treatment of metachromatic leukodystrophy (MLD) and Hurler syndrome (MPS-IH). Bone Marrow Transplant 2002;30:215–222.
25. Horwitz EM, Prockop DJ, Gordon PL, et al. Clinical responses to bone marrow transplantation in children with severe osteogenesis imperfecta. Blood 2001;97:1227–1231.
26. Horwitz EM, Gordon PL, Koo WWK, et al. Isolated allogeneic bone marrow-derived mesenchymal cells engraft and stimulate growth in children with osteogenesis imperfecta: Implications for cell therapy of bone. Proc Natl Acad Sci USA 2002;99:8932–8937.
27. Koc ON, Gerson SL, Cooper BW, et al. Rapid hematopoietic recovery after coinfusion of autologous-blood stem cells and culture-expanded marrow mesenchymal stem cells in advanced breast cancer patients receiving high-dose chemotherapy. J Clin Oncol 2000;18:307–316.
28. Kleinschmidt J, Hollinger JO. Animal models in bone research. In: Reddi MHaH, ed. Bone Grafts and Bone Substitutes. Philadelphia, W.B. Saunders, 1992, pp. 133–147.
29. Pan WT, Einhorn TA. The biochemistry of fracture healing. Curr Orthop 1992;6:207–213.
30. Cornell CN. Current assessment of fracture healing. In: Brighton CT, Freidlaender GE, Lane JM, eds. Bone Formation and Repair. Rosemont, IL, AAOS, 1994, pp. 499–504.
31. Einhorn TA. Enhancement of fracture healing by molecular or physical means: an overview. In: Brighton CT, Freidlaender GE, Lane JM, eds. Bone Formation and Repair. Rosemont, IL, AAOS, 1994, pp. 223–238.

32. Schenk RK, Hunziker EB. Histologic and ultrastructural features of fracture healing. In: Brighton CT, Freidlander GE, Lane JM, eds. Bone Formation and Repair. Rosemont, IL, AAOS, 1994, pp. 117–146.
33. Einhorn TA. Enhancement of fracture-healing. J Bone Joint Surg 1995;77A:940–956.
34. Hollinger JO, Wong MEK. The integrated processes of hard tissue regeneration with special emphasis on fracture healing. Oral Surg Oral Med Oral Pathol 1996;82:594–606.
35. Barnes GL, Kostenuik PJ, Gerstenfeld LC, Einhorn TA. Growth factor regulation of fracture repair. J Bone Min Res 1999;14:1805–1815.
36. Clark RAF. The Molecular and Cellular Biology of Wound Repair. New York, Plenum Press, 1996, pp. 1–611.
37. Hollinger JO, Buck DC, Bruder S. Biology of bone healing: its impact on clinical therapy. In: S. Lynch RG, R. Marx, ed. Tissue Engineering: Applications in Maxillofacial Surgery and Periodontics. San Diego, Quintessence, 1998, pp. 17–53.
38. Fitzpatrick LA, Bilezkian JP. Actions of parathyroid hormone. In: Bilezkian JP, Raisz LG, Rodan GA, eds. Principles of Bone Biology. New York, Academic Press, 1996, pp. 339–346.
39. Wang EA, Isreal DL, Luxenberg DP. Bone morphogenetic protein-2 causes commitment and differentiation in C3H10T1/2 and 3T3 cells. Growth Factors 1993;9:57–71.
40. Rosen V, Nove J, Song JJ, Thies S, Cox K, Wozney JM. Responsiveness of clonal limb bud cell lines to bone morphogenetic protein-2 reveals a sequential relationship between cartilage and bone cell phenotypes. J Bone Min Res 1994;9:1759–1768.
41. Rodan G. Control of bone formation and resorption: biological and clinical perspective. J Cell Biochem 1998;30:S55–S61.
42. Ducy P, Karsenty G. Genetic control of cell differentiation in the skeleton. Curr Opinion Cell Biol 1998;10:614–619.
43. Ng W, Romas E, Donnan L, Findlay D. Bone Biology. Bailliere's Clin Endocrin Metab 1997;11:1–22.
44. Ahrens M, Ankenbauer T, Schroder D, Hollnagel A, Mayer H, Gross G. Expression of human morphogenetic proteins-2 or -4 in murine mesenchymal progenitor C3H10T1/2 cells induces differentiation into distinct mesenchymal cell lineages. DNA Cell Biol 1993;12:871–880.
45. Reddi AH. Bone and cartilage differentiation. Curr Opin Gen De. 1994;4:737.
46. Yamaguchi A. Regulation of differentiation pathway of skeletal mesenchymal cells in cell lines by transforming growth factor-beta superfamily. Cell Biol 1995;6:165–173.
47. Asahina I, Sampath TK, Hauschka PV. Human osteogenic protein-1 induces chondroblastic, osteoblastic, and/or adipocytic differentiation. Exp Cell Res 1996;222:38–47.
48. Reissmann E, Ernsberger U, Francis-West PH, Rueger D, Brickell PM, Rohrer H. Involvement of bone morphogenetic protein-4 and bone morphogenetic protein-7 in the differentiation of the adrenergic phenotype in developing sympathetic neurons. Development 1996;122:2079–2088.
49. Dernyck R, Zhang Y, Feng XH. Smads: transcriptional activators of TGF-β responses. Cell 1998;95:737–740.
50. Sakou T, Onishi T, Yamamoto T, Nagamine T, Sampath TK, Dijke PT. Localization of Smads, the TGF-β family of intracellular signaling components during endochondral ossification. J Bone Min Res 1999;14:1145–1152.
51. Schmitt JM, Hwang K, Winn SR, Hollinger JO. Bone morphogenetic proteins: an update on basic biology and clinical relevance. J Orthop Re. 1999;17:269–278.
52. Mayer MH. Clinical perspectives on bone grafting: avoiding the complications of developmental malformations. In: Seyfer A, Hollinger J, eds. Bone Repair and Regeneration, vol. 21. Philadelphia, W.B. Saunders, 1994, pp. 365–376.

53. Mayer MH, Hollinger JO, Ron E, Wozney J. Repair of alveolar clefts in dogs with recombinant bone morphogenetic protein and poly(alpha-hydroxy acid). Plastic Reconstr Surg 1996;98: 247–259.
54. Urist MR. Fundamental and Clinical Bone Physiology. Philadelphia, J.B. Lippincott, 1980.
55. Goldberg VM, Stevenson S. Natural history of autografts and allografts. Clin Orthop Rel Res 1987;225:7–16.
56. Heiple KG, Goldberg VM, Powell AE, Bos GD, Zika JM. Biology of cancellous bone grafts. Orthop Clin North Am 1987;18:179–183.
57. Manson P. Facial bone healing and bone grafts. A review of clinical physiology. In: Seyfer AE, Hollinger JO, eds. Bone Repair and Regeneration, vol. 21. Philadelphia, W.B. Saunders, 1994, pp. 331–348.
58. Tomford W. Current concepts review. Transmission of disease through transplantation of musculoskeletal allografts. J. Bone Joint Surg 1995;77-A:1742–1754.
59. Stevenson S. Enhancement of fracture healing with autogenous and allogeneic bone grafts. Clin Orthop Rel Res 1998;355S:S239–S246.
60. Langer R, Vacanti JP. Tissue engineering. Science 1993;260:920–926.
61. Pittenger MF, Mackay AM, Beck SC, et al. Multilineage potential of adult human mesenchymal stem cells. Science 1999;284:143–147.
62. Bjornson CR, Rietze RL, Reynolds BA, Magli MC, Vescovi AL. Turning brain into blood: A hematopoietic fate adopted by adult neural stem cells in vivo. Science 1999;283:534–537.
63. Azizi S, Stokes D, Augelli B, DiGirolamo D, Prockop DJ. Engraftment and migration of human bone marrow stromal cells implanted in the brains of albino rats—similarities to astrocyte grafts. Proc Natl Acad Sci USA 1998;95:3908–3913.
64. Reyes M, Verfaillie CM. Turning marrow into brain: generation of glial and neuronal cells from adult bone marrow mesenchymal stem cells. Blood 1999;94:377a.
65. Woodbury D, Schwarz E, Prockop DJ, Black IB. Adult cell and human bone marrow stromal cells differentiate into neurons. J Neurosci Res 2000;61:364–370.
66. Mezey K, Key S, Vogelsang G, Szalayova I, Lange GD, Crain B. Transplanted bone marrow generates new neurons in human brains. Proc Natl Acad Sci USA 2003;1000:1364–1369.
67. Lagasse E, Connors H, Al-Dhalimy M. Purified hematopoietic stem cells can differentiate into hepatocytes in vivo. Nat Med 2000;6:1229–1234.
68. Austin TW, Lagasse E. Hepatic regeneration from hematopoietic stem cells. Mech Dev 2003;120:131–135.
69. Ferrari G, Ciusella-De Angelis G, Coletta M, et al. Muscle regeneration by bone marrow-derived myogenic progenitors. Science 1998;279:1528–1530.
70. Orlic D, Kajstura J, Chimenti S. Bone marrow cells regenerate infarcted myocardium. Nature 2001;410:701–705.
71. Jackson KA, Mi T, Goodell MA. Hematopoietic potential of stem cells isolated from murine skeletal muscle. Proc Natl Acad Sci USA 1999;96:14482–14486.
72. Hematti P, Sloand E, Carvallo C. Absence of donor-derived keratinocyte stem cells in skin tissues cultured from patients after mobilized peripheral blood hematopoietic stem cell transplantation. Exp Hematol 2002;30:943–949.
73. Badiavas EV, Abedi M, Butmarc J, Falanga V, Quesenberry P. Participation of bone marrow derived cells in cutaneous wound healing. J Cell Physiol 2003;196:245–250.
74. Caplan AI, Bruder SP. Mesenchymal stem cells: building blocks for molecular medicine in the 21st century. Trends Mol Med 2001;7:259.
75. Caplan AI. The mesengenic process. Clin Plastic Surg 1994;21:429–435.

76. Friedenstein AJ, Petrakova KV, Kurolesova AL, Frolova GP. Heterotopic transplants of bone marrow. Analysis of precursor cells for osteogenic and hematopoietic tissues. Transplantation 1968;6:230–247.
77. Friedenstein AJ, Deriglasova UF, Kulagina NN, et al. Precursors for fibroblasts in different populations of hematopoietic cells as detected by the in vitro colony assay method. Exp Hematol 1974;2:82–92.
78. Caplan AI. Mesenchymal stem cells. J Orthop Res 1991;9:641–650.
79. Haynesworth SE, Goshima J, Goldberg VM, Caplan AI. Characterization of cells with osteogenic potential from human marrow. Bone 1992;13:81–88.
80. Haynesworth SE, Baber MA, Caplan AI. Cytokine expression by human marrow-derived mesenchymal progenitor cells in vitro. J Cell Physiol 1996;166:585–592.
81. Majumdar MK, Thiede MA, Mosca JD, Moorman MA, Gerson SL. Phenotypic and functional comparison of cultures of marrow-derived mesenchymal stem cells (MSCs) and stromal cells. J Cell Physiol 1998;176:57–66.
82. Deans RJ, Moseley AB. Mesenchymal stem cells: biology and potential clinical uses. Exp Hematol 2000;28:875–884.
83. Devine SM. Mesenchymal stem cells: will they have a role in the clinic? J Cell Biochem Suppl 2002;38:73–79.
84. Reyes M, Verfaillie CM. Characterization of multipotent adult progenitor cells, a subpopulation of mesenchymal stem cells. Ann N Y Acad Sci 2001;938:231–233.
85. Reyes M, Lund T, Lenvik T, Aguiar D, Koodie L, Verfaillie CM. Purification and ex vivo expansion of postnatal human marrow mesodermal progenitor cells. Blood 2001;98:2615–2625.
86. Jiang Y, Jahagirdar BN, Reinhardt RL, et al. Pluripotency of mesenchymal stem cells derived from adult marrow. Nature 2002;418:41–49.
87. Verfaillie CM. Hematopoietic stem cells for transplantation. Nat Immunol 2002;3:314–317.
88. Jaiswal N, Haynesworth SE, Caplan AI, Bruder SP. Osteogenic differentiation of purified, culture-expanded human mesenchymal stem cells in vitro. J Cell Biochem 1997;64:295–312.
89. Dennis JE, Caplan AI. Differential potential of conditionally immortalized mesenchymal progenitor cells from adult marrow of a H-2Kb-tsA58 transgenic mouse. J Cell Physiol 1996;167:523–538.
90. Dennis JE, Merriam A, Awadallah A, Yoo JU, Johnstone B, Caplan AI. A quadripotential mesenchymal progenitor cell isolated from the marrow of an adult mouse. J Bone Miner Res 1999;14:1–10.
91. Jaiswal N, Haynesworth SE, Caplan AI, Bruder SP. Differentiation of human mesenchymal stem cells by transforming growth factor beta superfamily: expression of osteoblast phenotype by BMP-2 and BMP-4. J. Bone Miner Res 2000;14:20.
92. Bruder SP, Fink DJ, Caplan AI. Mesenchymal stem cells in bone development, bone repair, and skeletal regeneration therapy. J Cell Biochem 1994;56:283–294.
93. Lindholm TS, Gao TJ. Functional carriers for bone morphogenetic proteins. Ann Chir Gynaecol 1993;82:3–12.
94. Hollinger JO, Brekke J, Gruskin E, Lee D. The role of bone substitutes. Clin Orthop Rel Res 1996;324:55–65.
95. Winn SR, Uludag H, Hollinger JO. Sustained release emphasizing recombinant human bone morphogenetic protein-2. Adv Drug Deliv Rev 1998;31:303–318.
96. Urist MR. Bone: formation by autoinduction. Science 1965;150:893–899.
97. Urist MR, Silverman MF, Buring K, Dubuc FL, Rosenburg JM. The bone induction principle. Clin Orthop 1967;53:243.

98. Wozney J. The bone morphogenetic family: multifunctional cellular regulators in the embryo and adult. Eur J Oral Sci 1998;106:160–166.
99. Linkhart TA, Mohan S, Baylink DJ. Growth factors for bone growth and repair: IGF, TGF beta, and BMP. Bone 1996;19:1–12.
100. Urist MR. Bone morphogenetic proteins in biology and medicine. In: Lindholm TS, ed. Bone Morphogenetic Proteins: Biology, Biochemistry, and Reconstructive Surgery. New York, Academic Press, 1996, pp. 7–30.
101. Urist MR. Bone morphogenetic protein: The molecularization of the skeletal system. J Bone Min Res 1997;12:343–346.
102. Viljanen VV, Lindholm TS. The search for new members of the BMP/TGFbeta family. Genbank/genpept accession numbers and selected references. In: Lindholm TS, ed. Skeletal Reconstruction and Bioimplantation: Demineralized Bone Matrix, Non-Collagenous, Native, and Recombinant Bone Morphogenetic Proteins. New York, Academic Press, 1997, pp. 241–248.
103. Riedel GE, Valentin-Opran A. Preliminary report: new technology. Clinical evaluation of rhBMP-2/ACS in orthopedic trauma: a progress report. Orthopedics 1999;22:663–665.
104. Kingsley DM. The TGF-beta superfamily: new members, new receptors, and new genetic tests of function in different organisms. Genes Develop 1994;8:133–146.
105. Storm EE, Huynh TV, Copeland NG, Jenkins NA, Kingsley DM, Lee S. Limb alterations in brachypodism mice due to mutations in a new member of the TGF-beta superfamily. Nature 1994;368:639–643.
106. Tickle C. On making a skeleton. Nature 1994;368:587–588.
107. Kingsley DM. Genes that define the number and shape of bones in the mouse skeleton, Portland Bone Symposium, vol. 4. Portland, OR, 1995.
108. Song JJ, Celeste A, Kong FM, Jirtle RL, Rosen V, Thies RS. Bone morphogenetic protein-9 binds to liver cells and stimulates proliferation. Endocrinology 1995;136:4293–4297.
109. Tomizawa K, Matsui H, Kondo E, et al. Developmental alteration and neuron-specific expression of bone morphogenetic protein-6 (BMP-6) mRNA in rodent brain. Mol Brain Res 1995;28:122–128.
110. Vukicevic S, Helder MN, Luyten FP. The developing human lung and kidney are major sites of synthesis of bone morphogenetic protein-3. J Histochem Cytochem 1994;42:869–875.
111. Lindholm TS. Bone Morphogenetic Proteins: Biology, Biochemistry and Reconstructive Surgery. San Diego, Academic Press, Inc, 1996.
112. Vukicevic S, Kopp J, Luyton FP, Sampath K. Induction of nephrogenic mesenchyme by osteogenic protein 1 (bone morphogenetic protein 7). Proc Natl Acad Sci USA 1996;93: 9021–9026.
113. Winn SR, Uludag H, Hollinger JO. Carrier systems for bone morphogenetic proteins. Clin Orthop Rel Res 1999;367:95–106.
114. Marden LJ, Hollinger JO, Chaudhari A, Turek T, Schaub R, Ron E. Recombinant bone morphogenetic protein-2 is superior to demineralized bone matrix in repairing craniotomies defects in rat. J Biomed Mater Res 1994;28:1127–1138.
115. Bostrom M, Lane J, Tomin E, et al. Use of bone morphogenetic protein-2 in the rabbit ulnar nonunion model. Clin Orthop Rel Res 1996;327:272–282.
116. Boyne PJ, Marx RE, Nevins M, et al. A feasibility study evaluating rhBMP-2/absorbable collagen sponge for maxillary sinus augmentation. Int J Periodont Restor Dent 1997;17:11–25.

117. Zegzula HD, Buck D, Brekke J, Wozney J, Hollinger JO. Bone formation with use of rhBMP-2 (recombinant human bone morphogenetic protein-2). J Bone Joint Surg 1997;79-A:1778–1790.
118. Howell TH, Fiorellini J, Jones A, et al. A feasibility study evaluating rhBMP-2/absorbable collagen sponge device for local alveolar ridge preservation of augmentation. Int J Periodont Rest Dent 1997;17:125–139.
119. Geesink RG, Hoefnagels NH, Bulstra SK. Osteogenic activity of OP-1 bone morphogenetic protein (BMP-7) in a human fibular defect. J Bone Joint Surg 1999;81-B:710–718.
120. Bruder SP, Kurth AA, Shea M, Hayes WC, Jaiswal N, Kadiyala S. Bone regeneration by implantation of purified, culture-expanded human mesenchymal stem cells. J Orthop Res 1998;16:155–162.
121. Kadiyala S, Jaiswal N, Bruder SP. Culture-expanded, bone marrow-derived mesenchymal stem cells can regenerate a critical-sized segmental bone defect. Tissue Eng 1997;3:173–185.
122. Dayoub H, Dumont RJ, Zhong J, et al. Human mesenchymal stem cells transduced with recombinant bone morphogenetic protein-9 adenovirus promote osteogenesis in rodents. Tissue Eng 2003;9:347–356.
123. Khouri RK, Brown BK, Koudsi B. Repair of calvarial defects with flap tissue: role of bone morphogenetic proteins and competent responding tissues. Plast Reconstr Surg 1996;98: 103–109.
124. Young BH, Peng H, Huard J. Muscle-based gene therapy and tissue engineering to improve bone healing. Clin Orthop Rel Res 2002;403:S243–S251.
125. Balk ML. Effect of rhBMP-2 on the osteogenic potential of bone marrow stromal cells from an osteogenesis imperfecta mouse (oim). Bone 1997;21:7–15.
126. Caplan AI. Osteogenesis imperfecta, rehabilitation medicine and fundamental research. Conn Tissue Res 1995;31:S9–S14.
127. Lieberman JR, Le LQ, Wu L, et al. Regional gene therapy with a BMP-2 producing murine stromal cell line induces heterotopic and orthotopic bone formation in rodents. J Orthop Res 1998;16:330–339.
128. Lieberman JR, Daluiski A, Stevenson S, et al. The effect of regional gene therapy with bone morphogenetic protein-2-producing bone-marrow cells on the repair of segmental femoral defects in rats. J Bone Joint Surg 1999;81-A:905–917.
129. Breitbart AS, Grande DA, Mason JM, Barcia M, James T, Grant RT. Gene-enhanced tissue engineering: applications for bone healing using cultured periosteal cells transduced retrovirally with the BMP-7 gene. Ann Plast Surg 1999;42:488–495.
130. Allay JA, Dennis JE, Haynesworth SE, et al. LacZ and interleukin-3 expression in vivo after retroviral transduction of marrow-derived human osteogenic mesenchymal progenitors. Human Gene Ther 1997; 8:1417–1427.
131. Ono I, Gunji H, Kaneko F, Saito T, Kuboki Y. Efficacy of hydroxyapatite ceramics as a carrier for recombinant human bone morphogenetic protein. J Craniofac Surg 1995;6:238–244.
132. Bruder SP, Kraus KH, Goldberg VM, Kadiyala S. The effect of implants loaded with autologous mesenchymal stem cells on the healing of canine segmental bone defects. J Bone Joint Surg 1998;80-A:985–996.
133. Arinzeh TL, Peter SJ, Archambault MP, et al. Allogenic mesenchymal stem cells regenerate bone in a critical-sized canine segmental defect. J Bone Joint Surg Am 2003;85-A:1927–1935.
134. Chang SC-N, Wei FC, Chuang H, et al. Ex vivo gene therapy in autologous critical-size craniofacial bone regeneration. Plast Reconstr Surg 2003;112:1841.

135. Chang SC-N, Chuang HL, Chen YR, et al. Ex vivo gene therapy in autologous bone marrow stromal stem cells for tissue-engineered maxillofacial bone regeneration. Gene Ther 2003;10:2013–2019.
136. Lazarus HM, Haynesworth SE, Gerson SL, Rosenthal NS, Caplan AI. Ex vivo expansion and subsequent infusion of human bone marrow-derived stromal progenitor cells (mesenchymal progenitor cells): implications for therapeutic use. Bone Marrow Transplant 1995;16:557–564.
137. Koc ON, Lazarus HM. Mesenchymal stem cells: heading into the clinic. Bone Marrow Transplant 2001;27:235–239.
138. Bartholomew A, Sturgeon C, Siatskas M, et al. Mesenchymal stem cells suppress lymphocyte proliferation in vitro and prolong skin graft survival in vivo. Exp Hematol 2002;30:42–48.
139. Solter D, Gearhart J. Putting stem cells to work. Science 1999;283:1468–1470.

11 Spermatogenesis From Transplanted Spermatogenic Stem Cells

Michael D. Griswold and Derek McLean

CONTENTS

1. INTRODUCTION

Spermatogenesis is a biological process that results in the conversion of the relatively undifferentiated germ cell into the highly differentiated spermatozoan. In man, the process initiates at puberty and may be continuous for the adult life of the individual. The cells that replenish the differentiating cells are the spermatogenic stem cells. These male germ line stem cells can both self-renew and provide daughter cells that can differentiate into the terminal cell types *(1–4)*.

In mice, germ line stem cells can first be identified after 7–7.5 days of gestation as approximately 100 primordial germ cells (PGCs) in the embryonal ectoderm. PGCs multiply to about 20,000 cells while migrating to the genital ridges. After reaching the gonadal ridges, PGCs undergo meiosis and become oocytes in female mammals. After entering meiosis, these cells no longer have the potential to be stem cells. In the embryonic male mammal, after arrival at the gonadal ridge, primordial germ cells are encapsulated into seminiferous cords by embryonic Sertoli cells. This event results in the inhibition of the entry of these germ cells into meiosis and the preservation of their stem cell potential. Primordial germ cells complete their journey to the gonadal ridge on embryonic day 12 (E12) in the rat (all times are slightly earlier in the mouse) (for review, *see* refs. *5,6*). In the rat at day E12, the gonad is indifferent, but on day E13 the Sertoli cells

From: *Contemporary Endocrinology: Stem Cells in Endocrinology*
Edited by: L. B. Lester © Humana Press Inc., Totowa, NJ

differentiate and encompass the germ cells. The first identifiable seminiferous cords containing germ cells and Sertoli cells and surrounded by mesenchymal cells appear on day E14.

Primordial germ cells proliferate from day E12 to day E16, after which mitosis is arrested until birth. Spermatogenesis is initiated in the testes of postnatal mammals (shortly after birth in rodents) when quiescent primordial germ cells in the center of the cords resume proliferation, and migrate from the center to the periphery of the seminiferous cords and become gonocytes *(7,8)*. Pluripotent embryonic germ cells can be derived from PGCs *(9)*, but not from gonocytes, which are the first stem cells committed to the male germ line. After spermatogenesis is initiated the term *gonocyte* is replaced with the term *spermatogonia*.

The most widely accepted hypothesis is that spermatogonial cells of the type A_s (A single) are the stem cells of the adult testis *(10,11)*. They are present in low numbers and proliferate randomly to yield A_{pr} (A pair) and A_{al} (A-aligned) spermatogonia that are still considered to be undifferentiated cells but not stem cells. The A_{al} cells divide to form differentiated A_1 cells and, thereafter, there is a rapid succession of differentiated spermatogonial cell divisions that eventually yield spermatocytes. The spermatocytes undergo meiosis, first yielding round spermatids that transform into elongate spermatids that are finally released as spermatocytes.

2. SPERMATOGONIAL TRANSPLANTS

Identification of stem cells has required an assay that clearly shows the "renewal" function. Historically, spermatogenic stem cells have been difficult to identify because no functional assay existed and because there are no identifying markers. In 1994, Brinster and colleagues described a technique for the transplantation of germ cells from mouse to mouse, and, in 1996, they showed it could be done from rat to mouse *(12–14)*—referred to as syngeneic and xenogeneic transplants, respectively. These were the first successful transplantation experiments in which isolated germ cells could be shown to seed seminiferous tubules and the seeded tubules shown to continually produce sperm. In the initial studies by Brinster, although a complex mixture of cells was injected into the tubular lumen, it was assumed that the germ line stem cells were responsible for the renewed spermatogenesis. Thus it has become accepted that the stem cells in the preparation give rise to and replenish colonies of spermatogenic cells.

For maximum efficiency in the process, the testis of the recipient animal must lack virtually all germ cells *(15)*. In recipient animals the germ cells are depleted either by treatment of rodents with busulfan or by use of a murine strain genetically deficient in germ cells (W-locus mutants usually WW^v) *(16)*. Busulfan treatment does not eliminate all spermatogonia in recipient males, but does lower the number dramatically and suppresses spermatogenesis temporarily to allow seeding of transplanted cells. Some endogenous spermatogenesis in busulfan-treated animals does resume, eventually yielding sperm cells from both the host and the donor. Despite the injection of stem cells into an abnormal environment (the tubule lumen) the stem cells are able to make their way through layer of cells and junctional complexes to the basement membrane. Non-stem cells are flushed out of the tubule by normal fluid movements shortly after injection. The requirement to exclude endogenous cells in the recipient and the ability of the donor cell to find the right environment suggested to Brinster and colleagues that there was a spermatogenic stem cell niche in the testis *(15,17,18)*. There are additional studies that indicate a specific distribution of undifferentiated spermatogonia in mouse seminiferous tubules and, therefore, the niche position may be regulated *(19)*. What regulates the interaction between spermatogenic stem cell and niche is unknown.

To make donor cells identifiable, Brinster and others have used a transgenic strain of donor animals (Rosa 26) that expresses the *lac Z* gene in all cells, including the spermatogenic stem cells (for review, *see* ref. *20*). After incubation of recipient testes within the appropriate substrate, any cell that arose from the donor would stain a very characteristic blue color. Within a few days to a week after injection, the donor stem cells can be seen along the basement membrane of the recipient seminiferous tubules *(21)*. From 1 week to 1 month, donor cells on the basement membrane divided and formed an interconnected monolayer of cells. After 1 month, the cells in the center of the monolayer began to differentiate and, ultimately, established a region of spermatogenesis. The recipient was shown to pass the *lac Z* gene to progeny through normal breeding, thus establishing the biological success of the procedure *(13)*.

Since 1995, several laboratories have extended this technology and applied it to important biological problems. Advances include interspecies transplantation *(22–25)* and the development of techniques to enrich stem cells *(26–29)*. Some of the most important advances, however, have come in the techniques to culture stem cells and to transfect or transduct new genes in to cells via viral vectors. This technology offers the promise of a new technique for producing offspring with an engineered genome.

3. CELL CULTURE AND TRANSFECTION OF GERM CELLS

One of the major limitations in studies of male germ cells has been the inability to successfully maintain them in culture. Germ cell transplantation techniques provide a functional system to evaluate the success of long-term culture of germ cells. Using these techniques, mixtures of testicular germ cells maintained in culture from 19 to 132 days successfully generated donor-derived spermatogenesis following previous studies *(20,30,31)*. This was considered a major breakthrough because it was previously believed that germ cells did not survive in culture more than a few days. In this particular culture system, it was only necessary for the spermatogenic stem cells to survive. It was reported that the stem cells survived best when cultured on STO cell (mouse embryonic fibroblasts) feeder layers *(30,32)*.

More recently, successful transfection of spermatogonial stem cells was reported using a retroviral vector *(33,34)*. Several approaches were used to expose stem cells to retroviral particles expressing the bacterial β-galactosidase gene. Germ cells isolated from neonatal and cryptorchid testes were incubated with retroviral producing cells alone, with a STO feeder layer and retroviral producing cells, and with a STO feeder layer while being periodically exposed to retroviral particles. After infection, cultured cells were injected into recipient animals. After 2–3 months, blue colonies revealed donor-derived spermatogenesis by demonstrating development of sperm positive for the transfected gene, β-galactosidase. The periodic infection system produced the highest level of successful transfection. It was also shown that coinjection of retroviral particles and fresh germ cells into recipient testes could produce positive results. The colonies persisted and expressed the transgenes for at least 6 months after transplantation. It was reported that, under the most successful conditions, up to 71% (10 of 14) of the transplanted testes contained colonies expressing the transgene. When all of their in vitro data were analyzed, they found 71 blue areas in 171 testes. This was interpreted to be an infection rate of about 1 in 280 stem cells injected *(34)*. Stem cells must have been dividing in culture to achieve stable integration of the retroviral transgene. The efficiency of infection and stable integration is low, but the results demonstrate that genes can be directly introduced into the male germ line and have important future implications. Recently, other types of viral vectors and infection schemes have been used to achieve a high percentage of transduction in cultured spermatogonial stem cells *(35)*. These cells have been transplanted into recipients and gave rise to all stages of spermatogenesis expressing the transgene. In 2001, Nagano et al. revealed that they had produced transgenic offspring after retroviral transduction of cultured stem cells *(34)*. In 2002, Hamra et al. reported similar success using a lentivirus *(36)*.

A telomerase-immortalized mouse type A spermatogonial cell line, in the presence of stem cell factor, has been shown to go through meiosis and to form spermatocytes and spermatids in a continuous cell line *(37)*. This differentiation occurred in the absence of supportive cells. A reasonable interpretation is that the telomerase immortalized the seminiferous stem cells in this culture. This immortalized cell line is potentially a major breakthrough in elucidating the molecular mechanisms of spermatogenesis.

4. INFORMATION ABOUT TESTIS STEM CELLS GAINED FROM TRANSPLANTATION EXPERIMENTS

4.1. Number of Stem Cells

The most widely referenced number of spermatogenic stem cells in the mammalian testis is 0.02% of the total testis cell population (10^8) in the mouse *(38,39)*. This estimate is based on histological evaluation of spermatogonia in rodents. The spermatogonial stem cell transplantation technique has provided a functional assay for the presence of spermatogenic stem cells. Although the technique has dramatically enhanced the ability to investigate spermatogenic stem cell biology, estimation of the number of stem cells present in a cell suspension injected into recipient testes has relied on the previous estimate of 1 stem cell in every 5000 testicular cells in mice *(38,39)*.

The relative spermatogenic stem cell number increases during testis development *(18)*. This result was determined by transplantation of germ cells into recipient testes from neonate (days 0–4), pup (days 5–12), and cryptorchid adult. There are 39-fold more spermatogenic stem cells in adult cryptorchid testes than neonate testes. This result indicates that stem cell niches in the seminiferous tubules are continuously formed during testis development. However, the physical and biochemical characteristics of the spermatogenic stem cell niche have not been described. A stem cell niche can also be formed after elimination or lack of spermatogenic stem cells within a testis. This conclusion is based on the mere fact that the spermatogonial stem cell transplantation technique will result in donor-derived spermatogenesis in recipient testes (described previously).

The relative efficiency of spermatogenic stem cell colonization after transplantation can be determined by calculating the number of colonies that form after transplantation into a recipient testis. Likewise, the degree of spermatogenic stem cell enrichment can be evaluated using similar calculations. The efficiency of spermatogenic stem cell colonization in the testes of recipient mice has been reported to be 4–5% *(18)*, 12–15% *(40)*, and 9% *(41)*. Shinohara et al. *(18)* and Orwig et al. *(41)* based the colonization efficiency on the number of donor-derived spermatogenic colonies in recipient testes after transplantation and the approximation that 1 in 5000 cells in the testis is a spermatogenic stem cell *(38,39)*. In contrast, Nagano *(40)* estimated the colonization efficiency based on sequential transplantation of germ cells into multiple recipients. This strategy was used to analyze "homing efficiency" of spermatogenic stem cells after transplantation and required that germ cells are transplanted into one mouse, allowed to colonize for a period, and then transplanted into a second group of recipients. Using germ cells from cryptorchid and untreated controls as donors, Nagano *(40)* estimated there are 3500 and 3000 spermatogenic stem cells in mice testes, respectively. These numbers are significantly lower than previous estimates of 10,000 to 20,000 spermatogenic stem cells in the mouse testis depending on the number of stem cells recovered *(18,29,41)*.

The number of spermatogenic stem cells in rat testes was evaluated with the use of the spermatogonial stem cell transplantation technique. Interestingly, the number of spermatogenic stem cells that colonize recipient nude mice testes indicate there are 9.5-fold more stem cells in rat testes than mice testes *(41)*. Taking into account the number of Sertoli cells, type A isolated (A_{is}), and type A paired (A_{pr}) spermatogonia in the rat *(42)*, Orwig et al. *(41)* determined that the colonization efficiency of rat spermatogenic stem cells is 8.5% in recipient mice testes. Similarly, these researchers estimated there are approximately 830,000 spermatogenic stem cells in rat testes. The higher number of spermatogenic stem cells in rats when compared with mice raises interesting questions regarding the spermatogenic stem populations in similar and diverse species. The application of spermatogonial stem cell transplantation to other species will provide additional useful information about the spermatogenic stem cell population in a wide variety of species.

4.2. Timing of Stem Cell Differentiation

Spermatogenic stem cells are a stable population of cells in the adult testis that provide differentiating germ cells throughout life. This stable population must develop from undifferentiated gonocyte populations present in prenatal and neonatal animals. Because spermatogenic stem cells differentiate, a stem cell niche is formed that provides an environment that allows stem cells to function as progenitor cells. The exact timing by which these events occur has been examined with the use of spermatogonial stem cell transplantation.

At birth, a population of gonocytes is present in the seminiferous tubules, and these cells migrate to the periphery of the seminiferous tubule to initiate spermatogenesis (described in detail previously). The ability of mouse germ cells to establish donor-derived spermatogenesis is limited in the early neonatal period *(18,43)*. The innate ability of germ cells from the testes of neonatal animal to colonize recipient mice testes must be differentiated from the ability of colonized germ cells to initiate donor-derived spermatogenesis. Shinohara et al. *(18)* reported that neonate donors established very few colonies after transplantation. McLean et al. *(43)* demonstrated that a significant change occurs in the mouse spermatogenic stem cell population during the first 5 days postpartum. Germ cell donors ages 0–2 days postpartum colonized recipient testes as two to four cells that did not initiate donor-derived spermatogenesis. These cells did migrate to the basement membrane of the seminiferous tubules in recipient testes. Germ cells from the testes of day 3 postpartum and older mice colonize recipient testes and initiate areas of extensive donor-derived spermatogenesis. Apparently, at day 3 or 4 postpartum in mice, a population of spermatogenic stem cells capable of initiating donor-derived spermatogenesis has formed. This coincides with the migration of germ cells to the basement membrane of the seminiferous tubules and the postnatal initiation of mitosis in these cells.

The spermatogenic stem cell population continues to expand during testis development and puberty *(18)*. A dynamic relationship between the stem cell and the Sertoli cell of the seminiferous tubule leads to the formation of a niche and injected germ cells can compete with endogenous stem cells for these niches *(15)*. The identification of factors that may regulate the spermatogenic stem cell population and niche formation has been limited. Glial cell line-derived neurotrophic factor (GDNF) appears to affect the spermatogonial population in mice testes. Gene-targeted mice with one GDNF-null allele have depleted spermatogenic stem cell reserves, whereas mice in which Sertoli cells overexpress GDNF have an accumulation of undifferentiated spermatogonia *(44)*. The proliferation of undifferentiated spermatogonia has been stimulated in azoospermic mutant mice by GDNF *(45)*. Last, transplantation of germ cells from mice overexpressing GDNF results in recipient testes with a similar phenotype as is observed in the testes of GDNF-overexpressing donor animals *(46)*. These data suggest GDNF may regulate the accumulation of undifferentiated spermatogonia and the process in which these proceed into spermatogenesis. Further characterization of factors that regulate spermatogenic stem cell activity in vitro should provide important information on factors that influence spermatogenic stem cells and their niche in vivo.

4.3. Stem Cell Markers—Enrichment

The small number of spermatogenic stem cells in the testes and the lack of specific biochemical or physical characteristics have hampered the identification of these cells. Several techniques have been used to obtain an enriched population of spermatogenic stem cells. Information about other adult stem cell populations and testis biology has been used to successfully enrich spermatogenic stem cells. The ultimate goal of this research is to obtain a pure population of stem cells for complete characterization. The spermatogonial stem cell transplantation technique provides the only functional assay to test for enrichment of stem cells. This technique has dramatically accelerated the rate at which information about spermatogenic stem cells has been obtained.

Initial attempts to enrich for spermatogenic stem cells were based on stem cell properties. Laminin is a major extracellular matrix constituent of the basement membrane. Shinohara et al. *(26,47)* hypothesized spermatogonial stem cells will bind laminin because of their close contact with the basement membrane. Short-term culture of mouse germ cells on laminin-coated plates resulted in a fivefold to sevenfold enrichment for spermatogenic stem cells. Similarly, short-term culture of rat germ cells on laminin-coated plates resulted in 8.5-fold enrichment for spermatogenic stem cells *(33)*. Integrins are receptors present on cells that bind to integrins. Selection of testicular cells for β1- and α6-integrin with the use of fluorescent activated cell sorting (FACS) resulted in 5-fold and 10.2-fold enrichment of spermatogenic stem cells based on colonization following spermatogonial stem cell transplantation *(26)*. Interestingly, selection of testicular cell with FACS for cells positive for c-Kit, a receptor involved in spermatogonia proliferation and differentiation, did not lead to enrichment for spermatogenic stem cells *(26)*.

Exposing the testis to core body or slightly higher temperatures can reduce the number of differentiating germ cells. The experimental cryptorchid model in which testes are surgically secured in the body cavity leads to a 70% decrease in testis weight and a 40-fold reduction in testis cell number by 2 months. In mice, this leads to a 23-fold enrichment of spermatogonial stem cells *(47)*. Similarly, transplantation of germ cells from testes transiently exposed to 43°C (hyperthermia exposure) led to a 50% decrease in testis weight and a fivefold to sixfold enrichment of spermatogenic stem cells *(29)*.

Vitamin A is essential for normal spermatogenesis *(48)*. Vitamin A deficiency (VAD) in rodents results in multiple physiologic effects. One of these effects is a loss of mature germ cells in the testis, resulting in infertility. A single injection of retinol and the inclusion of vitamin A in the diet after a rat or mouse has developed VAD results in the resumption of spermatogenesis, indicating the spermatogenic stem cells remain viable in the testes of animals with VAD *(49)*. Transplantation of germ cells from the testes of mice with VAD indicated there was a 2.5-fold to 3-fold enrichment of spermatogenic stem cells. However, the testes in mice with VAD weighed 25% less than the testes from control animals. This degree of testicular regression, greater than experimental cryptorchidism or hyperthermia, suggests that spermatogenic stem cell enrichment would be greater than observed values. Therefore, vitamin A may be important in maintaining or activating the spermatogenic stem cell population in adult animals.

Selection of spermatogenic stem cells based on multiple parameters has been used for further enrichment beyond that achieved by single step enrichment. The highest levels of spermatogenic stem cell enrichment have been achieved with the use of experimental cryptorchism, along with FACS. Cryptorchid testis cells fractionated by FACS analysis based on light-scattering properties and the presence of cell-surface molecules has lead to dramatic enrichment of spermatogenic stem cells *(27)*. The most effective enrichment strategy selected germ cells from cryptorchid testes for low side scatter, a measure of cell complexity, positive staining for α6-integrin, and negative staining for αv-integrin. This resulted in a 166-fold enrichment of spermatogenic stem cells *(27)*. This level of enrichment leads to a cell suspension in which 1 of every 30–40 cells is a spermatogenic stem cell.

Identification of cell surface markers on spermatogenic stem cells has improved the understanding of how similar or different spermatogenic stem cells are to other adult stem cell populations. Spermatogenic stem cells in mice and rats can be enriched fivefold to sevenfold by selection of testis cells for CD9 as demonstrated by spermatogonial stem cell transplantation *(50)*. CD9 is expressed in multiple tissues including bone marrow cells, muscle, and brain. The expression of CD9 in the testis is not specific for spermatogenic stem cells. Immunohistochemical analysis of testis samples showed CD9 is expressed on cells near the basement membrane of the seminiferous tubule, including spermatogonia *(50)*.

Kubota et al. *(51)* conducted the most extensive characterization to date of the phenotypic and functional characteristics of spermatogenic stem cells. A combination of surface markers and FACS was used to identify spermatogenic stem cells as a distinctive population in the adult testis. First, spermatogonia do not express major histocompatibility complex (MHC) class I (MHC-I) molecules so these researchers hypothesized that spermatogenic stem cells do not express MHC-I. Negative selection of testis cells for MHC-I (MHC-I$^-$) resulted in a sixfold enrichment of spermatogenic stem cells. The cell population positive for MHC-I showed almost no stem cell activity *(51)*. The next step in this study used information about the hematopoietic stem cell (HSC) population to characterize spermatogenic stem cells. HSCs are positive for Thy-1 (CD90), a glycosyl phosphatidylinositol-anchored glycoprotein *(52)*. Testicular cells in the MHC-I$^-$ population were fractionated based on Thy-1 expression. In addition, the cells were fractionated based on *c-kit*$^-$ expression, which was previously shown to enrich for spermatogenic stem cells. Spermatogenic stem cell activity, based on colonization of recipient testes, was detected almost exclusively in the Thy-1$^+$ c-Kit$^-$ cell population *(51)*. Furthermore, this cell population, MHC-I$^-$ Thy-1$^+$c-Kit$^-$, is positive for other markers or characteristics previously used to enrich for spermatogenic stem cells including α6-integrin and low side scatter *(27)*. A final antigenic characterization of the MHC-I$^-$ Thy-1$^+$c-Kit$^-$ population demonstrated that cells in this population were positive for CD24 but not Sca-1 or CD34, which are all present on HSCs *(51)*.

Mouse HSCs can be isolated as a side population of cells based on the ability of the cells to rapidly efflux the fluorescent DNA-binding dye Hoechst 33342 *(53)*. Fractionation of testis cells into a side population characterized by Hoechst 33342 efflux was used to determine if spermatogenic stem cells share this characteristic with HSCs. Transplantation of testis cells in the side population did not have spermatogenic stem cell activity *(51)*. These results indicate the spermatogenic stem cells share several characteristics of HSCs such as being Thy-1^+-positive and CD24-positive but do not share other characteristics such as presence in a side population or the expression of Sca-1 or CD34. This strategy to identify phenotypic and functional characteristics of spermatogenic stem cells along with the spermatogonial stem cell transplantation assay provide a powerful means to identify unique properties of these cells, thereby accelerating the process of obtaining a pure population of spermatogenic stem cells. The surface phenotype for spermatogenic stem cells is side scatter^{low}, α6-integrin$^+$, β1-integrin$^+$, CD24$^+$, thy-1$^+$, αv-integrin$^-$, c-Kit$^-$, MHC-I$^-$, and CD9$^+$ and are not present in the side population.

In rats, spermatogenic stem cells seem to differentiate from a distinct population of gonocytes early in postnatal development. Rat gonocytes present in the testes of day 0–4 animals (day of birth = 0) form two distinct populations: pseudopod and round gonocytes *(54)*. Rat gonocytes at this age are larger than other testicular cells (12–15 mm) and have low intracellular complexity and prominent round nuclei. Pseudopod and round gonocytes represent 1.41% of the total number of cells in the testis isolated using a standard trypsin/DNase I digestion procedure *(54)*. In addition, pseudopod and round gonocytes are present in approximately the same numbers in the testis *(54)*. Round gonocytes were characterized with a round, smooth surface, whereas pseudopod gonocytes had distinct cytoplasmic extensions. Germ cell transplantation experiments demonstrated that the majority of spermatogonial stem cell activity was found in the pseudopod subpopulation of gonocytes. Specifically, 50 of 1001 pseudopod gonocytes produced and maintained colonies of spermatogenesis in recipient seminiferous tubules, whereas 1 of 579 round gonocytes produced a colony *(54)*. This represents a unique resource to characterize cells that have spermatogenic stem cell function.

Characterization and identification of spermatogenic stem cells may be further enhanced with the use of transgenic mouse lines in which promoters of spermatogonia-specific genes drive the expression of reporter genes. Selection of a reporter gene such as green fluorescent protein enables researchers to fractionate cells with positive expression with the use of FACS. This strategy has been used successfully to enrich for spermatogenic stem cells in two independent laboratories. Ohbo et al. *(55)* used an 18-kb genomic fragment of the Oct-4 promoter and enhancer to control the expression of green fluorescent protein. These researchers confirmed the spermatogenic stem cell population is characterized with low expression of *c-kit* and that activated leukocyte cell adhesion molecule is expressed transiently in gonocytes *(55)*. Another group used a 400-bp fragment of the spermatogonia-specific gene Stra8 *(56)* to regulate expression of reporter genes in spermatogonia and spermatogenic stem cells *(57)*. Germ cells positive for the reporter gene expression expressed α6- and β1-integrin and spermatogonial stem cell transplantation experiments indicated 700-fold enrichment for spermatogenic stem cell activity *(57)*. Transgenic models have great potential in the purification and characterization of spermatogenic stem cells. The biggest challenge with this approach is the identification of suitable promoters to control expression of reporter genes in spermatogenic stem cells.

REFERENCES

1. Dym M. Spermatogonial stem cells of the testis. Proc Natl Acad Sci USA 1994;91:11287–11289.
2. de Rooij DG, Grootegoed JA. Spermatogonial stem cells. Curr Opin Cell Biol 1998;10:694–701.
3. De Rooij DG, Van Dissel-Emiliani FM, Van Pelt AM. Regulation of spermatogonial proliferation. Ann N Y Acad Sci 1989;564:140–153.
4. Meachem S, von Schonfeldt V, Schlatt S. Spermatogonia: stem cells with a great perspective. Reproduction 2001;121:825–834.
5. McLaren A. Somatic and germ-cell sex in mammals. Philos Trans R Soc Lond [Biol] 1988;322:3–9.
6. McLaren A. Meiosis and differentiation of mouse germ cells. Symp Soc Exp Biol 1984;38:7–23.
7. Orth JM, Boehm R. Functional coupling of neonatal rat Sertoli cells and gonocytes in coculture. Endocrinology 1990;127:2812–2820.
8. McGuinness M, Orth J. Behavior of neonatal gonocytes (Gs) co-cultured with Sertoli cells (SCs). XIth North American Testis Workshop, Montreal, Canada, 1991.
9. Donovan PJ, de Miguel M, Cheng L, Resnick JL. Primordial germ cells, stem cells and testicular cancer. Apmis 1998;106:134–141.
10. Huckins C. The spermatogonial stem cell population in adult rats. 3. Evidence for a long-cycling population. Cell Tissue Kinet 1971;4:335–349.
11. Huckins C. The spermatogonial stem cell population in adult rats. II. A radioautographic analysis of their cell cycle properties. Cell Tissue Kinet 1971;4:313–334.
12. Brinster RL, Zimmerman JW. Spermatogenesis following male germ-cell transplantation. Proc Natl Acad Sc. USA 1994;91:11298–11302.
13. Brinster RL, Avarbock MR. Germline transmission of donor haplotype following spermatogonial transplantation. Proc Natl Acad Sci USA 1994;91:11303–11307.
14. Clouthier DE, Avarbock MR, Maika SD, Hammer RE, Brinster RL. Rat spermatogenesis in mouse testis. Nature 1996;381:418–421.
15. Shinohara T, Orwig KE, Avarbock MR, Brinster RL. Germ line stem cell competition in postnatal mouse testes. Biol Reprod 2002;66:1491–1497.
16. Mintz B. Embryological development of primordial germ cells in mouse, influence of a new mutation, W^I. J Embryol Exp Morphol 1957;5:396–403.
17. Ryu BY, Orwig KE, Avarbock MR, Brinster RL. Stem cell and niche development in the postnatal rat testis. Dev Biol 2003;263:253–263.
18. Shinohara T, Orwig KE, Avarbock MR, Brinster RL. Remodeling of the postnatal mouse testis is accompanied by dramatic changes in stem cell number and niche accessibility. Proc Natl Acad Sci USA 2001;98:6186–6091.
19. Chiarini-Garcia H, Homack JR, Griswold MD, Russell LD. Distribution of type A spermatogonia is not random. Biol Reprod 2001;65:1179–1185.
20. Brinster RL, Nagano M. Spermatogonial stem cell transplantation, cryopreservation and culture. Semin Cell Dev Biol 1998;9:401–409.

21. Nagano M, Avarbock MR, Brinster RL. Pattern and kinetics of mouse donor spermatogonial stem cell colonization in recipient testes. Biol Reprod 1999;60:1429–1436.
22. Dobrinski I, Avarbock MR, Brinster RL. Germ cell transplantation from large domestic animals into mouse testes. Mol Reprod Dev 2000;57:270–279.
23. Ogawa T, Dobrinski I, Avarbock MR, Brinster RL. Xenogeneic spermatogenesis following transplantation of hamster germ cells to mouse testes. Biol Reprod 1999;60:515–521.
24. Nagano M, McCarrey JR, Brinster RL. Primate spermatogonial stem cells colonize mouse testes. Biol Reprod 2001;64:1409–1416.
25. Nagano M, Patrizio P, Brinster RL. Long-term survival of human spermatogonial stem cells in mouse testes. Fertil Steril 2002;78:1225–1233.
26. Shinohara T, Avarbock MR, Brinster RL. beta1- and alpha6-integrin are surface markers on mouse spermatogonial stem cells. Proc Natl Acad Sci USA 1999;96:5504–5509.
27. Shinohara T, Orwig KE, Avarbock MR, Brinster RL. Spermatogonial stem cell enrichment by multiparameter selection of mouse testis cells. Proc Natl Acad Sci USA 2000;97:8346–8351.
28. Shinohara T, Brinster RL. Enrichment and transplantation of spermatogonial stem cells. Int J Androl 2000;23(Suppl. 2):89–91.
29. McLean DJ, Russell LD, Griswold MD. Biological activity and enrichment of spermatogonial stem cells in vitamin A-deficient and hyperthermia-exposed testes from mice based on colonization following germ cell transplantation. Biol Reprod 2002;66:1374–1379.
30. Nagano M, Avarbock MR, Leonida EB, Brinster CJ, Brinster RL. Culture of mouse spermatogonial stem cells. Tissue Cell 1998;30:389–397.
31. Kanatsu-Shinohara M, Ogonuki N, Inoue K, et al. Long-term proliferation in culture and germline transmission of mouse male germline stem cells. Biol Reprod 2003;69:612–616.
32. Nagano M, Ryu BY, Brinster CJ, Avarbock MR, Brinster RL. Maintenance of mouse male germ line stem cells in vitro. Biol Reprod 2003;68:2207–2214.
33. Orwig KE, Avarbock MR, Brinster RL. Retrovirus-mediated modification of male germline stem cells in rats. Biol Reprod 2002;67:874–879.
34. Nagano M, Brinster CJ, Orwig KE, Ryu BY, Avarbock MR, Brinster RL. Transgenic mice produced by retroviral transduction of male germ-line stem cells. Proc Natl Acad Sci USA 2001;98:13090–13095.
35. Jeong D, McLean DJ, Griswold MD. Long-term culture and transplantation of murine testicular germ cells. J Androl 2003;24:661–669.
36. Hamra FK, Gatlin J, Chapman KM, et al. Production of transgenic rats by lentiviral transduction of male germ-line stem cells. Proc Natl Acad Sci USA 2002;99:14931–14936.
37. Feng LX, Chen Y, Dettin L, et al. Generation and in vitro differentiation of a spermatogonial cell line. Science 2002;297:392–395.
38. Meistrich M, van Beek M. Spermatogonial stem cells. In: Desjardins C, Ewing L, eds. Cell and Molecular Biology of the Testis. New York, Oxford University Press, 1993, pp. 266–295.
39. Tegelenbosch RA, de Rooij DG. A quantitative study of spermatogonial multiplication and stem cell renewal in the C3H/101 F1 hybrid mouse. Mutat Res 1993;290:193–200.
40. Nagano MC. Homing efficiency and proliferation kinetics of male germ line stem cells following transplantation in mice. Biol Reprod 2003;69:701–707.
41. Orwig KE, Shinohara T, Avarbock MR, Brinster RL. Functional analysis of stem cells in the adult rat testis. Biol Reprod 2002;66:944–949.
42. Huckins C. The spermatogonial stem cell population in adult rats. I. Their morphology, proliferation and maturation. Anat Rec 1971;169:533–557.
43. McLean DJ, Friel PJ, Johnston DS, Griswold MD. Characterization of spermatogonial stem cell maturation and differentiation in neonatal mice. Biol Reprod 2003;69:2085–2091.

44. Meng X, Lindahl M, Hyvonen ME, et al. Regulation of cell fate decision of undifferentiated spermatogonia by GDNF. Science 2000;287:1489–1493.
45. Tadokoro Y, Yomogida K, Ohta H, Tohda A, Nishimune Y. Homeostatic regulation of germinal stem cell proliferation by the GDNF/FSH pathway. Mech Dev 2002;113:29–39.
46. Creemers LB, Meng X, den Ouden K, et al. Transplantation of germ cells from glial cell line-derived neurotrophic factor-overexpressing mice to host testes depleted of endogenous spermatogenesis by fractionated irradiation. Biol Reprod 2002;66:1579–1584.
47. Shinohara T, Avarbock MR, Brinster RL 2000;Functional analysis of spermatogonial stem cells in Steel and cryptorchid infertile mouse models. Dev Biol 220:401–11
48. Griswold MD, Bishop PD, Kim KH, Ping R, Siiteri JE, Morales C. Function of vitamin A in normal and synchronized seminiferous tubules. Ann N Y Acad Sci 1989;564:154–172.
49. van Pelt AM, de Rooij DG. Synchronization of the seminiferous epithelium after vitamin A replacement in vitamin A-deficient mice. Biol Reprod 1990;43:363–367.
50. Kanatsu-Shinohara M, Toyokuni S, Shinohara T. CD9 is a surface marker on mouse and rat male germline stem cells. Biol Reprod 2004;70:70–75.
51. Kubota H, Avarbock MR, Brinster RL. Spermatogonial stem cells share some, but not all, phenotypic and functional characteristics with other stem cells. Proc Natl Acad Sci USA 2003;100:6487–6492.
52. Randall TD, Weissman IL. Characterization of a population of cells in the bone marrow that phenotypically mimics hematopoietic stem cells: resting stem cells or mystery population? Stem Cells 1998;16:38–48.
53. Goodell MA, Brose K, Paradis G, Conner AS, Mulligan RC. Isolation and functional properties of murine hematopoietic stem cells that are replicating in vivo. J Exp Med 1996;183:1797–1806.
54. Orwig KE, Ryu BY, Avarbock MR, Brinster RL. Male germ-line stem cell potential is predicted by morphology of cells in neonatal rat testes. Proc Natl Acad Sci USA 2002;99:11706–11711.
55. Ohbo K, Yoshida S, Ohmura M, et al. Identification and characterization of stem cells in prepubertal spermatogenesis in mice small star, filled. Dev Biol 22003;58:209–225.
56. Oulad-Abdelghani M, Bouillet P, Decimo D, et al. Characterization of a premeiotic germ cell-specific cytoplasmic protein encoded by Stra8, a novel retinoic acid-responsive gene. J Cell Biol 1996;135:469–477.
57. Giuili G, Tomljenovic A, Labrecque N, Oulad-Abdelghani M, Rassoulzadegan M, Cuzin F. Murine spermatogonial stem cells: targeted transgene expression and purification in an active state. EMBO Rep 2002;3:753–759.

12 Hematopoietic Stem Cell Transplant in the Treatment of Autoimmune Endocrine Disease

Jody Schumacher and Ewa Carrier

CONTENTS

1. INTRODUCTION

The recent successful application of hematopoietic stem cell transplantation (HSCT) to the treatment of severe or refractory rheumatic autoimmune diseases has led to speculation of whether stem cell transplantation might benefit patients with endocrine autoimmune diseases. Autoimmune type 1 diabetes mellitus is a prime candidate for hematopoietic stem cell therapies because of both the severity of the disease and associated long-term complications of chronic hyperglycemia. HSCT in patients with recent-onset type 1 diabetes may prevent further autoimmune-mediated destruction of islet β cells and thus decrease acute and chronic risks of hyperglycemia. In patients with type 1 diabetes, however, pancreas or islet transplant is necessary to restore endogenous insulin production,

From: *Contemporary Endocrinology: Stem Cells in Endocrinology*
Edited by: L. B. Lester © Humana Press Inc., Totowa, NJ

and current protocols require the use of chronic immunosuppressive therapies to control autoimmunity and prevent allograft rejection. HSCT may overcome limitations associated with pancreas and islet transplant by inducing immunologic tolerance to islet β cells. Nevertheless, autologous HSCT is associated with autoimmune disease relapse, and correction of genetic susceptibility to the development of type 1 diabetes would require allogeneic HSCT with human leukocyte antigen (HLA)-DQ or DR (HLA class II) mismatched donors, which leads to a high risk of acute graft versus host disease. In this chapter, we examine both the potential therapeutic benefits and risks of HSCT for treatment of autoimmune type 1 diabetes mellitus as a model for HSCT in the treatment of endocrine autoimmune diseases.

2. HEMATOPOIETIC STEM CELL TRANSPLANTATION FOR AUTOIMMUNE DISEASES

Historically, HSCT was used to rescue hematopoiesis after myeloablative therapy for the treatment of nonresectable tumors and malignancies. Subsequently, improvements in induction and immunosuppressive therapies have allowed the use of myeloablative therapy as a supportive platform for replacement of defective hematopoietic stem cells in patients with congenital diseases. In the context of HSCT therapies, autoimmune diseases share aspects of both congenital diseases and malignancies, in that both immunosuppressive therapy and replacement of defective hematopoietic stem cells may be directly therapeutic. Recently, observed therapeutic resolution of coincidental autoimmune diseases in patients receiving HSCT for primary malignancies or hematopoietic failure suggested the possible application of HSCT in the treatment of primary autoimmune diseases (reviewed in ref. *1*).

Autoimmune diseases encompass a broad range of diseases with unique pathogeneses and manifestations. Criteria for classification of a disease as autoimmune include: (1) direct evidence of adoptive transfer of disease by immune cells or antibodies, (2) indirect evidence by reproduction of autoimmune disease in animal models, or (3) circumstantial evidence by clinical response to immunosuppressive therapy *(2)*. These criteria are functional, however, and do not implicate a specific mechanism in the pathogenesis of autoimmunity. To cure autoimmune disease, the mechanisms that promote autoimmunity must be altered; consequently, the potential of HSCT for treatment of these diseases differs with respect to the disease.

Allogeneic HSCT has the potential to cure autoimmune diseases in which genetic susceptibility to autoimmunity is expressed through hematopoietic stem cells. For example, allogeneic HSCT elicited durable disease remission in patients suffering from rheumatic autoimmune diseases coincidental to malignancy or marrow failure as indication for HSCT *(1)*. These observations led to the initiation of phase I/II clinical trials of HSCT for primary autoimmune diseases, and therapeutic resolution (durable remission) of autoimmune disease after allogeneic HSCT was observed (reviewed in ref. *3*). As a result, phase III clinical trials of HSCT for treatment of systemic lupus erythematosus, multiple sclerosis, rheumatoid arthritis, and systemic sclerosis are in development *(4)*.

Allogeneic HSCT is associated with significant morbidity and mortality from toxic conditioning therapies, graft-vs-host disease, graft loss, and infection secondary to chronic immunosuppressive therapies; therefore, allogeneic HSCT is limited to patients with life-threatening disease. Although the toxicity of conditioning regimens and the possibility of graft failure are limitations to the widespread application of allogeneic HSCT for the treatment of autoimmune diseases, recent research in animal models suggests that nonmyeloablative HSCT may cure autoimmune diseases *(5,6)*. In patients receiving HSCT for primary malignancies, donor immune cells preferentially target malignant cells, a phenomenon known as the "graft-vs-leukemia" effect *(7)*. Reduced toxicity of conditioning therapy often leads to the establishment of mixed hematopoietic chimerism after allogeneic HSCT, thus promoting therapeutic destruction of malignant cells while reducing the risks associated with graft loss and toxic conditioning therapies (reviewed in ref. *8*). In HSCT for primary autoimmune diseases, a similar phenomenon, that of "graft-vs-autoimmunity," led to resolution of autoimmune manifestations *(9)*. Therefore, allogeneic HSCT may cure autoimmune disease without the necessity for myeloablative conditioning, which reduces the risk of mortality resulting from severity of HSCT conditioning regimens and graft loss.

Autologous HSCT likewise may restore immunologic tolerance to self-antigens, thereby inducing autoimmune disease remission. Autologous HSCT for the treatment of autoimmune disease is based on the principle that dose escalation of immunosuppressive therapies may be necessary to fully ablate autoimmune-reactive cells, and hematopoietic stem cells necessary to restore hematopoiesis after immunosuppressive (or ablative) therapies. Autologous HSCT minimizes risks associated with allogeneic HSCT such as graft loss, graft-vs-host disease, and chronic immunosuppression; nevertheless, autologous HSCT carries increased risk of disease relapse or recurrence when compared with allogeneic HSCT because of both preexisting immunity to tissue antigens and genetic susceptibility to the (re)development of autoimmune reactivity to these antigens (reviewed in ref. *3*).

In general, diseases that are responsive to immunosuppressive therapy are candidates for dose escalation of immunosuppressive therapy followed by autologous hematopoietic stem cell rescue. For example, systemic lupus erythematosus and juvenile idiopathic arthritis respond to immunosuppressive therapy, and, in phase I/II clinical trials, long-term remission (>4 years) was induced in patients receiving autologous HSCT for these diseases *(10)*. Relapse was frequent after autologous HSCT for systemic lupus erythematosus and multiple sclerosis; nevertheless, patient sensitivity to standard clinical therapies was restored.

Although HSCT has the potential to cure or ameliorate symptoms of autoimmune diseases, the potential therapeutic benefit of HSCT in the treatment of autoimmune disease must not only justify the risks associated with transplant, but also must clearly demonstrate improved quality of life for patients when compared with available supportive therapies. HSCT has successfully induced disease remission in patients suffering from rheumatic autoimmune diseases, providing patients relief from debilitating illness. The success of HSCT in inducing remission of rheumatic autoimmune diseases has encouraged interest in the possible application of HSCT therapy to the treatment of endocrine autoimmune diseases.

3. AUTOIMMUNE ENDOCRINE DISEASES

The majority of autoimmune endocrine diseases are characterized by immune destruction of endocrine tissue leading to glandular dysfunction and hormonal imbalance. Endocrine autoimmune diseases include: hypophysitis, Graves' disease, thyroiditis, autoimmune disease of the adrenal gland (Addison's disease), hypoparathyroidism, autoimmune type 1 diabetes mellitus, and autoimmune polyendocrine syndromes. These diseases have complex etiologies, which are unique to each disease, and, to some extent, unique to each patient. With the exception of autoimmune polyendocrine syndrome type I, genetic susceptibility to the development of endocrine autoimmune diseases is associated with multiple polymorphisms in the major histocompatibility complex genes *(11)*. Genetic susceptibility alone, however, is insufficient to elicit autoimmune disease. Studies of autoimmune disease manifestation in identical twins show a lack of concordance, suggesting that specific (environmental or stochastic) immune triggering events are essential to pathogenesis of autoimmune disorders in patients with genetic susceptibility *(12)*.

The potential of HSCT for treatment of autoimmune diseases is dependent on both the pathogenesis and severity of the underlying disorder. For example, hormone replacement therapy is both effective and well tolerated in patients with thyroiditis and (after destruction or removal of the thyroid gland) Graves' disease. Prognosis for these diseases is excellent, and complications related to hormone therapy are minimal; therefore, HSCT for these diseases cannot be justified. Moreover, HSCT is effective only for diseases in which the primary defect is expressed through hematopoietic stem cells. For example, autoimmune polyendocrine syndrome type 1 results from a defect in central (thymic) tolerance, which allows for the clonal expansion of self-reactive T cells *(13)*. HSCT in patients with autoimmune polyendocrine syndrome type 1, whether autologous or allogeneic, might restore immunologic tolerance to autologous tissue antigens; however, in the absence of therapy to correct the defect in central tolerance mechanisms, autoimmune pathology will recur. Nevertheless, therapies to cure autoimmune polyendocrine syndrome type 1 must also address existing immunologic reactivity toward auto-antigens, and thus HSCT might be used as supportive therapy to thymic transplantation.

Stem cell therapies should be considered, however, for autoimmune type 1 diabetes mellitus, Addison's disease, and autoimmune polyendocrine syndromes types II and III, because these diseases are both clinically severe and potentially amenable to HSCT. Autoimmune type 1 diabetes mellitus is strongly associated with both types II and III autoimmune polyendocrine syndromes *(14)*. Moreover, autoimmune type 1 diabetes is representative of the difficulties associated with HSCT for endocrine autoimmune diseases. The remainder of this chapter, therefore, will focus on the potential therapeutic benefit of HSCT for autoimmune type 1 diabetes mellitus as a model for the potential of HSCT in the treatment of endocrine autoimmune diseases.

3.1. Autoimmune Type 1 Diabetes Mellitus

Of the endocrine autoimmune diseases, autoimmune type 1 diabetes mellitus (hereafter referred to as type 1 diabetes) is the most extensively studied because of both disease prevalence and severity. In 2002, approximately 13 million people in the United States (6.3% of the population) suffered from diabetes, and approximately 5–10% of these cases were diagnosed as type 1 diabetes *(15)*. Furthermore, in the year 2000, diabetes was the sixth leading cause of death listed on death certificates in the United States *(15)*. Thus, despite supportive therapy, diabetes mellitus causes significant morbidity and mortality.

Type 1 diabetes is characterized by insulin deficiency secondary to progressive T-cell-mediated destruction of insulin-producing pancreatic β cells within the islets of Langerhans. Clinical therapy is supportive; blood glucose is controlled by insulin injections, diet, and exercise. Nevertheless, homeostatic maintenance of blood glucose through shifting physiologic conditions is clearly unrealistic, and long-term complications of chronic hyperglycemia, including retinopathy, peripheral neuropathy, stroke, cardiovascular disease, and nephropathy, frequently develop. Although tight glycemic control delays the development of chronic complications *(16)*, the incidence of acute, life-threatening episodes of hypoglycemia is more than three times higher with this treatment *(17)*.

The pathogenesis of type 1 diabetes has yet to be unequivocally identified. Genetic predisposition to the development of type 1diabetes is associated with multiple alleles both within and outside the major histocompatibility complex

(MHC) (reviewed in ref. *18*). Penetrance, however, is variable, and may be associated with specific autoimmune-triggering events. A variety of environmental or random (stochastic) events may lead to the abrogation of immunologic tolerance to islet β cells. Viral infection has been associated with the development of type 1 diabetes through the process of molecular mimicry of islet antigens or bystander T-cell activation *(19–21)*. Alternatively, antigenic similarities between islet cell antigens and antigens in cow's milk have been proposed to induce type 1 diabetes in genetically susceptible individuals *(20)*. Loss of tolerance to islet β cells in genetically susceptible individuals likewise could occur through stochastic processes involving determinant spreading of cryptic epitopes *(22)*.

Although there is a lack of consensus regarding autoimmune-triggering events, it is clear that autoimmunity toward islet β cells is T cell-mediated and, at least primarily, results from failure of peripheral tolerance mechanisms. A dual checkpoint peripheral tolerance failure model has been proposed to explain the pathogenesis of type 1 diabetes in genetically susceptible individuals *(23)*. Progression through the first checkpoint suggested peripheral tolerance leads to autoreactive T-cell infiltration of pancreatic islets (a pathologic process known as insulitis), whereas progression to active destruction of islet β cells occurs after the second peripheral tolerance checkpoint. The dual checkpoint model may explain variable penetrance; a series of autoimmune-triggering events, whether stochastic or environmental, may lead to peripheral tolerance failure in genetically susceptible individuals. Therapeutic intervention at either of the peripheral tolerance regulatory checkpoints may prevent or halt the progression to type 1 diabetes. Ideally, patients with genetic susceptibility to type 1 diabetes could be identified in early infancy and the development of diabetes prevented. Unfortunately, early trials of preventive therapy have been unsuccessful *(24)*. Moreover, in the majority of patients autoimmunity is developed at the time of clinical presentation, and thus therapeutic benefit must derive from reversal of active autoimmunity.

Hematopoietic stem cell transplantation may reverse autoimmunity in patients with type 1 diabetes. In mouse models of type 1 diabetes, autoimmunity can be adoptively transferred to nondiabetic hosts via allogeneic HSCT; conversely, allogeneic HSCT of healthy donor cells into diabetic recipients halts autoimmune disease progression *(25)*. Likewise, transfer of type 1 diabetes from human donor to recipient was observed after a sibling HLA-identical bone marrow transplant *(26)*. Genetic susceptibility to acquired immunity in type 1 diabetes thus appears to be expressed through immune cells, and defects inherent in hematopoietic cells can be corrected by allogeneic HSCT. Likewise, development of autoimmunity is dependent, to some extent, on environmental influences or stochastic events, and therefore autologous HSCT may restore self-tolerance by recapitulating hematopoiesis.

4. AUTOLOGOUS HSCT IN RECENT-ONSET AUTOIMMUNE TYPE 1 DIABETES MELLITUS

Loss of islet β cells occurs over a time span of 3–5 years and is initially balanced by regeneration; however, persistent autoimmunity eventually exhausts or overwhelms the regenerative capacity of pancreatic stem cells *(27)*. Clinical symptoms manifest when the number of islet β cells falls below the threshold necessary to maintain glycemic control, but before complete ablation of islet β cells. Patients with residual islet β cells have better metabolic control, are less likely to experience acute hypoglycemic or ketotic episodes, and are less likely to develop chronic complications *(28)*. Therapeutic intervention designed to control autoimmunity in patients with recent onset type 1 diabetes may preserve remaining islets and thus improve disease management.

Autologous HSCT has the potential to restore self tolerance to islet β cells, and thus preserve remaining pancreatic islets. The rationale for autologous HSCT is based on the observations that (1) development of type 1 diabetes in genetically susceptible individuals is dependent on environmental or stochastic immune-triggering events and (2) type 1 diabetes is responsive to immunosuppressive therapy. Although autologous HSCT would not alter genetic susceptibility to the development of type 1 diabetes, genetic susceptibility alone does not induce type 1 diabetes in susceptible individuals. Therefore, restoration of self-tolerance may result in durable disease remission. Likewise, type 1 diabetes is transiently responsive to immunosuppressive therapy, which suggests that dose-escalation of immunosuppressive therapies, although requiring stem cell rescue, may result in greater therapeutic benefit.

In patients with recent-onset type 1 diabetes, immunosuppressive therapy with corticosteroids or cyclosporine delays the onset of insulin-dependency; nevertheless, chronic immunosuppressive therapy slows but does not halt autoimmune disease progression *(29–33)*. Lack of long-term benefits of chronic immunosuppressive therapy in patients with recent-onset type 1 diabetes may be due to inadequate immunosuppression resulting in low-level, persistent autoimmune reactivity or cumulative diabetogenic effects of immunosuppressive agents. Both cyclosporine and corticosteroids are associated with the development of insulin resistance and inhibition of insulin secretion by pancreatic islet β cells *(34–37)*. Nevertheless, dose reduction or withdrawal of corticosteroids or cyclosporine may reverse impaired insulin secretion *(38)*; therefore, intensive, short-term therapy with immunosuppressive agents may minimize toxic effects. Dose escalation of immunosuppressive therapies followed by stem cell rescue (autologous HSCT) might overcome the limitations of low-dose, chronic immunosuppressive therapies and restore self-tolerance to islet β cells. Relief from autoimmunity would preserve remaining islet β cells and potentially allow for complete restoration of glycemic control as a result of islet β-cell regeneration. Nevertheless, the likelihood of autoimmune relapse or recurrence after autologous HSCT may outweigh the possible benefits of short-term remission or extended insulin-independence.

Autologous HSCT does not correct genetic predisposition to development of autoimmunity, and thus the mechanisms that trigger autoimmunity in type 1 diabetes profoundly affect whether autologous HSCT can provide therapeutic benefit (durable disease remission). For example, if autoimmunity is triggered by exposure to specific pathogens, then autologous HSCT could provide therapeutic benefit in the absence of reexposure to the inducing pathogen. Alternatively, in the event that autoimmunity develops as a consequence of nonspecific immune processes such as inflammation or pancreatic damage, then autologous HSCT might accelerate recurrent type 1 diabetes because of both preexisting autoimmune-mediated damage as well as the diabetogenic effects of many of the available immunosuppressive drugs. Although autologous HCT followed by chronic immunosuppressive therapy to prevent disease recurrence may be more effective than immunosuppressive therapy alone, the necessity for chronic immunosuppressive therapy negates many of the benefits to autologous versus allogeneic HSCT.

One of the more compelling arguments for autologous HSCT in the treatment of type 1 diabetes is the number of monozygotic twins that do not share type 1 diabetes. Concordance among identical twins is typically estimated at 30–50% *(39,40)*; however, long-term studies show that lifetime concordance rates may be as high as 50–70% *(41,42)*. Moreover, in a long-term study of diabetes concordance of monozygotic twins, 8 of 12 nondiabetic twins tested showed evidence of damage to pancreatic β cells or autoimmunity in the absence of diabetes (based on the presence of autoantibodies or functional insulin release tests *(41)*). The genetic influence toward development of type 1 diabetes thus may be higher than previously assumed; moreover, susceptibility toward (re)development of autoimmunity may be higher in patients with preexisting pancreatic endocrine damage than in nondiabetic twins.

The possibility of autoimmune disease relapse or recurrence and benefit of relief from hyperglycemia must be balanced against the risks of autologous HSCT. The acute risk of mortality resulting from induction toxicity and infections after autologous HSCT is approximately 1–2% *(43)*. Although the potential for durable disease remission in patients with debilitating autoimmune disease favors autologous HSCT in spite of the risk of acute mortality, recent-onset type 1 diabetes can be controlled with exogenous insulin therapy in the majority of patients. The potential benefit of autologous HSCT thus does not balance the risk of HSCT in patients with recent-onset type 1 diabetes because (1) high probability of disease recurrence after autologous HSCT, (2) toxicity of induction therapies, and (3) acute risk of mortality from infection after HSCT.

The benefit-to-risk ratio of autologous HSCT would favor autologous HSCT, however, with the development of gene therapy or successful pre-autoimmune vaccination protocols. If autologous HSCT could correct genetic predisposition to the development of type 1 diabetes, then the potential for long-term disease remission (or cure) would negate the necessity for chronic post-HSCT immunosuppressive therapies and offset the acute risk of mortality.

5. ALLOGENEIC HSCT IN RECENT-ONSET AUTOIMMUNE TYPE 1 DIABETES MELLITUS

In contrast to autologous HSCT, allogeneic HSCT may cure autoimmunity, and consequently preserve remaining pancreatic islets in patients with recent-onset type 1 diabetes. The rationale for allogeneic HSCT for patients with recent-onset type 1 diabetes is based on the following observations: (1) allogeneic HSCT will halt autoimmune-mediated destruction of islet β cells; (2) preservation of intact islet β cells is beneficial to the patient even in the absence of full metabolic control; (3) because hyperglycemia is more easily managed in patients with functional islet β cells, chronic complications are less likely to develop; and (4) there is a low probability of disease relapse or recurrence after allogeneic HSCT.

Allogeneic HSCT is difficult to justify in recently diagnosed patients, however, because chronic effects of hyperglycemia are unlikely to manifest before complete loss of islet β cells. In patients likely to receive maximum therapeutic benefit from allogeneic HSCT, therefore, lack of life-threatening disease manifestations argues against high-risk, aggressive therapies. This conundrum is not unique to type 1 diabetes; for example, in patients with the congenital disease β-thalassemia, HSCT early in the course of disease (before peripheral organ involvement) results in a higher rate of disease-free survival, and a correspondingly lower incidence of transplant-related mortality (approximately 3% in patients younger than age 16) *(44)*. The potential benefit of allogeneic HSCT differs, however, with respect to the indicating disease. In patients with type 1 diabetes, potential therapeutic benefit of relief from hyperglycemia and associated chronic complications must be balanced against the risks associated with allogeneic HSCT.

Donor selection will increase the comparable risk of allogeneic HSCT for early-onset type 1 diabetes. Although the incidence of type 1 diabetes in the general population of Western countries is approximately 1 in 300, the incidence for first-degree relatives of affected individuals is approximately 1 in 20 *(45)*.

The strongest genetic determinants of type 1 diabetes are particular polymorphisms of the MHC class II DQ and DR alleles; approximately 20–50% of familial aggregation is associated with specific DQ and DR haplotypes *(45)*. Because genetic susceptibility to the development of type 1 diabetes is associated with MHC loci, allogeneic HSCT from an HLA-identical sibling donor might not correct genetic susceptibility to the development of autoimmunity. Although genes outside the MHC complex may influence genetic susceptibility to the development of type 1 diabetes, these associations are unclear, and likely contributory rather than causal *(18)*. Selection of a related donor with a disparate DQ or DR haplotype would correct genetic susceptibility toward development of type 1 diabetes; however, MHC class II DR or DQ loci disparity between donor and recipient is associated with an increased incidence of acute graft versus host disease following HSCT *(46)*. Therefore, to correct genetic susceptibility, allogeneic HSCT would require at least a single loci donor-recipient mismatch, which is a negative indication for allogeneic HSCT in low-risk patients *(47)*.

Although donor selection increases the risk of allogeneic HSCT in patients with recent-onset type 1 diabetes, the balance of risk versus benefit to HSCT still may be shifted in favor of HSCT. Identification of patients with increased risk for developing severe complications would increase the perceived benefit of allogeneic HSCT; for instance, specific genetic polymorphisms are associated with increased risk of proliferative retinopathy *(48)*, nephropathy *(49)*, and coronary heart disease *(50)*. Furthermore, demonstration of islet regeneration and consequent resumption of full metabolic control after allogeneic HSCT would favor allogeneic HSCT. Although differentiation of donor hematopoietic stem cells into pancreatic islets is unlikely, allogeneic HSCT in mice led to homing and engraftment of donor bone marrow-derived endothelial cells in the exocrine pancreas *(51)*. Increased angiogenesis may promote autologous islet regeneration, particularly if therapy with growth factors known to promote islet neogenesis were initiated after HSCT *(52)*.

A concomitant decrease in risks associated with allogeneic HSCT likewise would favor clinical use of HSCT in patients with recent-onset type 1 diabetes. Nonmyeloablative HSCT reduces the toxicities of induction therapies, allows for recovery of autologous hematopoiesis in the event of graft loss, and preserves immunologic responsiveness to novel immune challenges (reviewed in ref. *8*). In actively diabetic nonobese diabetic (NOD) mice, nonmyeloablative HSCT resulted in mixed donor-recipient hematopoietic chimerism that restored tolerance to autologous islet β cells *(53)*. Similar observations of a graft-vs-autoimmunity effect after clinical transplantation would increase the potential benefit of HSCT. Additionally, ex vivo manipulation of donor grafts to induce recipient-specific tolerance and the potential for donor-specific immunotherapy in the event of recurrent β cell-specific autoimmune reactivity may further reduce the risks associated with allogeneic HSCT (reviewed in ref. *54*). Finally, if allogeneic HSCT in patients with severe, life-threatening complications of chronic hyperglycemia successfully cured autoimmunity and demonstrated low risk of acute mortality, then these therapies could be extended to patients with recent-onset type 1 diabetes.

In summary, allogeneic HSCT before complete loss of pancreatic islets may cure type 1 diabetes, and the risks of HSCT may be justified in patients with acute, life-threatening hypoglycemic episodes or patients at increased risk of developing life-threatening complications of chronic hyperglycemia. Nevertheless, patients with recent onset type 1 diabetes are at low risk for immediate disease-related mortality, and thus HSCT with MHC class II DQ or DR mismatched donor grafts carries unacceptable risk with available therapies.

6. PANCREAS AND ISLET TRANSPLANT FOR AUTOIMMUNE TYPE 1 DIABETES MELLITUS

In contrast to HSCT for rheumatic autoimmune diseases, HSCT for patients with type 1 diabetes cannot provide relief from clinical symptoms of chronic disease. Frequently, clinical presentation of type 1 diabetes is subsequent to autoimmune-mediated damage to islet β cells; therefore, damaged or destroyed endocrine tissue must be regenerated or replaced in order to alleviate clinical manifestations of disease. Conversely, islet or pancreas transplant may lead to recurrent autoimmune-mediated destruction of donor tissue, and thus HSCT may be necessary to cure autoimmunity before endocrine tissue replacement.

Pancreatic transplantation has been used to correct insulin deficiency in patients with type 1 diabetes, and is performed most often in conjunction with renal transplantation in patients with diabetic nephropathy *(55)*. Solid-organ transplantation for type 1 diabetes is limited to patients with life-threatening disease; however, because of the risks associated with invasive surgical procedures and toxicity of immunosuppressive therapies, it is necessary to induce and maintain allograft tolerance *(55)*. Nevertheless, in a review of more than 2000 pancreas transplants performed in the United States, functional survival of transplanted pancreas was observed in greater than 70% of patients 1 year after transplant, although this rate declined to 66% at 2 years, and 59% at 3 years *(55)*.

Transplantation of pancreatic islets alone may be as effective as pancreas transplant in reversing insulin dependence, and pancreatic islets can be implanted into the portal vein without resort to invasive surgery. Until recently, islet transplantation for type 1 diabetes was largely unsuccessful in the clinical setting; only 8% of patients receiving allogeneic islet transplants remained insulin independent for more than 1 year *(56)*. Recently, a small number of patients received islet allografts from cadaveric donors with immunosuppressive therapy modified to omit corticosteroids, and with procedural modifications in islet preparation (known as the Edmonton protocol) *(57)*. Successful engraftment of cadaveric pancreatic islets was achieved in 15 of 21 patients (71%) with the Edmonton protocol *(58)*, and 1 year after transplant, 12 of these 15 patients were insulin-independent *(59)*. In a more recent report, 82% of 40 patients accepting cadaver islet transplants with the Edmonton protocol at the University of Alberta remained insulin-independent at 1 year posttransplant *(60)*.

The improved success of islet transplantation with the Edmonton protocol may be explained, in part, by procedural modifications in donor islet preparation, the large number of viable islets transplanted (>9,000 islet equivalents/kilogram body weight of the patient), and the modifications made to the immunosuppressive therapy. The Edmonton protocol uses a corticosteroid-free immunosuppressive regimen consisting of daclizumab (Zenapax), low-dose tacrolimus (Prograf), and sirolimus (Rapamune). The omission of corticosteroids, particularly in light of the possible synergy in diabetogenic effect between tacrolimus and corticosteroids *(61)*, may allow for improved outcome of allogeneic islet transplants by controlling immune response toward allogeneic cells while suppressing autoimmune response.

Although the markedly improved success of islet transplantation with the Edmonton protocol is promising, both the high number of donor islets (requiring two to three donor pancreases per transplant recipient) and the necessity for chronic immunosuppressive therapy remain barriers to widespread clinical application. Also, although indications for islet transplant include severe hypoglycemia unawareness or severe metabolic instability, intrahepatic islet transplant does not restore hypoglycemic hormonal counterregulation *(62)*. Finally, risk of recurrent autoimmune disease after pancreas or islet transplantation has yet to be adequately addressed.

Consistent with the finding that autoimmune T-cell reactivity toward islet antigens may persist up to 26 years after disease onset *(63)*, autoimmune destruction of donor islets (as opposed to allogeneic graft rejection) has been observed in a subset of patients after cadaveric pancreas transplants *(64)*. Likewise, antibodies specific to islet β-cell antigens have been observed after pancreas transplant, despite continued graft function and immunosuppressive therapies *(65)*. Furthermore, of the three patients transplanted with the Edmonton protocol who had initially successful islet grafts but that subsequently failed, two patients had antibodies specific to glutamic acid decarboxylase and islet cell antigen after islet transplant, suggesting that graft failure resulted from recurrent autoimmunity.

The incidence of recurrent autoimmunity after islet or pancreas transplant may be dependent on the extent of immunosuppression. In one clinical study, autoimmune reactivity toward islet β cells of donor pancreas was associated with decreased immunosuppressive therapies in recipients of HLA-matched sibling and identical twin donor organs *(66)*. Whereas patients receiving reduced immunosuppressive therapy following HLA-matched sibling and identical twin organs showed recurrent autoimmunity toward transplanted islet β cells, patients receiving sibling-matched donor pancreas transplant with aggressive immunosuppressive therapy did not manifest recurrent autoimmune destruction of islet β cells. If pseudo-autologous (identical twin) or HLA-matched sibling organs are protected from autoimmune-mediated destruction after aggressive immunosuppressive therapy, then dose escalation of immunosuppressive therapy with subsequent autologous HSCT to recapitulate hematopoieses is a promising approach to inducing tolerance to islet β cells. Nevertheless, alternative explanations for the observed autoimmune recurrence are possible. For instance, cumulative effects of chronic immunosuppressive agents such as tacrolimus may contribute to the loss of insulin independence. Another explanation is that patients with autoimmune recurrence following allogeneic islet or pancreas transplantation may represent a specific subset of patients with unique disease severity or manifestation (perhaps resulting from impaired renal function or specific genetic susceptibility loci). Finally, studies in the NOD mouse model suggest that MHC class II matching favors recurrent destruction of transplanted islet cells *(67)*.

Ultimately, the possibility of recurrent autoimmune destruction of transplanted islets or allograft rejection after islet or pancreas transplant necessitates use of chronic immunosuppressive therapy. Chronic immunosuppressive therapies are associated with organ toxicity, opportunistic infections, and an increased incidence of cancer (reviewed in ref. *43*). Clearly, therapies designed to induce immunologic tolerance to transplanted islet β-cell antigens (both autoimmune stimulating and allograft associated antigens) would improve the quality of life of transplant recipients, and likewise may improve rates of both engraftment and function of transplanted pancreatic islets.

7. COMBINED ENDOCRINE TISSUE REPLACEMENT AND HSCT

A combined islet/hematopoietic stem cell transplant may both restore glycemic control and induce sustained immunologic tolerance to transplanted islets. In contrast to patients with recent-onset type 1 diabetes, hematopoietic stem cell transplantation may be justified in patients with labile diabetes or severe hypoglycemic episodes that qualify them for islet transplant. Dose-escalated immunosuppressive therapies followed by autologous stem cell rescue may increase the success of islet transplant; alternatively, allogeneic HSCT combined with islet transplant would allow for cessation of chronic immunosuppressive therapy after transplant. Although the procedures and methods for such combined transplants are in preliminary research stages, successful combined transplants could potentially overcome the islet transplant-associated limitations of the need for both multiple donor organs and chronic immunosuppressive therapies.

There are four models for the combined HSCT/islet transplant paradigm: (1) combined autologous HSCT/allogeneic islet transplant, which is a modification of existing procedures; (2) combined autologous HSCT/autologous islet transplant, which is dependent on the development of methods to produce autologous islets in vitro; (3) combined allogeneic HSCT/allogeneic islet transplant, which is dependent on the ability to harvest both hematopoietic stem cells and sufficient islets for transplant from a single donor; and (4) combined allogeneic HSCT/autologous islet transplant, which is dependent on the induction and maintenance of stable hematopoietic chimerism and the development of methods to produce autologous islets in vitro.

Combined autologous HSCT/islet transplant might overcome immunologic barriers to successful islet transplant. As previously discussed, transplanted islets are subject to both autoimmune-mediated destruction as well as allograft rejection. Dose escalation of immunosuppressive therapies may decrease the incidence of recurrent autoimmune-mediated destruction of islet β cells, and likewise prevent acute allograft rejection of transplanted islets. The drawback of this approach is that the possibility of autoimmune disease relapse or recurrence necessitates the use of chronic immunosuppressive therapies. Nevertheless, clinical islet or pancreas transplants require chronic immunosuppressive therapy to maintain allografts; therefore, autologous HSCT may result in higher rates of successful islet transplant with minimal acute risks related to induction toxicities.

Allogeneic HSCT can potentially cure autoimmunity in patients with type 1 diabetes. In the combined allogeneic HSCT/islet transplant models, if hematopoietic chimerism were established with nonmyeloablative HSCT induction therapies, then either autologous or allogeneic pancreatic islets could be implanted without the need for further immunosuppressive therapies. Hematopoietic chimerism is dynamically maintained by interaction of functional immune cells of both recipient and donor origin, and thus the use of chronic immunosuppressive therapies is not only unnecessary, but also may lead to the loss of hematopoietic chimerism. If, in fact, autoimmunity were suppressed by donor lymphocytes (graft-vs-autoimmunity effect), then transplant with autologous islet cells could restore glycemic control. Likewise, reciprocal graft/recipient tolerance would allow for successful engraftment of pancreatic islets from the HSCT donor.

The model closest to possible clinical application is combined allogeneic transplant from a single donor. The potential use of HSCT as immunotherapy in solid-organ transplant has become more acceptable with the development of nonmyeloablative HSCT induction therapies and lack of adverse effects in preliminary clinical trials *(68,69)*. Immunologic tolerance to donor organ grafts has been induced with nonmyeloablative HSCT, and immunologic tolerance was maintained despite subsequent loss of hematopoietic chimerism *(70)*. In combined HSCT/liver transplant, hematopoietic stem cells obtained from the iliac crest of cadaveric donors induced hematopoietic microchimerism in matched-cadaveric liver recipients. Combined hematopoietic stem cell and renal transplant resulted in a lower incidence of chronic rejection and concomitant increased survival of organ allografts in this study *(71)*. Likewise, mixed renal/hematopoietic stem cell transplant from living donors induced microchimerism in recipients, which led to immunologic unresponsiveness to donor alloantigen *(71)*. To date, sufficient pancreatic islet cells cannot be safely harvested from living donors, and thus combined allogeneic HSCT/allogeneic islet transplant from cadaveric donors is the only currently available therapy option. To meet the goals of this therapy, however, sufficient islets for transplant must be obtained from a single cadaveric donor. Nevertheless, while the Edmonton protocol calls for transplantation of more than 9000 islet equivalents per kilogram, allograft tolerance induced by allogeneic HSCT may allow successful engraftment of a higher number of donor islets and thus provide therapeutic benefit with fewer transplanted islet equivalents. A phase II clinical trial of combined HSCT/islet transplant is under way at the University of Miami Diabetes Research Institute (National Library of Medicine Identifier NCT00021801); however, results have not yet been published.

The development of methods to produce islet cells in vitro would allow for the use of living, related donors for combined allogeneic HSCT/islet transplants, which would greatly expand the available donor pool. The ideal model for allogeneic transplant would involve the identification and enrichment of adult stem cells capable of producing pancreatic islets. Pancreatic ductal epithelial cells from both mice *(72)* and humans *(73)* have been stimulated to produce functional islets in culture. Furthermore, islets produced from mouse pancreatic ductal epithelium reversed insulin dependence when implanted into NOD mice *(72)*. Nevertheless, islets generated in vitro produced less insulin than freshly extracted islets, which is a concern in the context of islet replacement therapy for type 1 diabetes. Moreover, when in vitro generated murine islets were implanted into the subcapsular region of the kidney of diabetic NOD mice, islet morphology was lost and insulin-producing β cells were observed as a contiguous cell mass *(72)*. Thus, although preliminary research into the generation of functional islet β cells from ductal epithelium is promising, much more information is needed to assess the possibilities of this approach. Nevertheless, if human pancreatic stem cells were identified and could be stimulated to produce fully functional islet cells in vitro, then the possibility of combined HSCT/islet transplant from living donors could be realized. Moreover, although speculative, if the conditions necessary to stimulate islet cell neogenesis were identified, it might be possible to transplant pancreatic stem cells into tolerant recipients and encourage in vivo islet neogenesis rather than depending on in vitro expansion of pancreatic islets.

Alternatively, therapeutic cloning of embryonic stem cells may provide a readily available source of pancreatic islets for transplantation. Pancreatic islets generated from embryonic stem cells have the potential to fulfill the requirements of all four models of combined HSCT/islet transplants. In the autologous transplant model, recipient cells would be cloned from embryonic stem cells and induced to differentiate into islet cells in vivo, and implantation would be combined with standard hematopoietic stem cell recruitment, induction, and transplant. Similarly, a sufficiently broad collection of embryonic stem cell lines would allow for the selection of suitably matched donor cells that could be induced to differentiate into both islet cells and hematopoietic stem cells. Potential complications of these transplants are similar to those indicated for HSCT in patients with recent-onset type 1 diabetes; autologous transplant carries increased risk of autoimmune disease relapse or recurrence despite chronic immunosuppressive therapies, and allogeneic transplant poses similar risks for an HLA-identical donor. However, additional complications are associated with the therapeutic transplant of tissue derived from embryonic stem cells or germ cells.

Embryonic stem cells produce teratomas when injected into immunodeficient mice *(74,75)*. Moreover, transplant of undifferentiated embryonic stem cells may lead to uncontrolled or inappropriate proliferation. Further, factors that control commitment to a particular cell type are not yet fully understood *(76)*. Nevertheless, mouse embryonic stem cells were induced to differentiate into islet-like structures that produced insulin, secreted insulin in response to glucose, and retained cluster-like morphology and insulin production when injected into streptozotocin *(77)*. However, islet-like structures derived from embryonic stem cells, like those derived from adult ductal epithelium, had 50 times less insulin per cell than normal islet β cells *(77)*. Thus, although the therapeutic use of embryonic stem cells holds enormous potential, much more information is needed before embryonic stem cells can be used in the treatment of patients with type 1 diabetes.

8. CONCLUSION

HSCT has the potential to restore self-tolerance and prevent further destruction of islet β cells in patients with recent-onset type 1 diabetes. Autologous HSCT, however, is associated with risk of recurrent autoimmunity, and although allogeneic HSCT may cure autoimmunity to islet β cells in patients with recent-onset type 1 diabetes, the risks associated with allogeneic HSCT outweigh the known potential benefits of this therapy. Nevertheless, hematopoietic stem cell transplantation as immunosuppressive therapy or tolerance induction therapy may contribute to successful engraftment and maintenance of pancreatic islets in patients with chronic disease. As sources of functional pancreatic islets are developed, the possibilities for therapy are likewise expanded. Identification and differentiation of pancreatic stem cells or embryonic stem cells may alleviate the limitations caused by lack of available donors; moreover, allogeneic HSCT may cure autoimmunity, and thus allow for resumption of glycemic control without the necessity for chronic immunosuppressive therapies. Moreover, these conclusions may be extrapolated to the treatment of patients with type 1 diabetes as a component of autoimmune polyendocrine syndromes type II and III.

REFERENCES

1. Carrier E, Burt R. Stem cell transplantation for autoimmune diseases: pros and cons. Current Opinion in Organ Transplantation 2000;5:343–351.
2. Rose NR, Bona C. Defining criteria for autoimmune diseases (Witebsky's postulates revisited). Immunol Today 1993;14:426–430.
3. Burt RK, Slavin S, Burns WH, Marmont AM. Induction of tolerance in autoimmune diseases by hematopoietic stem cell transplantation: getting closer to a cure? Int J Hematol 2002;76(Suppl. 1):226–247.
4. Carrier E, Burt RK. Mobilization and conditioning regimens in stem cell transplant for autoimmune disease. In: Burt RK, Marmont A, eds. Stem Cell Therapy for Autoimmune Disease. Landes Bioscience, Georgetown, TX, 2004, pp. 253–261.
5. Nikolic B, Takeuchi Y, Leykin I, Fudaba Y, Smith RN, Sykes M. Mixed hematopoietic chimerism allows cure of autoimmune diabetes through allogeneic tolerance and reversal of autoimmunity. Diabetes 2004;53:376–383.
6. Wang B, Yamamoto Y, El-Badri NS, Good RA. Effective treatment of autoimmune disease and progressive renal disease by mixed bone-marrow transplantation that establishes a stable mixed chimerism in BXSB recipient mice. Proc Natl Acad Sci USA 1999;96:3012–3016.
7. Nash RA, Storb R. Graft-versus-host effect after allogeneic hematopoietic stem cell transplantation: GVHD and GVL. Curr Opin Immunol 1996;8:674–680.
8. Slavin S. Graft-versus-host disease, the graft-versus-leukemia effect, and mixed chimerism following nonmyeloablative stem cell transplantation Int J Hematol 2003;78:195–207.
9. Hinterberger W, Hinterberger-Fischer M, Marmont A. Clinically demonstrable anti-autoimmunity mediated by allogeneic immune cells favorably affects outcome after stem cell transplantation in human autoimmune diseases. Bone Marrow Transplant 2002;30:753–759.
10. Van Laar JM, Tyndall A. Intense immunosuppression and stem-cell transplantation for patients with severe rheumatic autoimmune disease: a review Cancer Control 2003;10:57–65.
11. Tait KF, Gough SC. The genetics of autoimmune endocrine disease. Clin Endocrinol (Oxf) 2003;59:1–11.
12. Hawkes CH. Twin studies in medicine—what do they tell us? QJM 1997;90:311–321.
13. Zuklys S, Balciunaite G, Agarwal A, Fasler-Kan E, Palmer E, Holländer GA. Normal thymic architecture and negative selection are associated with *Aire* expression, the gene defective in the autoimmune-polyendocrinopathy-candidiasis-ectodermal dystrophy (APECED). J Immunol 2000;165:1976–1983.

14. Meyerson J, Lechuga-Gomez EE, Bigazzi PE, Walfish PG. Polyglandular autoimmune syndrome: current concepts. Can Med Assoc J 1988;138:605–612.
15. National Institute of Diabetes and Digestive and Kidney Diseases. National Diabetes Statistics fact sheet: general information and national estimates on diabetes in the United States, 2003. Bethesda, MD, U.S. Department of Health and Human Services, National Institutes of Health, 2003.
16. The Diabetes Control and Complications Trial Research Group. The effect of intensive treatment of diabetes on the development and progression of long-term complications in insulin-dependent diabetes mellitus. N Engl J Med 1993;329:977–986.
17. The Diabetes Control and Complications Trial Research Group. Hypoglycemia in the diabetes control and complications trial. Diabetes 1997;46:271–286.
18. Sheehy MJ. HLA and insulin-dependent diabetes. A protective perspective. Diabetes 2001;41:123–129.
19. Horwitz MS, Bradley LM, Harbertson J, Krahl T, Lee J, Sarvetnick N. Diabetes induced by Coxsackie virus: initiation by bystander damage and not molecular mimicry Nat Med 1998;4:781–785.
20. Oldstone MBA. Molecular mimicry and immune-mediated diseases. FASEB J 1998;12: 1255–1265.
21. Albert LJ, Inman RD. Molecular mimicry and autoimmunity. N Engl J Med 1999;341: 2068–2074.
22. Goodnow CC. Balancing immunity and tolerance: deleting and tuning lymphocyte repertoires. Proc Natl Acad Sci USA 1996;93:2264–2271.
23. André I, Gonzalez A, Wang B, Katz J, Benoist C, Mathis D. Checkpoints in the progression of autoimmune disease: lessons from diabetes models. Proc Natl Acad Sci USA 1996;93:2260–2263.
24. Diabetes Prevention Trial-Type 1 Diabetes Study Group. Effects of insulin in relatives of patients with type 1 diabetes mellitus. N Engl J Med 2002;346:1685–1691.
25. LaFace DM, Peck AB. Reciprocal allogeneic bone marrow transplantation between NOD mice and diabetes-nonsusceptible mice associated with transfer and prevention of autoimmune diabetes. Diabetes 1989;38:894–901.
26. Lampeter EF. Homberg M, Gries FA, Kolb H, Quabeck K, Schaefer UW, P. Wernet P, Grosse-Wilde H, Bertrams J. Transfer of insulin-dependent diabetes between HLA-identical siblings by bone marrow transplantation. Lancet 1993;341:1243–1244.
27. Foulis AK, Liddle CN, Farwuharson MA, Richmond JA, Weir RS. The histopathology of the pancreas in Type 1 diabetes (insulin dependent) mellitus: a 25-year review of deaths in patients under 20 years of age in the United Kingdom. Diabetologia 1986;29:267–274.
28. The Diabetes Control and Complications Trial Research Group. Effect of intensive therapy on residual beta-cell function in patients with type 1 diabetes in the Diabetes Control and Complications Trial: a randomized, controlled trial. Ann Intern Med 1998;128:517–523.
29. Goday A, Pujol-Borrell R, Fernandez J, et al. Effects of a short prednisone regime at clinical onset of type 1 diabetes. Diabetes Res Clin Pract 1993;20:39–46.
30. Eisenbarth GS, Srikanta S, Jackson R, et al. Anti-thymocyte globulin and prednisone immunotherapy of recent onset type 1 diabetes mellitus Diabetes Res 1985;2:271–276.
31. Silverstein J, Maclaren N, Riley W, Spillar R, Radjenovic D, Johnson S. Immunosuppression with azathioprine and prednisone in recent-onset insulin-dependent diabetes mellitus. N Engl J Med 1988;319:599–604.
32. Bougneres PF, Carel JC, Castano L, et al. Factors associated with remission of type 1 diabetes in children treated with cyclosporine. N Engl J Med 1988;318:663–670.

33. Martin S, Schernthaner G, Nerup J, et al. Follow-up of cyclosporine A treatment in type 1 (insulin-dependent) diabetes mellitus: lack of long-term effects. Diabetologia 1991;34:429–434.
34. Delaunay F, Khan A, Cintra A, et al. Pancreatic beta cells are important targets for the diabetogenic effects of glucocorticoids. J Clin Invest 1997;100:2094–2098.
35. Krentz AJ, Dousset B, Mayer D, et al. Metabolic effects of cyclosporin A and FK 506 in liver transplant recipients. Diabetes 1993;42:1753–1759.
36. Nielsen JH, Mandrup-Poulsen T, Nerup J. Direct effects of cyclosporin A on human pancreatic β-cells. Diabetes 1986;35:1049–1052.
37. Dufer M, Krippeit-Drews P, Lembert N, Idahl LA, Drews G. Diabetogenic effect of cyclosporin A is mediated by interference with mitochondrial function of pancreatic B-cells. Mol Pharmacol 2001;60:873–879.
38. Gunnarsson R, Klintmalm G, Lundgren G, et al. Deterioration in glucose metabolism in pancreatic transplant recipients after conversion from azathioprine to cyclosporine Transplant Proc 1984;16:709–712.
39. Kaprio J, Tuomilehto J, Koshenvuo M, et al. Concordance for type 1 (insulin-dependent) and type 2 (non-insulin-dependent) diabetes mellitus in a population-based cohort of twins in Finland Diabetologia 1993;35:1060–1067.
40. Kumar D, Gemayel NS, Deapen D, et al. Genetic, etiological, and clinical significance of disease concordance according to age, zygosity, and the interval after diagnosis in first twin. Diabetes 1993;42:1351–1363.
41. Verge CF, Gianani R, Yu L, et al. Late progression to diabetes, evidence for chronic beta cell autoimmunity in identical twins of patients with type I diabetes. Diabetes 1995;44:1176–1179.
42. Kyvik KO, Green A, Beck-Nielsen H. Concordance rates of insulin dependent diabetes mellitus: a population based study of young Danish twins. BMJ 1995;311:913–917.
43. Niethammer D, Kümmerle-Deschner J, Dannecker GE. Side-effects of long-term immunosuppression versus morbidity in autologous stem cell rescue: striking the balance. Rheumatology 1999;38:747–750.
44. Lucarelli G, Galimberti M, Giardini C, et al. Bone marrow transplantation in thalassemia. The experience of Pesaro. Ann NY Acad Sci 1998;850:270–275.
45. Slover RH, Eisenbarth GS. Prevention of type 1 diabetes and recurrent β cell destruction of transplanted islets. Endocrine Rev 1997;18:241–258.
46. Petersdorf EW, Longton GM, Anasetti C, et al. Definition of HLA-DQ as a transplantation antigen. Proc Nat Acad Sci 1996;93:15358–15363.
47. Kanda Y, Chiba S, Hirai H, et al. Allogeneic hematopoietic stem cell transplantation from family members other than HLA-identical siblings over the last decade (1991–2000). Blood 2003;102:1541–1547.
48. Mimura T, Funatsu H, Uchigata Y, et al. Relationship between human leukocyte antigen status and proliferative diabetic retinopathy in patients with younger-onset type 1 diabetes mellitus. Am J Ophthalmol 2003;135:844–848.
49. Yang B, Cross DF, Ollerenshaw M, Millward BA, Demaine AG. Polymorphisms of the vascular endothelial growth factor and susceptibility to diabetic microvascular complications in patients with type 1 diabetes mellitus. J Diabetes Complications 2003;17:1–6.
50. Tarnow L, Stehouwer CD, Emeis JJ, et al. Plasminogen activator inhibitor-1 and apolipoprotein E gene polymorphisms and diabetic angiopathy. Nephrol Dial Transplant 2000;15:625–630.
51. Mathews V, Hanson PT, Ford E, Fujita J, Polonsky KS, Graubert TA. Recruitment of bone marrow-derived endothelial cells to sites of pancreatic beta-cell injury. Diabetes 2004;53:91–98.
52. Brand SJ, Tagerud S, Lambert P, et al. Pharmacological treatment of chronic diabetes by stimulating pancreatic beta-cell regeneration with systemic co-administration of EGF and gastrin. Pharmacol Toxicol 2002;91:414–420.

53. Nikolic B, Takeuchi Y, Leykin I, Fudaba Y, Smith RN, Sykes M. Mixed hematopoietic chimerism allows cure of autoimmune diabetes through allogeneic tolerance and reversal of autoimmunity. Diabetes 2004;53:376–383.
54. Domenick MA, Ildstad ST. Impact of bone marrow transplantation on type 1 diabetes. World J Surg 2001;25:474–480.
55. Remuzzi G, Ruggenenti P, Mauer SM. Pancreas and kidney/pancreas transplants: experimental medicine or real improvement? Lancet 1994;343:27–31.
56. Brendel MD, Hering BJ, Schulz AO, Bretzel RG. Int Islet Transpl Reg ITR Newsletter 1999;9:1–20.
57. Shapiro AM, Lakey JR, Ryan EA, et al. Islet transplantation in seven patients with type 1 diabetes mellitus using a glucocorticoid-free immunosuppressive regimen. N Engl J Med 2000;343:230–238.
58. Immune Tolerance Network. Preliminary results of ITN Multicenter Islet Transplant Trial confirm potential patient benefits, underscore steep learning curve. Available online at http://www.immunetolerance.org/news/articles/itn_news/article_255.html. Accessed March 10, 2004.
59. Ryan EA, Lakey JRT, Paty1 BW, et al. Successful islet transplantation: continued insulin reserve provides long-term glycemic control. Diabetes 2002;51:2148–2157.
60. Shapiro J. Eighty years after insulin: parallels with modern islet transplantation Can Med Assoc J 2002;167:1398–1400.
61. Shapiro AM, Geng Hao E, Lakey JR, Finegood DT, Rajotte RV, Kneteman NM. Diabetes mellitus and islet cell specific autoimmunity as adverse effects of immunosuppressive therapy by FK506/tacrolimus. Exp Clin Endocrinol Diabetes 2000;108:347–352.
62. Paty BW, Ryan EA, Shapiro JAM, Lakey JR, Robertson RP. Intrahepatic islet transplantation in type 1 diabetic patients does not restore hypoglycemic hormonal counterregulation or symptom recognition after insulin independence. Diabetes 2002;51:3428–3434.
63. Dosch H, Cheung RK, Karges W, Pietropaolo M, Becker DJ. Persistent T cell anergy in human type 1 diabetes. J Immunol 1999;163:6933–6940.
64. Tydén G, Reinholt FP, Sundkvist G, Bolinde J. Recurrence of autoimmune diabetes mellitus in recipients of cadaveric pancreatic grafts. N Engl J Med 1996;335:860–863.
65. Esmatjes E, Rodriguez-Villar C, Ricart MJ, et al. Recurrence of immunological markers for type 1 (insulin-dependent) diabetes mellitus in immunosuppressed patients after pancreas transplantation. Transplantation 1998;66:128–131.
66. Sutherland DER, Goetz FC, Sibley RK. Recurrence of disease in pancreas transplants. Diabetes 1989;38(Suppl. 1):85–87.
67. Makhlouf L, Kishimoto K, Smith RN, et al. The role of autoimmunity in islet allograft destruction: major histocompatibility complex class II matching is necessary for autoimmune destruction of allogeneic islet transplants after T-cell costimulatory blockade. Diabetes 2002;11:3202–3210.
68. Rifle G, Mousson C. Donor-derived hematopoietic cells in organ transplantation: a major step toward allograft tolerance? Transplantation 2003;75(9 Suppl.):3S–7S.
69. De Pauw L, Toungouz M, Goldman M. Infusion of donor-derived hematopoietic stem cells in organ transplantation: clinical data. Transplantation 2003;75(9 Suppl.):46S–49S.
70. Spitzer TR, Delmonico F, Tolkoff-Rubin N, et al. Combined histocompatibility leukocyte antigen-matched donor bone marrow and renal transplantation for multiple myeloma with end stage renal disease: the induction of allograft tolerance through mixed lymphohematopoietic chimerism. Transplantation 1999;68:480–484.

71. Mathew JM, Garcia-Morales RO, Carreno M, et al. Immune responses and their regulation by donor bone marrow cells in clinical organ transplantation. Transplant Immunol 2003;11:307–321.
72. Ramiya VK, Maraist M, Arfors KE, Schatz DA, Peck AB, Cornelius JG. Reversal of insulin-dependent diabetes using islets generated in vitro from pancreatic stem cells. Nat Med 2000;6:278–282.
73. Bonner-Weir S, Taneja M, Weir GC, et al. In vitro cultivation of human islets from expanded ductal tissue. Proc Natl Acad Sci USA 2000;97:7999–8004.
74. Rosenthal N. Prometheus's vulture and the stem-cell promise. N Engl J Med 2003;349:267–274.
75. Smith AG. Embryo-derived stem cells: of mice and men. Annu Rev Cell Dev Biol 2001;17:435–462.
76. Sipione S, Eshpeter A, Lyon JG, Korbutt GS, Bleackley RC. Insulin expressing cells from differentiated embryonic stem cells are not beta cells. Diabetologia 2004;47:499–508.
77. Lumelsky N, Blondel O, Laeng P, Velasco I, Ravin R, McKay R. Differentiation of embryonic stem cells to insulin-secreting structures similar to pancreatic islets [erratum, Science 2001;293:428]. Science 2001;292:1389–1394.

13 Preclinical Trials for Stem Cell Therapy

Linda B. Lester, K. Y. Francis Pau, and Don P. Wolf

CONTENTS

1. INTRODUCTION

Stem cell-based therapy holds great promise for the treatment of human diseases attributable to the loss or dysfunction of a single cell type. However, before stem cells can be used clinically, their safety and efficacy must be clearly established. This is particularly important for endocrine applications in which hormone replacement treatments are available. Indeed, new stem cell-based treatments must meet or exceed the gold standard already established for safety and efficacy *(1)*. Traditional hormone replacement therapies are, however, frequently inadequate, either overtreating or undertreating the respective disorder. Stem cell therapies could offer the significant advantage of linking hormone release to physiologic stimuli resulting in improved hormonal control. This potential must be established and the risks assessed through rigorous preclinical testing before stem cell-based therapies are applied to humans.

The initial intent of preclinical studies is to develop safety and efficacy information that will facilitate future clinical trials. This is critical for stem cell therapies in which a number of unique risks must be investigated *(2–5)* including toxicities associated with ex vivo culturing, induction of genetic mutations,

From: *Contemporary Endocrinology: Stem Cells in Endocrinology*
Edited by: L. B. Lester © Humana Press Inc., Totowa, NJ

misdirected cell migration, tumor formation, and immunologic rejection. Model systems must be developed to test stem cell therapies and evaluate these risks and identify other unexpected problems *(4)*. These model systems should also provide key insights into the effectiveness of stem cell based therapies.

A major consideration in the development of preclinical in vivo models is the system to use, which in turn will be dependent on the disease of interest and the testing methods. Investigation of many human diseases is often constrained by a lack of in vitro models; therefore, most preclinical trials use in vivo testing in animals *(6,7)*. Ideally, these animal models address numerous questions/considerations with the potential for extrapolation to human physiology, including potential toxicity assessment. Because it is critical to determine the stability of stem cell grafts in an in vivo environment similar to humans, we believe that for most disease states the nonhuman primate will be superior to murine models for the final preclinical trials because of anatomic and physiologic similarities between monkeys and humans. Unfortunately, primate models of spontaneous autoimmune disease including many endocrine disorders are not available.

In this chapter, we will review specific concerns that pertain to the potential use of stem cell therapies for the treatment of human endocrine disorders. Furthermore, we will discuss the role of preclinical trials using different animal models to assess safety and efficacy concerns. By focusing on preclinical trials, this chapter will summarize the themes of earlier chapters centered on basic and applied research in an attempt to bridge the transition from research to therapy.

2. ASSESSING POTENTIAL STEM CELL RISKS AND COMPLICATIONS

2.1. Tumorigenicity

The most pressing issue regarding the use of stem cells for cell-based therapies, particularly pluripotent embryonic stem cells, is their capacity to generate tumors after transplantation *(8)*. Thus a characteristic of undifferentiated embryonic stem cells is their ability to give rise to teratoma formation after transplantation *(9,10)*; this capacity must clearly be prevented if they are to be used as therapies.

How does one assess the tumorigenic potential of a particular cellular therapy? The risk of tumor formation likely follows the risk of teratoma formation, which correlates with the number of pluripotent or partially differentiated cells in the population of transplanted cells. Pluripotency in primate embryonic stem (ES) cells can be determined by identifying a unique repertoire of cell surface molecules associated with the undifferentiated phenotype. These markers include the stage-specific embryonic antigens 3 and 4, the glycoproteins TRA-1-60 and TRA-1-81, and the activities of specific enzymes such as alkaline phosphatase and telomerase *(11)*. Additional molecular markers, Oct4 and Rex1, are expressed in

Table 1
Markers of Pluriopotency and Risk of Teratoma Formation

Source of stem cells	*Markers*	*Teratoma formation*	*Reference*
Mouse embryonic germ line stem cells	Oct4, SSEA-1, alkaline phosphatases	Yes	*76,89*
Human embryonic stem cells	Oct4, SEEA-3/4, alkaline phosphatase	Yes	*30,89*
Human embryonic germ line stem cells	Oct4?, alkaline phosphatases, SSEA-1, SSEA-3/4	No	*89,90*
Human mesenchymal stem cell	Major histocompatibility complex class I and II negative SSEA-1, Oct4	No	*89,91*

early development and then rapidly downregulated on differentiation *(12–14)*. One method, therefore, to determine the presence of pluripotent cells in vitro is to identify the persistent expression of these markers (Table 1).

After cells are transplanted, teratoma formation can be monitored by following serum levels of germ cell tumor markers including α-fetoprotein, human chorionic gonadotropin, and lactate dehydrogenase *(15)*. Such monitoring will provide an important safety net for assessing stem cell therapy risks in preclinical studies. Before these therapies can be used for human experimentation, however, undifferentiated, pluripotent cells almost certainly will need to be removed from the cell transplants or rendered nonfunctional producing a more homogenous, terminally differentiated cell implant with a decreased risk for teratoma formation. As an example, Hori et al. recently described an approach in which they treated mouse ES-derived cells with a growth factor signaling inhibitor *(9)* that prevented teratoma formation after the transplantation of insulin-producing cells. An alternative method could use markers of a mature phenotype to select differentiated cells from the population. This could produce a purified cell population and eliminate or diminish the presence of undifferentiated cells. ES cells could be genetically modified to heterologously express a foreign marker protein *(16–19)*. These techniques could be employed to tag ES-derived cells to allow ex vivo purification and in vivo identification of ES cell progeny after transplantation into a host. For example, rhesus monkey ES cells or ES-derived cells could be tagged with a reporter gene such as green fluorescent protein (GFP) *(20)* or directly with iron nanoparticles such as CLIO *(21,22)* . The use of GFP as a reporter molecule has several advantages over other reporter genes: fluorescence does not depend on cofactors or substrates; the protein product is stable and not subject to rapid photobleaching; and visualization of living cells can be performed usually without detriment to cell viability *(23)*. We have fused the human insulin promoter to the GFP gene, such that, cells expressing this construct that differentiate into insulin-expressing, β-like cells can be identified by their GFP fluorescence *(24)*. The selection of GFP-positive cells by fluorescent cell sorting could produce a purified, homogenous cell population that is less likely to result in teratoma formation *(25)*. An added benefit to this approach is that purifying the cell population before transplantation minimizes the size of the tissue transplant increasing the likelihood of adequate angiogenesis after grafting.

Independent of the method used to diminish the pluripotent or undifferentiated cell populations, cell stability must be assessed after transplantation. It is unclear what environmental cues or niches are necessary to maintain the in vitro differentiated state posttransplantation. As described for mouse ES cell transplants, this can be accomplished by the removal and histologic evaluation of cell transplants, at least for cells at the site of transplantation. However, if cell migration occurs after transplantation, teratoma formation may be missed. Cells will, therefore, have to be tracked to determine the stability of their location and their phenotype after transplantation. Tracking stem cell transplants is discussed in Subheading 2.4.

2.2. Stem Cell Genetic Mutations

Concern over spontaneous genetic mutation continues to trouble scientists working on stem cell therapies, particularly for prolonged culture of embryonic stem cells in which DNA mutations may occur every three cell divisions *(26–28)*. Despite this tendency, ES cells may be more stable than previously thought. First, late-passage (>250 doublings) or cloned murine ES cells can colonize embryos without signs of damage or transformation. Second, early- and late-passage somatic cells, from fetal or adult donors, can be used to create cloned animals by nuclear transfer at about equal efficiencies, and normal ES cells can be generated from clones. Third, telomerase-immortalized human somatic cells are viable and nontransformed *(29)* with the ability to retain differentiated function after several hundred divisions. Finally, human ES cells are telomerase positive, immortal, clonable, pluripotent cells that form mature tissues containing cells derived from all three embryonic germ layers when injected into immune-compromised mice, even after 250 doublings in culture *(30)*.

Despite these findings, it is imperative that cell cultures destined for transplantation be screened for genetic mutations. For human therapeutic applications, good medical practice regulations will require qualification of cell banks or individual, stem cell-derived lines *(31)*. Given the need to expand cell populations for banking purposes, there is ample time to perform genetic manipulation, clonal selection, quality testing, and creation of working cell banks for subsequent differentiation under standardized conditions.

The type of stem cell may also influence the risk of genetic mutation. The best available candidates as a source of safe, effective, and expandable replacement cells are ES cells. Most somatic stem cells appear to be telomerase-negative, are usually difficult to isolate, and senesce within about 50 divisions, limiting their expandability. Hematopoietic and mesenchymal stem cells have had limited success, in part because of their ability to be easily cloned, manipulated, and expanded. These are important features that limit the usefulness of somatic stem cells for the development of safe, efficacious, and cost-effective cell therapies for the millions of patients with chronic degenerative diseases. Whether embryonic or other stem cells are involved, screening for genetic stability including karyotyping will be a critical part of the safety evaluation necessary for the implementation of stem cell-based therapies.

2.3. Toxicities From Ex Vivo Culturing

Transplantation of tissues from a foreign species carries the risk of infectious disease transmission from the donor to the recipient. Use of animal proteins or cells to grow human stem cells effectively transforms the human transplant into a xenotransplant. Of the potential risks, most concerning is exposure of the transplant recipient to animal retroviruses such as the porcine endogenous retrovirus (PERV) *(32)*. Past experiments have shown that PERV can infect human cell lines in vitro *(33)*. Recently, cross-species infection occurred from the transplantation of PERV-infected pig pancreatic islet cells into NOD/SCID (nonobese diabetic, severe combined immunodeficiency) mice *(34)*. This risk effectively eliminates animal stem cells for therapeutic application and it also greatly limits the use of human stem cells that have been exposed to animal proteins.

Until recently, human embryonic stem cells had to be propagated on mouse embryonic fibroblast-feeder layers to maintain the undifferentiated state *(35)*. These culture techniques exposed the cells to murine proteins and pathogens, making them xenographs if transplanted. As noted previously, xenographs carry the risk of transferring animal pathogens but can also result in significant anaphylactic responses to the foreign proteins after transplantation. Several breakthroughs have recently demonstrated the ability to culture human ES cells without the need for animal cells or proteins. Initially, cells were maintained in xeno-free culture systems using human fetal fibroblast feeder layers *(35)*. Although this step represented an improvement over growth on mouse tissues, these cultures still required the use of fetal calf serum, thus exposing human cells to bovine contaminants. Further modifications now allow human ES cells to be grown on fibronectin matrices with a serum substitute and a combination of growth factors including transforming growth factor-β1, leukemia inhibitory factor, and basic fibroblast growth factor *(36)*. This ongoing evolution of culture techniques has dramatically reduced stem cell exposure to animal proteins, improving their safety for transplantation.

These recent advances in culturing human stem cells have mostly eliminated the possibility of transmitting endogenous retroviruses from the animal to the patient. However, there will be an ongoing need to develop methods to monitor production of stem cells for therapeutic use, similar to the current Food and Drug Administration guidelines for bone marrow transplantation *(37)*.

2.4. Monitoring Cell Fate After Transplantation

Monitoring cell stability in vivo requires isolation or tracking of all transplant-derived cells and if cell migration occurs, which appears inevitable, tissues from multiple sites will need to be evaluated. Existing evidence for stem cell migration can be found in studies of mesenchymal stem cell migration to sites of myocardial infarction *(38)*. Most techniques to study the fate of stem cells after transplantation involve histological evaluation of the whole animal or cell explant requiring many animals per experiment since each can only be used for a single time or data point. Although fluorescent protein tagging provides an efficient means to identify and purify cells ex vivo, the signals cannot currently be identified in vivo, which limits their utility in monitoring stem cell migration. However, tagging cells with magnetic nanoparticles, such as CLIO, allows both ex vivo purification by magnetic sorting and in vivo identification through noninvasive magnetic resonance imaging *(39)*. Although the stability, toxicity, and propagation of the nanoparticle signal must be evaluated extensively in vivo, this technique has been successfully employed to track stem cell transplants in mice *(21,22)*. Use of these tracking methods could provide essential information on the stability of the cell transplant and the effects of any cell migration on cell phenotype or vice versa. With regard to the latter, a frequent concern with the use of stem cells in vivo is the loss of cell phenotype and more importantly the development of unstable, transformed tissues. In addition to general tumorigenicity or teratoma formation, altered and excessive cellular function could occur. In vivo assays will be required to test the stability of all stem cell-derived progeny. Excessive or irregular cellular activity postimplantation could result from unanticipated hyperplasia or unusually high pharmacological, electrical, or metabolic activity of the cells. Genetic mutations could predispose to all of these. To date, animal trials have not suggested that such alterations will occur; however, the length of these in vivo trials has been limited *(8,40–42)*. Therefore, along with cell migration and tumorigenicity, the propensity to develop excessive or disregulated cellular function must be assessed in adequately designed preclinical trials.

2.5. Immune Rejection

A major concern for stem cell-based therapies is the possible destruction of transplanted cells through activation of the host immune response. For endocrine-based stem cell transplants, this could occur through one of two possible mechanisms; allogenic rejection through the expression of foreign proteins on the transplanted cell surfaces or autoimmune rejection of the functional endocrine tissue.

Allogenic graft rejection is a concern for all transplants containing any source of genetically dissimilar tissue including those of embryonic origin or adult stem cells isolated from cadavers or unrelated tissue banks. The major alloantigens responsible for activating the host immune response include the minor and major histocompatibility complex (MHC) proteins and the ABO blood group proteins, all expressed on cell surfaces *(43)*. When these alloantigens differ between graft and host, host T-lymphocytes will recognize the tissue as foreign, resulting in allograft rejection. This response can be prevented or modulated using broad-spectrum immunosuppressant agents similar to the management of whole-organ transplantation. However, these agents carry significant risks, including end-organ dysfunction, systemic infections, and malignancy *(44,45)*. In conjunction with research on stem cell biology and the development of stem cell therapies, approaches that prevent allogenic immune rejection of stem cells and stem cell-derived tissues should be actively pursued.

To ensure that stem cell-based therapies can be broadly applicable for many conditions and individuals, means to overcome tissue rejection must be found. Use of embryonic stem cells may minimize the allogenic response because they express low levels of the MHC proteins *(46,47)*. However, because the ES cells are differentiated to mature cell types, expression of MHC molecules increases, making allogenic rejection of ES derived tissues likely *(48)*. Methods to minimize allogenic rejection include genetic manipulation of the stem cells and the development of large banks of embryonic stem cell lines. Gene knockouts of the β2-microglobulin to reduce expression of MHC molecules or expression of FasL to induce apoptosis of T-lymphocytes could protect stem cell lines from allogenic rejection and thereby creating universally accepted stem cell lines *(46,49,50)*. Although controversial, somatic cell nuclear transfer, a technique that produces a lineage of stem cells that are genetically identical to the donor, promises such an advantage *(51)*. This technique, called therapeutic cloning, would allow for development of self-embryonic cell lines from which tissues for autologous transplantation could be grown. Recently, proof of principle experimentation was reported resulting in the development of a cloned human embryonic stem cell line *(52)*, but the impractical nature of this approach makes widespread applicability unlikely. Furthermore, development of isogenic self-embryonic cell lines will not prevent or modify autoimmune responses.

Autoimmune rejection is a particular concern for stem cell therapies for endocrine disorders because many of these disorders occur through autoimmune destruction of the endocrine organ *(53)*. Methods to block the autoimmune and the allogenic response will be necessary to harness the full capacity of cell-based endocrine therapies. As discussed in Chapter 12, hematopoietic cell transplants may be used to block or minimize ongoing autoimmune destruction through tolerance induction *(54–56)*. This approach can reverse autoimmune diabetes in mice by allowing endogenous islet precursors to replace lost β cells *(56)*. Using donor-derived bone marrow and stem cells to avoid immune rejection of transplant tissue requires human leukocyte antigen matching of both cell types between the donor and recipient before the organ transplant. This procedure can now be performed under nonmyeloablative conditions in rodents *(56)*. If similar techniques can be replicated in humans, then mixed hematopoietic chimerism will likely become an important method in treating human endocrine disease.

Finally, stem cell-based transplants could be placed in immune privileged sites to prevent immunologic rejection. The eye, brain, and testis have all demonstrated immunologic tolerance to MHC-unmatched grafts *(57)*. Human fetal neurons transplanted into the central nervous system of adult humans survived for years without immune rejection suggesting that transplantation of stem cell-derived tissues into immune-privileged sites will improve their survival. Whether or not this approach will be adequate or applicable to multiple cell types must be carefully evaluated.

Although it is unclear which of the described approaches will be used for stem cell-based transplants, their multiplicity and their success in rodent models provides optimism for their use in human studies. Allogenic hematopoietic stem cell transplants are under evaluation in the treatment of autoimmune disorders in humans *(58)*. Nevertheless, the efficacy of these techniques to suppress immune rejection of stem cell-based therapies must be confirmed in preclinical trials. As discussed in the next section, the choice of animal model to study the immunology of stem cell transplants will be critical to the translation of results to human trials.

3. ASSESSING STEM CELL THERAPEUTIC EFFICACY AND STABILITY

Of equal importance in evaluating the risks of stem cell-based therapies is establishing their efficacy. In vitro testing of cellular function is the appropriate starting point, but a progression through a carefully defined, stepwise series involving in vivo testing will be critical (Fig. 1). Preclinical animal models will be essential to assess stem cell therapeutic efficacy and determine the longevity of their function.

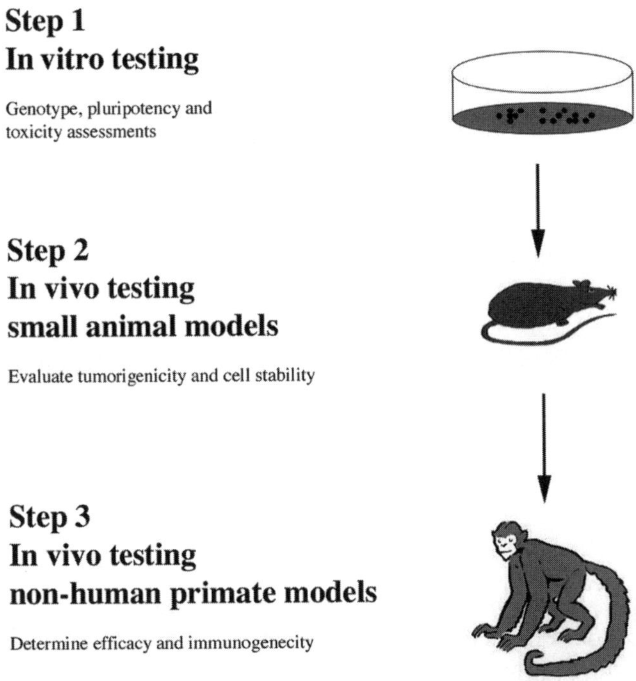

Fig. 1. Schematic for preclinical testing of stem cell-based therapies. Preclinical testing of therapies derived from stem cells should be initiated in vitro and include genotype and phenotype assessments along with general toxicology assessment. Transplantation studies should begin in rodent models to assess general cell stability and tumorigenicity. Finally, transplantation studies in nonhuman primates should be performed to assess cell therapy efficacy and immunogenicity.

3.1. In Vitro Testing

The initial step in evaluating stem cell therapeutic efficacy for endocrine disorders is to establish cell lines with the appropriate phenotype; criteria for a specific phenotype may differ so developing clear goals for monitoring cell function is critical *(59)*. For example, considerable debate has arisen on how to define a β-cell phenotype from ex vivo-derived cells; some believe this should be based on genetic determinants, others on detailed histologic markers. Ultimately, it will be cellular function at the graft site, specifically cell responses to physiologic stimuli that will be the ultimate measure of their therapeutic potential. In the case of β cells, stem cell progeny may give rise to cells that release insulin in response to glucose but may not express all other attributes of a β cell. Such cells could be potentially used to treat patients with diabetes, even if they fail to share all of the characteristics of a β cell.

Interfering or interacting substances in the growth media can complicate assessing the functional status of stem cell progeny. Again using β-cell differentiation as an example, insulin present as a growth factor interferes with the use of insulin as a marker for the cell phenotype. Alternative approaches are, therefore, necessary to identify β-like cells, one of which is to use C-peptide as a marker for *de novo* insulin synthesis, allowing for the identification of hormone production without inference from exogenous insulin *(60)*. In addition, electrophysiology may support cell identification because endocrine cells often have altered membrane electrical currents in response to stimuli or vesicle fusion. Although this approach could allow the undisputed identification of cellular responsiveness, only individual cells and not large cell populations can be readily assessed. Therefore, identification of a desired phenotype remains problematic requiring improved methods of assessment before using stem cell-derived cells for in vivo testing.

3.2. In Vivo Testing

After the functional capacity of cells destined for transplantation have been established with in vitro systems, cell safety and efficacy must be established in vivo. The goal for stem cell-based therapy is to match or improve on current exogenous therapeutic options. To establish this standard, stem cell-based therapies must be tested in appropriate animal models, assessing the animals' physiologic responses and evaluating cell phenotype stability.

To improve on current exogenous hormonal approaches, stem cell therapies must accurately couple metabolic stimuli to hormonal release. This will require appropriate responses to primary stimuli and integration of other modifying signals. β-cell therapy, for example, will require insulin secretion in grafted cells to respond not only to appropriate levels of glucose and other nutrients but also to modification by signaling from incretions (GLP-1, GIP), neurotransmitters, and paracrine factors *(61–63)*. Although all of these capabilities may not be needed before using cells for therapy, the more physiologic the cellular response, the more efficacious the therapy is likely to be. Critical to assessing efficacy will be the identification of appropriate animal models.

4. GOALS FOR PRECLINICAL ANIMAL MODEL DEVELOPMENT

To understand and integrate the risks and the physiologic benefits, stem cell transplants must be studied in vivo. The primary intent of preclinical studies is to acquire this experience (i.e., conduct safety, feasibility, and efficacy testing). There are numerous questions that should be asked during these preclinical studies, including: Which animal models best mimic the target human population and disease process? Are stem cells stabile and physiologically active following transplantation? What is the best site and developmental stage for stem cell transplantation? Should the transplanted population include both progenitor and terminally differentiated cells? Do tumors form? Do the grafted cells survive in high efficiency? Selection of the most appropriate animal model will depend on the questions being asked as well as the disease state being studied. Here, we have included some considerations for developing a preclinical model to evaluate stem cell therapies to treat certain endocrine diseases.

4.1. Animal Species for the Model

To answer all preclinical questions the model should manifest the human disease process under evaluation and possess immunologic characteristics similar enough to humans to allow an estimation of autoimmune and allogenic rejection. Models for many human endocrine diseases have been established in mice, including type 1 diabetes mellitus (DM) *(64–67)*, type 2 DM, thyroiditis *(68)*, and osteoporosis (Table 2) *(69,70)*. But nonhuman primates, who share similar immune systems to humans, do not spontaneously develop all of the human diseases of interest, in particular type 1 DM. Because there is not a single animal model that is ideally suited to answer all preclinical questions, careful integration of the results collected from multiple animal models into a coherent framework may be the only viable alternative.

Even though representative animal models do not exist for every human disease, several are represented, among them genetically based diseases, several species of cancer, and autoimmune conditions. Rodents are typically the first choice for a model as they have a very high reproduction rate, a short life-span, and mature quickly. This makes it possible to follow the effect of an intervention over many generations and to develop genetic models of disease with the help of molecular biologic techniques including transgenics and gene knockouts. One mouse model is the SCID mouse, which models have been used to identify pluripotent stem cells *(41)*. Intravenous injection of irradiated SCID mice with human bone marrow, cord blood, or granulocyte-colony stimulating factor (G-CSF) cytokine-mobilized peripheral blood mononuclear cells resulted in the engraftment of a human hematopoietic system in the murine recipient demonstrating uniform donor acceptance in these animals. The SCID mice model will be used in the first critical stem cell transplant experiments allowing evaluation of the stem cells in the absence of immuno-modulatory drugs.

Rodent models for genetic diseases have also originated through spontaneous mutations as opposed to genetic manipulation. The NOD mouse model represents a naturally occurring model genetically predisposed to autoimmune diseases including type 1 DM *(64)*. NOD mice generally develop diabetes between 12 and 16 weeks of age. Given the reliable and early onset of diabetes and the

Table 2
Animal Models for Endocrine Diseases

Disease state	*Animal model*	*Benefits*	*Limitations*	*Reference*
Type 1 DM, spontaneous	BB-DP rat NOD mouse	Autoimmune; lower maintenance costs	Increased non-insulin-mediated glucose disposal; ease in reversing disease; differences in immune system	*64,66,67*
Type 1 DM, experimentally induced	STZ-monkey	Glucose disposal similar to humans; onset of disease regulated	No autoimmunity	*92,93*
Type 2 DM	GK rat ZDF rat	Obesity, insulin resistance		*94,95*
	Ob/ob mouse Db/db mouse	Obesity, insulin resistance		*96*
	Rhesus and cynomolgus monkeys	Obese, spontaneous DM Spontaneous, amyloid	No transgenic approach	*97–99*
	Baboons	Spontaneous amyloid deposition in islets		*100*
Thyroiditis	Dog (beagles)	Spontaneous lymphocytic infiltration		*68*
	BALB/c mice TSH-R cDNA	Th2 thyroiditis Graves disease model		*7,101*
Osteopenia/osteoporosis	OVX rat	Popular Increased sensitivity to loss of estrogen	Weight gain suppress loss of cancellous bone On-going longitudinal growth	*69,102, 103*
	OVX baboon	Closes model to humans	Increased bone turnover at 6 months	*104*
	Glucocorticoid-treated sheep	Drug induced decrease in bone turnover	Doesn't mimic all aspects of human pathophysiology	*105,106*
	Aging cynomolgus and rhesus monkey	Similar pathophysiology to humans	Length of time to manifest disease (10–30 years) Difficulty in handling	*107,108*

DM, diabetes mellitus.

autoimmune nature of the disease process, this model is ideal for beginning in vivo testing of stem cell therapies for autoimmune-based endocrine diseases. However, there are substantial differences between rodent and primate physiology that limit the translation of information from any murine model to humans. Differences in β-cell physiology have been noted between species, which could be important in assessing the β-cell phenotype *(71)*. In the case of diabetic therapies, rodents have much higher non-insulin-dependent glucose disposal; thus, the use of a rodent model may over estimate the clinical benefit of cell therapy.

Primates and rodents also have notable differences in their immune responsiveness that could affect the transplantation of stem cells *(72)*. Such differences have been noted in prior testing of autologous transplantation and, along with differences in islet isolation, have contributed to significant delay in the development of successful human islet transplantation protocols *(73)*. The use of nonhuman primates, including the rhesus macaque, has provided invaluable, clinically relevant information including tissue quantities, graft sites, and immune responsiveness not available from the rodent model *(74,75)*. These results have contributed to the development of successful whole islet transplantation protocols.

Finally, primate (monkey and human) ES cells differ from mouse ES cells in their morphology, cell-surface marker expression, and sensitivity to leukemia inhibitory factor *(76)*. Moreover, the nonhuman primate shares genetic diversity in MHC proteins demonstrated by humans but not by rodents. As such, the immune sensitivity to donor tissue is similar between nonhuman and human primates. For these reasons, it will be necessary to reassess the clinical efficacy of these therapies established in rodent studies, in nonhuman primates before beginning clinical trials in humans.

Nonhuman primates such as baboons and Old World macaques have long been used as animal models for basic and preclinical studies *(74,75,77–81)*. By virtue of their anatomic, physiological, and genetic similarities to humans, studies have been performed during the entire spectrum of development from embryonic to pubertal and from adult to aging. For the most part, the research results can be translated readily to human biology, and in some cases to clinical trials. However, only a few nonhuman primate models are available for therapeutic studies limiting the potential needs of stem cell-based trials. For example, a monkey model of autoimmune (type 1) DM has not been established; therefore, it will not be possible at the present time to perform allogenic transplantation of insulin-producing phenotypes derived from monkey embryonic stem cells into monkeys with this form of diabetes. Development of a primate model of autoimmune diseases would greatly strengthen the preclinical trials of stem cell therapies for endocrine disorders. Short of developing an autoimmune primate model, surrogate primate models using chemically induced, β-cell failure can be used.

In addition, an obese monkey model is available to evaluate cell-based therapy as a type 2 DM preclinical model.

There are other nonhuman primate models established for research in cell-based replacement therapies, including a model of radiation-induced myelosuppression (ablation of hematopoiesis and blood cells) for bone marrow or hematopoietic stem cell transplantation *(82,83)*, a model of Parkinson's disease (loss of dopaminergic neurons in the midbrain and striatum) induced by MPTP (1-methyl-4-phenyl-1,2,3,6-tetrahydropyridine) for preclinical trials of striatal transplantation of fetal mesencephalic neurons *(84–86)*, and a model of Huntington's disease (loss of GABAergic and cholinergic neurons in the striatum and thalamus) induced by quinolinic acid administration is also available *(87)*. Monkey models have also been used for AIDS research and vaccine development *(77)* and for myoblast transplantation for the treatment of myopathies *(88)*. Therefore, given the strengths and drawbacks of nonhuman primates and other animal models, it will be necessary to perform in vivo testing in a progressive, stepwise manner beginning with rodent studies and progressing to nonhuman primates studies (*see* Fig. 1). Integration of results from all animal and in vitro studies will be essential to understand and define the risks and the benefits of stem cells transplantation before clinical trials in humans

5. LENGTH OF PRECLINICAL STUDIES

Determining the appropriate length of the preclinical study will be an important component of experimental design. Initially, relatively short studies involving several weeks or 1–2 months in duration could be performed in small animal models to test variables including transplantation sites, cell stability and migration. Such short-term studies will inevitably be followed by studies of several months' duration to determine therapeutic efficacy, viability, and stability of the transplanted stem cells and will have to be performed in both small and large animals.

6. SUMMARY

Stem cell therapy offers the potential to treat a myriad of human diseases, including endocrine diseases. Ongoing activities with primate ES cells include identifying the cell type or types that are appropriate for each therapeutic application and perfecting the methodology to produce highly enriched populations of specific phenotypes. Progress is occurring on a daily basis, leading to optimism that breakthroughs in stem cell therapy will likely occur in the near future. Before these findings can be translated to clinical therapies, preclinical testing is necessary. We believe that a stepwise approach, beginning in vitro with genotype and phenotype characterization, followed by in vivo testing of transplant protocols in animal models, will provide critical information to ensure the eventual success of stem cell-based therapies for endocrine diseases.

REFERENCES

1. Halban P, Kahn SE, Lernmark A, Rhodes CJ. Gene and cell-replacement therapy in the treatment of type 1 diabetes: how high must the standards be set? Diabetes 2001;50:2181–2192.
2. Weissman IL. Translating stem and progenitor cell biology to the clinic: barriers and opportunities. Science 2000;287:1442–1447.
3. Dawson L, Baetman-House AS, Agnew DM, et al. Safety issues in cell-based intervention trials. Fert Sterility 2003;80:1077–1085.
4. Ginis I, Rao MS. Toward cell replacement therapy: promises and caveats. Exp Neurol 2003;184:61–77.
5. Passier R. Potential of human embryonic stem cells in regenerative medicine. Hormone Res 2003;60:11–14.
6. Mandel TE. Fetal Islet xenotransplantation in rodents and primates. J Mol Med 1999;77:155–160.
7. Many MC, Costagliola S, Detrait M, Denef F, Vassart G, Ludgate MC. Development of an animal model of autoimmune thyroid eye disease. J Immunol 1999;162:4966–4974.
8. Asano T, Ageyama N, Takeuchi K, et al. Engraftment and tumor formation after allogenic in utero transplantation of primate embryonic stem cells. Transplantation 2003;76:1011–1014.
9. Hori Y, Rulifson I, Tsal BC, Helt JJ, Cahoy JD, Kim SK. Growth inhibitors promote differentiation of insulin-producing tissue from embryonic stem cells. Proc Natl Acad Sci USA 2002;99:16105–16110.
10. Thomson JA, Itskovitz-Eldor J, Shapiro SS. Embryonic stem cell lines derived from human blastocysts. Science 1998;282:1145–1147.
11. Thomson JA. Pluripotent cell lines derived from common marmoset (Cllithrix jacchus) blastocyst. Biol Reprod 1996;55:254–259.
12. Pesce M, Gross MK, Scholer HR. In line with our ancestors: Oct-4 and the mammalian germ. Bioessays 1998;20:722–732.
13. Niwa H, Miyazaki J, Smith AG. Quantitative expression of Oct-3/4 defines differentiation, dedifferentiation or self-renewal of ES cells. Nat Genet 2000;24:372–376.
14. Nichols J, Zevnik B, Anastassiadis K, et al. Formation of pluripotent stem cells in the mammalian embryo depends on the POU transcription factor Oct4. Cell 1998;95:379–391.
15. DeBrujin HWA, Sleijfer DTH, Koops HS, Suurmeijer AJH, Marrink J, Ockhuizen R. Significance of human chorionic gonadotrophin, alpha-fetoprotein, and pregnancy-specific beta 1 glycoprotein in the detection of tumor relapse and partial remission in 126 patients with nonseminomatous testicular germ cell tumors. Cancer 1985;55:829–835.
16. Eiges R, Schuldiner M, Drukker M, Yanuka O, Itskovitz-Eldor J, Benveniste H. Establishment of human embryonic stem cell-transfected clones carrying a marker for undifferentiated cells. Curr Biol 2001;11:514–518.
17. Meyer K, Irminger JC, Moss LG, et al. Sorting human beta-cells consequent to targeted expression of green fluorescent protein. Diabetes 1998;47:1974–1977.
18. Ma Y, Ramezani A, Lewis R, Hawley RG, Thomson JA. High-level sustained transgene expression in human embryonic stem cells using lentiviral vectors. Stem Cells 2003;21:111–117.
19. Zwaka TP, Thomson JA. Homologous recombination in human embryonic stem cells. Nat Biotech 2003;21:319–321.

20. Coffin RS, Thomas SK, Thomas NSB, et al. Pure populations of transduced primary human cells can be produced using GFP expressing herpes virus vectors and flow cytometry. Gene Ther 1998;5:718–722.
21. Bulte JWM, Douglas T, Witwer B, et al. Magnetodendrimers allow endosomal magnetic labeling and in vivo tracking of stem cells. Nat Biotech 2001;19:1141–1145.
22. Bulte JWM, Zhang SC, Gelderen PV, et al. Neurotransplantation of magnetically labeled oliodendrocyte progenitors: Magnetic resonance tracking of cell migration and myelination. Proc Natl Acad Sci USA 1999;96:15256–15261.
23. Chalfie M, Tu Y, Euskirchen G, Ward WW, Prasher DC Green fluorescent protein as a marker for gene expression. Science 1994;263:802–805.
24. Lester LB, Kuo HC, Andrews L, Nauert B, Wolf DP. Directed differentiation of rhesus monkey ES cells into pancreatic cell phenotypes. Reprod Biol Endocrinol 2004;2:42.
25. Kume A, Hashiyama M, Suda T, Ozawa K Green. Fluorescent protein as a selectable marker of retrovirally transduced hematopoietic progenitors. Stem Cells 1999;17:226–232.
26. Roccanova L, Ramphal P, Rappa R Mutation in embryonic stem cells. Science 2001;292:438–440.
27. Buzzard JJ, Gough NM, Crook JM, Colman A. Karyotype of human ES cells during extended culture. Nat Biotechnol 2004;22:381–382.
28. Cervantes RB, Stringer JR, Shao C, Tischfield JA, Stambrook PJ. Embryonic stem cells and somatic cells differ in mutation frequency and type. Proc Natl Acad Sci USA 2002;99:3586–3590.
29. Ouellette MM, McDaniel LD, Wright WE, Shay JW, Schultz RA. The establishment of telomerase-immortalized cell lines representing human chromosome instability syndromes. Human Mol Genet 2000;9:403–411.
30. Amit M, Carpenter MK, Inokuma MS, et al. Clonally derived human embryonic stem cell lines maintain pluripotency and proliferative potential for prolonged periods of culture. Dev Biol 2000;227:271–278.
31. Preti RA. Challenges associated with the development, manufacturing, and delivery of cellular medicines. Cancer J 2001;7:S62–S66.
32. Patience C, Takeuchi Y, Weiss RA. Infection of human cells by an endogenous retrovirus of pigs. Nat Med 1997;3:282–286.
33. Wilson CA, Wong S, Muller J, Davidson GE, Rose TM, Burd P. Type C retrovirus released from porcine primary peripheral blood mononuclear cells infects human cells. J Virol 1998;72:3082–3082.
34. Van der Lawn LJ, Lockey C, Griffeth BC, Frasier FS, Wilson CA, Onions DE. Infection by porcine endogenous retrovirus after islet xenotransplantation in SCID mice. Nature 2000;407:90–94.
35. Richards M, Fong CY, Chan WK, Wong PC, Bongso A. Human feeders support prolonged undifferentiated growth of human inner cell masses and embryonic stem cells. Nature Biotechnol 2002;20:933–936.
36. Amit M, Shariki C, Margulets V, Itskovitz-Eldor J. Feeder layer- and serum-free culture of human embryonic stem cells. Biol Reprod 2004;70:837–845.
37. Shpall EJ, Warkentin P, Gee A, et al. ASBMT raises concerns about FDA draft rules for "good tissue practices." Biol Blood & Marrow Transplant 2001:400–407.
38. Kraitchman DL, Heldman AW, Atalar E, et al. In vivo magnetic resonance imaging of mesenchymal stem cells in myocardial infarction. Circulation 2003;107:2290–2293.
39. Modo M, Cash D, Mellodew K, et al. Tracking transplanted stem cell migration using bifunctional contrast agent-enhanced, magnetic resonance imaging. NeuroImage 2002;17:803–811.
40. D'Amour KA, Gage FH. Genetic and functional differences between multipotent neural and pluripotent embryonic stem cells. Proc Natl Acad Sci USA 2003;100:11866–11872.

41. Greiner DL, Hesselton RA, Shultz LD. SCID mouse models of human stem cell engraftment. Stem Cells 1998;16:166–177.
42. Min J-Y, Yang Y, Converso KL, et al. Transplantation of embryonic stem cells improves cardiac function in postinfarcted rats. J Appl Physiol 2002;92:288–296.
43. Watkins WM. The ABO blood group system: historical background. Transfus Med 2001;11:243–285.
44. Abraham RT, Wiederrecht GJ. Immunopharmacology of rapamycin. Annu Rev Immunol 1996;14:483–510.
45. DeFranco AL. Immunosuppressants at work. Nature 1991;352:754–755.
46. Drukker M, Benvenisty N. The immunogenicity of human embryonic stem-derived cells. Trends Biotechnol 2004;22:136–141.
47. Drukker M, Katz G, Urbach A, et al. Characterization of the expression of MHC protein in human embryonic stem cells. Proc Natl Acad Sci USA 2002;99:9864–9869.
48. Draper JS, Pigott C, Thomson JA, Andrews PW. Surface antigens of human embryonic stem cells: changes upon differentiation in culture. J Anat 2002;200:249–258.
49. Griffith TS, Brunner T, Fletcher SM, Green DR, Ferguson TA. Fas ligand-induced apoptosis as a mechanism of immune privilege. Science 1995;270:1158–1159.
50. Zijlstra M, Bix M, Simister NE, Loring JM, Raulet DH, Jaenisch R. Beta 2 microglobulin deficient mice lack CD4–8+ cytolytic T cells. Nature 1990;344:742–746.
51. Wakayama T, Tabar V, Rodriguez I, Perry ACF, Studer L, Mombaerts P. Differentiation of embryonic stem cell lines generated from adult somatic cells by nuclear transfer. Science 2001;292:740–743.
52. Hwang WS, Ryu YJ, Park JH, et al. Evidence of a pluripotent human embryonic stem cell line derived from a cloned blastocyst. Science 2004;303:1669–1674.
53. Baker JRJ. Autoimmune endocrine disease. JAMA 1997;278:1931–1937.
54. LaFace DW, Peck AB. Reciprocal allogeneic bone marrow transplantation between NOD mice and diabetes-nonsusceptible mice associated with transfer and prevention of autoimmune diabetes. Diabetes 1989;38:894–899.
55. Mathieu C, Casteels K, Bouilon R, Waer M. Protection against autoimmune diabetes in mixed bone marrow chimeras. Immunobiology 1997;194:1453–1457.
56. Nikolic B, Takeuchi Y, Leykin I, Fudaba Y, Smith RN, Sykes M. Mixed hematopoietic chimerism allows cure of autoimmune diabetes through allogeneic tolerance and reversal of autoimmunity. Diabetes 2004;53:376–383.
57. Ferguson TA, Griffith TS. A vision of cell death: insights into immune privilege. Immunol Rev 1997;156:167–184.
58. Marmont AM, Gualandi R, Van Lint MT, Bacigalupo A. Refractory Evan's syndrome treated with allogeneic SCT followed by DLI. Demonstration of a graft-versus-autoimmunity effect. Bone Marrow Transplant 2003;31:399–402.
59. Clark SA, Quaade C, Constandy H, et al. Novel insulinoma cell lines produced by iterative engineering of Glut2, glucokinase, and human insulin expression. Diabetes 1997;46:958–967.
60. Kemmler W, Peterson J, Rubenstein A, Steiner D. On the biosynthesis, intracellular transport and mechanism of conversion of proinsulin to insulin and C-peptide. Diabetes 1972;21:572–581.
61. Garcia-Flores M, Zueco JA, Alvarez E, Blazquez E. Expression of glucagon-like peptide-1 (GLP-1) receptor and the effect of GLP-1-(7–36) amide on insulin release by pancreatic islets during rat ontogenic development. Eur J Biochem 2001;268:514–520.
62. Prasadan K, Daume E, Preuett B, et al. Glucagon is required for early insulin-positive differentiation in the developing mouse pancreas. Diabetes 2002;51:3229–3236.

63. Tourrel C, Bailbe D, Meile M-J, Kergoat M, Portha B. Glucagon-like Peptide-1 and Exendin-4 stimulate β-cell neogenesis in streptozotocin-treated newborn rats resulting in persistently improved glucose homeostasis at adult age. Diabetes 2001;50:1562–1570.
64. Atkinson M, Leiter EH. The NOD mouse model of type 1 diabetes: as good as it gets? Nat Med 1999;5:601.
65. Greiner DL, Rossini AA, Mordes JP. Translating data from animal models into methods for preventing human autoimmune diabetes mellitus: caveat emptor and primum non nocere. Clin Immunol 2001;100:134–143.
66. Lam-Tse WK, Lernmark A, Drexhage HA. Animal models of endocrine/organ-specific autoimmune diseases; do they really help us to understand human autoimmunity? Springer Semin Immunopathol 2002;24:297–321.
67. Polychronakos C. Animal models of spontaneous autoimmune diabetes: notes on their relevance to the human disease. Curr Diab Rep 2004;4:151–154.
68. Benjamin SA, Stephens LC, Hamilton BF, et al. Associations between lymphocytic thyroiditis, hypothyroidism and thyroid neoplasia in beagles. Vet Pathol 1996;33:486–494.
69. Wronski TJ, Schenck PA, Cintron M, Walsh CC. Effect of body weight on osteopenia in ovariectomized rats. Calcif Tissue Int 1987;40:155–159.
70. Turner AS. Animal models of osteoporosis–necessity and limitations. Eur Cell Materials 2001;1:66–81.
71. Schuit FC. Is GLUT2 required for glucose sensing? Diabetologia 1997;40:104–111.
72. Ginis I, Luo Y, Miura T, et al. Differences between human and mouse embryonic stem cells. Dev Biol 2004;269:360–380.
73. Kenyon NS, Ranuncoli A, Masetti M, Chatzipetrou M, Ricordi C. Islet transplantation: present and future prospectives. Diabetes Metab Rev 1998;14:303–313.
74. Hirshberg B, Mog S, Patterson N, Leconte J, Harlan DM. Histopathological study of intrahepatic islets transplanted in the nonhuman primate model using Edmonton protocol immunosuppression. J Clin Endocrinol Metab 2002;87:5424–5429.
75. Hirshberg B, Montgomery S, Wysoki MG, et al. Pancreatic islet transplantation using the nonhuman primate (rhesus) model predicts that the portal vein is superior to the celiac artery as the islet infusion site. Diabetes 2002;51:2135–2140.
76. Sato N, Sanjuan IM, Heke M, Uchida M, Naef F, Brivanlou AH. Molecular signature of human embryonic stem cells and its comparison with the mouse. Dev Biol 2003;260:404–413.
77. Amado RG, Mitsuyasu RT, Zack JA. Gene therapy for the treatment of AIDS: animal model and human clinical experience. Front Biosci 1999;15:D468–D475.
78. Carlisle KS, Montagna W. Aging model for unexposed human dermis. J Invest Dermatol 1979;73:54–58.
79. Crawford DH, Janossy G, Hetherington CM, et al. Immunological characterization of hemopoietic cells in the common marmoset, rhesus monkey, and man. Transplantation 1981;31:245–250.
80. Jampel HD, Leong KW, Dunkelburger GR, Quigley HA. Glaucoma filtration surgery in monkeys using 5-fluorouridine in polyanhydride disks. Arch Ophthalmol 1990;108:430–435.
81. Dunbar CE. The use of nonhuman primate models to improve gene transfer into haematopoietic stem cells. J Intern Med 2001;249:329–338.
82. Donahue RE, Dunbar CE. Update on the use of nonhuman primate models for preclinical testing of gene therapy approaches targeting hematopoietic cells. Human Gene Ther 2001;12:607–717.
83. Farese AM, Casey DB, Smith WG, Vigneulle RM, McKearn JP, MacVittie TJ. Leridistim, a chimeric dual G-CSG and IL-3 receptor agonist, enhances multilineage hematopoietic

recovery in a nonhuman primate model of radiation-induced myelosuppression: effect of schedule, dose, and route of administration. Stem Cells 2001;19:522–533.
84. Lindvall O, Brundin P, Widner H, et al. Grafts of fetal dopamine neurons survive and improve motor function in Parkinson's disease. Science 1990;247:574–577.
85. Kordower JH, Freeman TB, Snow BJ, et al. Neuropathological evidence of graft survival and striatal reinnervation after the transplantation of fetal mesencephalic tissue in a patient with Parkinson's disease. N Engl J Med 1995;332:1118–1124.
86. Freed CR, Greene PE, Breeze RE, et al. Transplantation of embryonic dopamine neurons for severe parkinson's disease. N Engl J Med 2001;344:710–719.
87. Emerich DF, Winn SR, Hantraye PM, et al. Protective effect of encapsulated cells producing neurotrophic factor CNTF in a monkey model of Huntington's disease. Nature 1997;386:395–399.
88. Skuk D, Tremblay JP. Myoblast transplantation: the current status of a potential therapeutic tool for myopathies. J Muscle Res Cell Motil 2003;24:285–300.
89. Pera MF, Reubinoff B, Trounson A. Human embryonic stem cells. J Cell Sci 2000;113:5–10.
90. Shamblott MJ, Axelman J, Littlefield JW. Human embryonic germ cell derivatives express a broad range of developmentally distinct markers and proliferate extensively in vitro. Proc Natl Acad Sci USA 2001;98:113–118.
91. Jinag Y, Jahagirdar BN, Reinhardt RL, et al. Pluripotency of mesenchymal stem cells derived from adult marrow. Nature 2002;418:41–49.
92. Thomas JM, Contreras JL, Smyth CA, et al. Successful reversal of streptozotocin-induced diabetes with stable allogeneic islet function in a preclinical model of type 1 diabetes. Diabetes 2001;50:1227–12236.
93. Kenyon NS, Chatzipetrou M, Masetti M, et al. Long-term survival and function of intrahepatic islet allografts in rhesus monkey treated with humanized anti-CD154. Proc Natl Acad Sci USA 1999;96:8132–8137.
94. Young AA, Gedulin BR, Bhavsar S, et al. Glucose-lowering and insulin-sensitizing actions of exendin-4: studies in obese diabetic (ob/ob, db/db) mice, diabetic fatty Zucker rats and diabetic rhesus monkeys (Macaca mulatta). Diabetes 1999;48:1026–1034.
95. Wang MY, Shimabukuro M, Lee Y, et al. Adenovirus-mediated overexpression of uncoupling protein-2 in pancreatic islets of Zucker diabetic rats increases oxidative activity and improves beta-cell function. Diabetes 1999;48:1020–1025.
96. Yoon JW, Leiter EH, Coleman DL, et al. Genetic control of organ-reactive autoantibody production in mice by obesity (ob) diabetes (db) genes. Diabetes 1988;37:1287–1293.
97. Hansen BC. Pathophysiology of obesity-associated type II diabetes (NIDDM): implications from longitudinal studies of non-human primates. Nutrition 1989;51:48–50.
98. de Koning EJ, Bodkin NL, Hansen BC, Clark A. Diabetes mellitus in Macaca mulatta monkeys is characterized by islet amyloidosis and reduction in beta-cell population. Diabetologia 1993;36:378–384.
99. O'Brien TD, Wagner JD, Litwak KN, et al. Islet amyloid and islet amyloid polypeptide in cynomolgus macaques (Macaca fascicularis): an animal model of human non-insulin-dependent diabetes mellitus. Vet Pathol 1996;33:479–485.
100. Hubbard GB, Steele KE, Davis KJI, Leland MM. Spontaneous pancreatic islet amyloidosis in 40 baboons. J Med Primatol 2002;31:84–90.
101. Costagliola S, Many MC, Stalmans-Falys M, Vassart G, Ludgate MC. Transfer of thyroiditis, with syngeneic spleen cells sensitized with the human thyrotropin receptor, to naive BALB/c and NOD mice. Endocrinology 1996;137:4637–4643.

102. Miller SC, Bowman BA, Miller MA, Bagi CM. Calcium absorption and osseous organ-tissue, and envelope-specific changes following ovariectomy in rats. Bone 1991;12:439–446.
103. Miller SC, Bowman BM, Jee WSS. Available animal models of osteopenia—small and large. Bone 1995;17:117S-123S.
104. Jerome CP, Kimmel DB, McAlister JS, Weaver DS. Effects of ovariectomy on iliac trabecular bone in baboons (Papio anubis). Calc Tissue Int 1986;39:206–208.
105. Chavassieux P, Pastoureasu P, Chapuy MC, Delmas PD, Meunier PJ. Glucocorticoid-induced inhibition of osteoblastic bone formation in ewes. a biochemical and histomorphometric study. Osteoporosis Int 1993;3:97–102.
106. O'Connell SL, Tresham J, Fortune CL, et al. Effects of prednisolone and deflazacort on osteocalcin metabolism in sheep. Calcif Tissue Int 1993;53:117–121.
107. Pope NS, Gould KS, Anderson DC, Mann DR. Effects of age and sex on bone density in rhesus monkey. Bone 1989;10:109–112.
108. Jayo MJ, Jerome CP, Lees CJ, Rankin SE, Weaver DS. Bone mass in female cynomolgus macaques: a cross-sectional and longitudinal study by age. Calcif Tissue Int 1994;54:231–236.

Index

D